GA.007EMQ

EM
for Surgical Finals

D1579525

EMQs and MCQs for Surgical Finals

Hye-Chung Kwak
Bariatric Surgical Research Fellow, Derby Hospitals NHS Foundation Trust

Imran Bhatti
Pancreatic Surgical Research Fellow, Derby Hospitals NHS Foundation Trust

Jaskarn Rai
Urology Surgical Research Fellow, Derby Hospitals NHS Foundation Trust

Farhan Rashid
Upper GI Surgical Research Fellow, Derby Hospitals NHS Foundation Trust

Bachittar Singh Jassar
Neurosurgical Registrar, Barts and the London NHS Trust

Murthy Nyasavajjala
Colorectal Surgical Research Fellow, Derby Hospitals NHS Foundation Trust

Viren Asher
Gynaecology Research Fellow, Derby Hospitals NHS Foundation Trust

Jon Lund
Clinical Associate Professor, University of Nottingham and Consultant Colorectal Surgeon, Derby Hospitals NHS Foundation Trust

Mike Larvin
Professor of Surgery, University of Nottingham and Honorary Consultant Surgeon, Derby Hospitals NHS Foundation Trust

⊛WILEY-BLACKWELL

A John Wiley & Sons, Ltd., Publication

This edition first published 2011, © 2011 by Hye-Chung Kwak, Imran Bhatti, Jaskarn Rai, Farhan Rashid, Bachittar Singh Jassar, Murthy Nyasavajjala, Viren Asher, Jon Lund and Mike Larvin

Blackwell Publishing was acquired by John Wiley & Sons in February 2007. Blackwell's publishing program has been merged with Wiley's global Scientific, Technical and Medical business to form Wiley-Blackwell.

Registered Office
John Wiley & Sons Ltd, The Atrium, Southern Gate, Chichester, West Sussex, PO19 8SQ, UK

Editorial Offices
9600 Garsington Road, Oxford, OX4 2DQ, UK
The Atrium, Southern Gate, Chichester, West Sussex, PO19 8SQ, UK
111 River Street, Hoboken, NJ 07030-5774, USA

For details of our global editorial offices, for customer services and for information about how to apply for permission to reuse the copyright material in this book please see our website at www.wiley.com/wiley-blackwell

Library of Congress Cataloging-in-Publication Data

EMQs and MCQs for surgical finals / Hye-Chung Kwak ... [et al.].
     p. ; cm.
   Includes bibliographical references.
   ISBN 978-1-4051-9941-4 (pbk. : alk. paper)
   1. Surgery–Examinations, questions, etc.   I. Kwak, Hye-Chung.
   [DNLM: 1. Surgical Procedures, Operative–Examination Questions. WO 18.2]
   RD37.2.E47 2011
   617.0076–dc22

                                   2010039155

A catalogue record for this book is available from the British Library.

Set in 8/10.5pt Meridien by SPi Publisher Services, Pondicherry, India.
Printed and bound in Singapore by Fabulous Printers Pte Ltd

1   2011

Contents

Acknowledgements, ix

Preface, x

Abbreviations, xi

Notation used in this book, xvi

PART 1 ESSENTIAL SKILLS IN SURGERY, 1
 1 Preoperative assessment, 1
  History and physical examination, 1
  Static investigations: non-invasive diagnostic testing, 1
  Dynamic investigations: functional capacity
   investigations, 2

PART 2 HEAD AND NECK, 4
 2 Neurosurgery, 4
  Head injury, 4
  Extradural haematoma, 5
  Subdural haematoma, 5
  Subarachnoid haemorrhage, 7
  Cerebrospinal fluid, 9
  Hydrocephalus, 10
  Cauda equina syndrome, 11

 3 Ear, nose and throat, 19
  Epistaxis, 19
  Earache (otalgia), 20
  Foreign bodies, 22
  Tonsillitis, 23
  Quinsy, 24
  Parotid swelling, 25
  Parotid pleomorphic adenoma, 25

 4 Endocrine, 34
  Thyroid swellings, 34
  Thyroid cancers, 35
  Parathyroid gland and hyperparathyroidism, 36

PART 3 CHEST, 43
 5 Thorax, 43
  Penetrating thoracic trauma, 43
  Blunt thoracic/cardiac trauma, 44

Rib fracture, 44
Tension pneumothorax, 45

6 Breast, 52
Mastitis, 52
Fat necrosis, 53
Benign breast lumps, 53
Breast cancer, 54

PART 4 ABDOMEN, 60

7 Acute abdomen, 60
Overview, 60
Necrotizing fasciitis, 61
Sigmoid volvulus, 62
Shock, 62
ATLS, 67

8 Foregut, 76
Dysphagia, 76
Gastro-oesophageal reflux disease (heartburn), 78
Barrett's oesophagus, 79
Malignant oesophageal tumours, 79
Gastric cancer, 80

9 Hepato-pancreato-biliary disease, 88
Pancreatic cancer, 88
Liver abscess, 89
Hepatocellular carcinoma, 90
Cholangiocarcinoma, 90
Acute pancreatitis, 91
Chronic pancreatitis, 93
Pancreatic pseudocyst (advanced topic), 94
Gallstones, 95

10 Spleen, 111
Anatomy, 111
Functions, 111

11 Midgut, 115
Acute appendicitis, 115
Small bowel obstruction, 115
Meckel's diverticulum, 116

12 Colorectal, 122
Diverticular disease, 122
Colorectal cancer, 123
Inflammatory bowel disease, 125
Lower gastrointestinal bleeding, 127
Haemorrhoids, 128
Fissure in ano, 129
Fistula in ano, 129

13 Nutrition in surgical patients, 140

14 Hernias, 144
Overview, 144
Inguinal hernia, 145
Femoral hernia, 145
Umbilical hernia, 146
Incisional hernia, 146

PART 5 PELVIS, 148

15 Gynaecology, 148
Ectopic pregnancy, 148
Pelvic inflammatory disease, 149
Ovarian cyst, 151

16 Urology, 157
Urinary tract infection, 157
Renal colic, 157
Prostate cancer, 158
Benign prostatic hypertrophy, 159
Renal cell carcinoma, 160
Bladder cancer, 161

PART 6 VASCULAR, 168

17 Vascular, 168
Abdominal aortic aneurysm, 168
Popliteal artery aneurysm, 169
Carotid artery disease, 170
Amputations, 171
Varicose veins of the lower limbs, 172
Diabetic foot, 173
Peripheral vascular disease, 175
Acutely ischaemic limb, 176

PART 7 ORTHOPAEDIC, 188

18 Orthopaedics, 188
Brachial plexus injury, 188
Radial nerve injury or entrapment, 189
Ulnar nerve palsy, 190
Carpal tunnel syndrome, 191
Shoulder dislocation, 191
Colles' fracture, 192
Fractured neck of femur, 193
Osteoarthritis of knee, 194

PART 8 BURNS AND PLASTICS, 205

19 Burns and plastics, 205
Burns, 205
Plastics, 207

PART 9 USEFUL PROCEDURES, 212

20 Useful procedures, 212

Abscess, 212

Urinary catheter insertion, 213

Examining stomas, 214

21 Clinical scenarios, 218

ANSWERS, 225

Appendix 1: Commonly used surgical equipment, 327

Appendix 2: Normal ranges for blood tests, 328

Appendix 3: Orthopaedic examination, 329

Further reading and useful websites, 331

Acknowledgements

The authors would like to thank Ms Mallicka M. Chakrabarty, MBBS, DNB (Gen Surg), MRCS Edinburgh, for her contribution to the section on burns and plastics, and for reviewing five of the chapters; Dr Sharmilee Gnanapavan, MBBS, BMedSci, MRCP, for reviewing the book; and Chris Towlson for his help with the photographs.

Preface

Of all the hurdles in a medical career, passing 'Finals' seems the most daunting. It is the first high-stakes assessment undertaken, and rightly so as it leads to a provisional licence to practise medicine. The surgical aspects of summative medical course assessments are important. Around half of all hospital inpatients may be classified as surgical, and GPs are usually first to see and refer such patients. GPs also undertake minor surgical procedures, as well as increasing amounts of aftercare given the shorter hospital stays resulting from increased day-case surgery and enhanced recovery programmes. Physicians need to know who to refer their patients to if they develop surgical problems, and are increasingly involved with the care of patients within the wider surgical team.

This book will help you to prepare for finals by providing a succinct but comprehensive revision guide, focusing on the clinical aspects of surgery. It is subdivided into sections covering the main sub-specialties. A concise summary is provided for each section, followed by a range of different question techniques to allow you to self-assess your own knowledge. It cannot substitute for seeing patients and reading about them throughout the clinical years, but it will help you to decide whether some additional reading is needed. Ideally, this book should be used well before finals, while you are still undertaking surgical rotations. However, final-year students will find it an excellent revision aid for finals, and will gain confidence from working through it from cover to cover.

Abbreviations

+/−	With or without
<	Less than
=	Equates to
>	Greater than
≈	Approximately equal to
AAA	abdominal aortic aneurysm
ABCDE	Airways, Breathing, Circulation, Disabilities, Exposure/Environment
ABG	arterial blood gas
ABPI	ankle–brachial pressure index
ADH	antidiuretic hormone
A&E	accident and emergency department
AF	atrial fibrillation
AFP	alpha-fetoprotein
AJCC	American Joint Committee on Cancer
AKA	above-knee amputation
ALP	alkaline phosphatase
ALT	alanine transaminase
AP	anteroposterior
APACHE	Acute Physiology and Chronic Health Evaluation
APTT	activated partial thromboplastin time
5-ASA	5-Acetylsalicylic acid
ASA	American Society of Anesthesiologists
AST	aspartate transaminase
ATLS	advanced trauma life support
AVM	arteriovenous malformation
AVN	avascular necrosis
AXR	abdominal X-ray
BiPAP	bi-level positive airway pressure ventilation
BKA	below-knee amputation
BMI	body mass index [weight (kg)/height (m^2)]
BP	blood pressure
BPH	benign prostatic hypertrophy
bpm	beats per minute
BRCA1, BRCA2	breast cancer genes
BSA	body surface area
BSG	British Society of Gastroenterology
BTS	British Thoracic Society
CBD	common bile duct
CCF	congestive cardiac failure

CD	Crohn's disease
CEA	carcinoembryonic antigen
CES	cauda equina syndrome
CFU	colony-forming units
CIS	carcinoma *in situ*
Cl	chloride
CMV	cytomegalovirus
CN	cranial nerve
CNS	central nervous system
CP	chronic pancreatitis
CPAP	continuous positive airway pressure ventilation
CPP	cerebral perfusion pressure
CRC	colorectal cancer
CRP	C-reactive protein
CSF	cerebrospinal fluid
C-spine	cervical spine
CT	computed tomography
CTA	computed tomography angiogram
CVA	cerebrovascular accident
CVS	cardiovascular system
CXR	chest X-ray
DCIS	ductal carcinoma *in situ*
DEXA	dual-energy X-ray absorptiometry
DHS	dynamic hip screw
DHT	dihydrotestosterone
DIC	disseminated intravascular coagulation
DKA	diabetic ketoacidosis
DM	diabetes mellitus
DRE	digital rectal examination
DSA	digital subtraction angiography/angiogram
DVT	deep vein thrombosis
EBV	Epstein–Barr virus
ECG	electrocardiogram
EDH	extradural haematoma
EPVD	end-stage peripheral vascular disease
ER	estrogen receptor
ERCP	endoscopic retrograde cholangiopancreatography
ESR	erythrocyte sedimentation rate
ESWL	extracorporeal shock-wave lithotripsy
EUA	examination under anaesthesia
EUS	endoscopic ultrasound; endoluminal ultrasonography
EVAR	endovascular repair
EVD	external ventricular drain
F	female
FAP	familial adenomatous polyposis
FAST	focused assessment with sonography for trauma
FB	foreign body
FBC	full blood count
FDG	fluorodeoxyglucose

FDP	flexor digitorum profundus
FNA	fine needle aspiration biopsy
FNAC	fine needle aspiration cytology
FNH	focal nodular hyperplasia
Fr	French (gauge)
G&S	group and save
GA	general anaesthesia
GALT	gut-associated lymphoid tissue
GCS	Glasgow Coma Scale
GGT	gamma-glutamyltransferase
GI	gastrointestinal
GIT	gastrointestinal tract
GOJ	gastro-oesophageal junction
GOO	gastric outlet obstruction
GORD	gastro-oesophageal reflux disease
GTN	glyceryl trinitrate
GUM	genitourinary medicine
H_2 blockers	histamine H_2 receptor blockers
Hb	haemoglobin
HCC	hepatocellular carcinoma
HCG	human chorionic gonadotrophin
Hct	haematocrit
HER2	human epidermal growth factor receptor 2
HHD	hand-held Doppler
HI	head injury
HIFU	high-intensity focused ultrasound
HIV	human immunodeficiency virus
HL	Hodgkin's lymphoma
HLD	herniated lumbar disc
HNPCC	hereditary non-polyposis colorectal cancer
HPV	human papillomavirus
HT	hormone therapy
IABP	intra-aortic balloon pump
IBD	inflammatory bowel disease
ICA	internal carotid artery
ICP	intracranial pressure
ICS	intercostal space
IDDM	insulin-dependent diabetes mellitus
IM	intramuscular
INR	international normalized ratio
IUCD	intrauterine contraceptive device
IV	intravascular/intravenous
IVC	inferior vena cava
IVDU	intravenous drug user
IVF	*in vitro* fertilization
IVU	intravenous urogram
JVP	jugular venous pressure
KUB	kidney, ureter, bladder
K-wire	Kirschner wire

LA	local anaesthesia
LBP	lower back pain
LCIS	lobular carcinoma *in situ*
LFTs	liver function tests
LOC	loss of consciousness
LP	lumbar puncture
LT	leukotriene
LUQ	left upper quadrant
M	male
MALT	mucosa-associated lymphoid tissue
MAP	mean arterial pressure
MCP	metacarpophalangeal
MC&S	microscopy, culture and sensitivity
MCV	mean corpuscular volume
MEN I, II	multiple endocrine neoplasia type I and II
MI	myocardial infarction
MMA	middle meningeal artery
MND	motor neurone disease
MODS	multiorgan dysfunction syndrome
MRA	magnetic resonance angiogram
MRCP	magnetic resonance cholangiopancreatography
MRI	magnetic resonance imaging
MSU	mid-stream urine
MUST	Malnutrition Universal Screening Tool
Na	sodium
NaCl	sodium chloride
NBM	nil by mouth
neuro obs	neurological observations
NGT	nasogastric tube
NHL	non-Hodgkin's lymphoma
NJT	nasojejunal tube
NOS	not otherwise specified
NSAID	non-steroidal anti-inflammatory drug
OA	osteoarthritis
OCP	oral contraceptive pill
OGD	oesophagogastroduodenoscopy
PAA	popliteal artery aneurysm
PCR	polymerase chain reaction
PEG	percutaneous endoscopic gastrostomy
PET	positron emission tomography
PG	prostaglandin
PID	pelvic inflammatory disease
PP	pulse pressure
PPI	proton pump inhibitor
PR	progesterone receptor
PSA	prostate-specific antigen
PSC	primary sclerosing cholangitis
PTC	percutaneous transhepatic cholangiography
PTFE	polytetrafluoroethylene

PTH	parathyroid hormone
PVD	peripheral vascular disease
RAAA	ruptured abdominal aortic aneurysm
RBC	red blood cell
RCC	renal cell carcinoma
RDI	recommended daily intake
RR	respiratory rate
RS	respiratory system
RUQ	right upper quadrant
SAH	subarachnoid haemorrhage
SBO	small bowel obstruction
SC	subcutaneous
SDH	subdural haematoma
SFJ	saphenofemoral junction
SIRS	systemic inflammatory response syndrome
SLE	systemic lupus erythematosus
SMA	superior mesenteric artery
SMV	superior mesenteric vein
SOB	shortness of breath
STI	sexually transmitted infection
T_4	thyroxine
TIA	transient ischaemic attack
TNM	tumour (size of tumour), node (lymph node involvement), metastasis (spread)
TPN	total parenteral nutrition
TSH	thyroid-stimulating hormone
TURBT	transurethral resection of bladder tumour
TURP	transurethral resection of prostate
TVU	transvaginal ultrasound
Tx	thromboxane
U&E	urea and electrolytes
UC	ulcerative colitis
UICC	Union Internationale Contre le Cancer (International Union Against Cancer)
UO	urine output
URTI	upper respiratory tract infection
USS	ultrasound/ultrasonography
UTI	urinary tract infection
VHL	von Hippel–Lindau (syndrome)
VP	ventriculoperitoneal
vs.	versus
WBC	white blood cell
WCC	white cell count

Notation used in this book

The following list outlines the format of this revision book. There may be extra sections added or deleted depending on the topic.

D: Definition/description

I & S: Incidence and prevalence, and sex

A & P: Aetiology and pathology

CF & D: Clinical features and diagnosis. This section also includes investigations.

T & M: Treatment and management

P: Prognosis

Followed by helpful hints and mnemonics

Part 1 Essential skills in surgery
1 Preoperative assessment

D : Assessing the individual patient's risk to minimize the morbidity and mortality associated with elective surgery.

I & S : All patients should have preoperative assessment, in particular the elderly patient.

CF&D: Patient evaluation is broadly divided into historical review, static investigations and dynamic investigations of function. The investigations are ordered based on the American Society of Anesthesiologists (ASA) grade and level of surgery.

History and physical examination

A full and detailed history is vital to establish an individual's cardiorespiratory functional capacity, providing benefits to any further management of perioperative events. It helps aid the identification of any significant diseases that would place the patient in a high surgical risk category. The history should also highlight symptoms that require further investigation.

Examine the patient for skin lesions and bony abnormalities; examine the CVS for murmurs and arrhythmias; listen to the chest for abnormal breath sounds; examine the abdomen for masses.

Based on the history, the ASA grade determines the need for further investigations.

Grade I	A normal healthy patient. The process for which the operation is being performed is localized and causes no systemic upset.
Grade II	Mild systemic disease. This category includes all patients over 80 years old.
Grade III	Severe systemic disease.
Grade IV	Incapacitating systemic disease that is a constant threat to life.
Grade V	A moribund patient unlikely to survive 24 hours with or without surgery.

Static investigations: non-invasive diagnostic testing

Most routine investigations provide a snapshot of the events taking place at the time of the test.

EMQs and MCQs for Surgical Finals, 1st edition. © Hye-Chung Kwak, Imran Bhatti, Jaskarn Rai, Farhan Rashid, Bachittar Singh Jassar, Murthy Nyasavajjala, Viren Asher, Jon Lund and Mike Larvin. Published 2011 by Blackwell Publishing Ltd.

- CXR: rule out pneumonia, cardiomegaly
- ECG: identify arrhythmias and silent MI
- Spirometry: respiratory physiology
- LFTs: assess liver protein synthesis
- Renal function testing
- Hb/haematocrit on FBC: anaemia
- Pregnancy testing
- Coagulation testing: for patients on anticoagulation, identify clotting disorders
- Urine analysis: proteinuria, diabetes, infection.

Dynamic investigations: functional capacity investigations

- Ambulatory and exercise ECG
- Echocardiography (static and stress)
- Ventriculography
- Radioisotope scanning
- Coronary angiography
- Lung function tests.

T & M : Optimize any pre-existing comorbidities preoperatively.
P : Reduced length of hospital stay, reduced last-minute cancellations, reduced morbidity and mortality.

MCQs (Answers, see p. 225)

1 A 65-year-old man was scheduled for hernia repair under GA. He was found to have a significant dynamic cardiac murmur on auscultation. Further preoperative assessment of this murmur would include:
a Troponin.
b Transthoracic echocardiogram studies.
c Transoesophageal echocardiogram studies.
d Bubble study.
e Coronary angiogram.

2 A 24-year-old man found to be otherwise fit and healthy on detailed history and examination is listed for circumcision under GA. His preoperative assessment would include:
a Chest X-ray.
b ECG and echocardiogram.
c Routine FBC and electrolytes.
d Abdominal ultrasound.
e CT chest and abdomen.

3 A 75-year-old woman is scheduled for a bowel resection due to diverticulitis as an acute emergency admission. During detailed history, she was found to be using a sublingual spray to alleviate chest tightness, started by her GP

last week. Her preoperative assessment would include at least the following investigations:

a Chest X-ray.
b 12-lead ECG.
c Echocardiogram.
d Routine FBC and electrolytes.
e Abdominal ultrasound.

4 A 60-year-old man is scheduled for a laparoscopic cholecystectomy and on-table cholangiogram. He is on warfarin for chronic AF. How many days prior to surgery should he stop his warfarin?

a 2 days.
b 3 days.
c 4 days.
d 5 days.
e 6 days.

5 A 72-year-old woman is due to have trans-sphenoidal pituitary surgery for a pituitary adenoma. On clinical examination, there is a new ejection systolic murmur noticed over the atrial region. What investigation is required?

a Chest X-ray.
b LFTs.
c Echocardiogram.
d Lung function tests.
e Abdominal ultrasound.

6 A fit and healthy 25-year-old man is scheduled for a hernia repair under local anaesthetic. What investigations does he require?

a Chest X-ray.
b 12-lead ECG.
c Echocardiogram.
d Routine blood test.
e No investigations are required.

Part 2　Head and neck

2　Neurosurgery

Head injury

D :　HI refers to trauma that leads to injury of the scalp, skull or brain, categorized as closed (no skull fracture) and penetrating (skull penetrated).

I & S :　Every year in the UK there are 1 million attendees to A&E and 150 000 admissions to hospital. More common in young males.

A & P :　RTA, falls, assaults. Frequency varies between age groups and geography.

Types of injury

- Primary (impact) injury occurs at time of trauma (cortical contusions, lacerations, diffuse axonal injury).
- Secondary injury (potentially avoidable): hypoxia, ischaemia (as a result of raised ICP and shock), oedema, intracranial haematoma, infection.

There is disruption of cerebral autoregulation, and as a result the ICP increases and the CPP reduces (CPP = BP − ICP). A drop in CPP is more likely to reduce cerebral blood flow and cause ischaemia.

C F & D :　Includes history, examination, GCS, and imaging. Assess evidence of injury, basal fracture sign, conscious level, pupil response, limb weakness and eye movements. Head injuries are graded: mild (GCS 14–15); moderate (GCS 9–13); severe (GCS ≤ 8).

Glasgow Coma Scale

GCS points	Best eye	Best verbal	Best motor
6	–	–	Obeys
5	–	Orientated	Localizes pain
4	Spontaneous	Confused	Normal flexion
3	To speech	Inappropriate	Abnormal flexion
2	To pain	Incomprehensible	Extensor
1	None	None	None

T & M :　Patients need a CT scan, resuscitation to minimize secondary brain damage +/− surgery.

EMQs and MCQs for Surgical Finals, 1st edition.　© Hye-Chung Kwak, Imran Bhatti, Jaskarn Rai, Farhan Rashid, Bachittar Singh Jassar, Murthy Nyasavajjala, Viren Asher, Jon Lund and Mike Larvin. Published 2011 by Blackwell Publishing Ltd.

General

- Prevent primary injury: better engineering (seatbelts, crash helmets), education (road safety), enforcement (speed limits).
- Prevent secondary injury: resuscitation (ABC), measures to lower ICP, avoid hypoxia and hypotension.

Specific

- Mild HI (GCS 14–15): discharge or admit for 24 hours for neuro obs.
- Moderate HI (GCS 9–13): admit, resuscitate, neuro obs, look for drop in GCS. Urgent CT scan (<1 hour). Inform neurosurgeon.
- Severe HI (GCS ≤ 8): intubate, resuscitate, neuro obs, look for pupil size. Immediate CT scan; do NOT waste time. Inform neurosurgeon.

Neurosurgical management

- 30° head up, oxygenation, mannitol, seizure prophylaxis, surgery (decompression, CSF diversion).

P: Mild HIs usually recover quickly and fully; severe HIs often have permanent physical and mental disabilities such as epilepsy. Generally, patients with persistently high ICP in the first 24 hours and those requiring surgery have poorer outcomes.

Extradural haematoma

D : EDH is a collection of blood in the potential space between the dura and the bone, associated with a fractured skull, traumatic lumbar puncture.

I & S : It occurs in about 2% of all cases of head injury. M/F ratio 4 : 1.

A & P : Commonly, there is an underlying skull fracture associated with a rupture of the middle meningeal artery (MMA).

C F & D : Typically involves young patients in a low-speed injury. There is initial alertness which declines, known as the 'lucid interval'. A unilateral fixed dilated pupil is a late sign. Diagnosis involves history, examination, GCS and CT scan.

Radiological features (see images)

- Biconvex appearance or 'lentiform'
- Temporo-parietal site commonest
- No brain abnormality

T & M : Urgent craniotomy for large EDH especially if located in temporal fossa.

P : The outcome of therapy is directly determined by the GCS before surgery. Can be rapidly fatal if not treated promptly.

Subdural haematoma

D : SDH is a collection of blood in the potential space between the dura mater and the arachnoid.

I & S : Acute SDH (<72 hours old) occurs in about one-third of people with a severe HI. Chronic SDH (>3 weeks old) often occurs in the elderly following a trivial fall. Both are commoner in males.

SAH

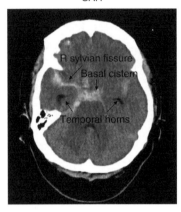

EDH

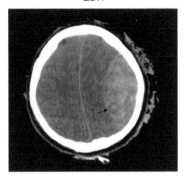

There is presence of blood in the subarachnoid spaces, in particular the right sylvian fissure and the basal cisterns. Prominence of temporal horns in keeping with hydrocephalus.

Large acute extradural haematoma over the left parietal convexity, with areas of low attenuation (arrow) within this haematoma suggestive of ongoing acute bleeding. There is marked midline shift to the right.

CSDH

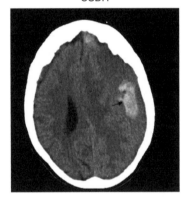

Large left acute-on-chronic subdural haematoma with mass effect. There is hyperdensity (arrow) within isodense/hypodense area. There is compression of the left lateral ventricle, and midline shift.

A & P: Dural bridging vein rupture.

CF & D: Most patients cannot even recall the injury that caused the bleed. Diagnosis involves history, examination, GCS and CT head.

Radiological features (see images)

- 'Moon-crescent' between the skull and brain
- Crosses suture lines
- Injury is trivial in chronic SDH
- Rare to find skull fractures in chronic SDH

T & M : Surgical evacuation if there is significant mass effect. Urgent craniotomy is required for large acute SDH, burr hole evacuation for chronic SDH.

P : Mortality is high in acute SDH. Prognosis is better if there is no damage to the brain.

Subarachnoid haemorrhage

D: Subarachnoid space lies under subarachnoid membrane which surrounds the brain, filled with CSF; within this space are major arteries supplying the brain.

I & S : Occurs in 8000 people per year in the UK, commoner in middle-aged persons, F > M.

A & P : SAH occurs when blood leaks into the subarachnoid space on the surface of the brain, usually secondary to trauma.

Causes of SAH

- Aneurysm (75%): causes spontaneous (primary) SAH as a result of ruptured congenital saccular or berry aneurysms in up to 85% of patients.
- AVM (5%): abnormal connections between arteries of unknown cause.
- Other causes (5%): tumour, cavernoma, trauma, clotting abnormalities.
- No cause (15%): 'angio-negative SAH'. Much lower incidence of further bleeding.

C F & D : There is usually no warning.

- Headache: sudden severe headache, described as like an explosion the head.
- Consciousness: immediate or delayed LOC, altered GCS with agitation and restlessness.
- Neurological deficits: motor deficit, dysphasia.
- Chemical meningitis: neck stiffness, vomiting and photophobia, and ongoing meningismus.

The World Federation of Neurosurgeons (WFNS) grading system for SAH

WFNS grade	GCS	Motor deficit
1	15	Absent
2	14–13	Absent
3	14–13	Present
4	12–7	Present or absent
5	6–3	Present or absent

Investigations for diagnosis

- CT brain (see images): usually shows blood around the brain, which may be intraventricular or intracerebral.
- LP: if scans are negative, an LP will be performed. CSF may be blood-stained or show xanthochromia (yellow).

Having established the diagnosis, further tests are needed to define the cause of the bleed.

- Angiography (best test): under LA, a thin tube is passed into the femoral artery; the tip of the tube is passed into the arteries of the brain, dye injected and serial X-rays taken. This should outline the arteries with any abnormality.
- Alternatives: CTA or MRA.

T&M: The primary aim is to prevent a potentially catastrophic second bleed.

Management

- ABC: oxygen, analgesia, laxatives, calcium channel blocker (nimodipine).
- Patient admitted to neurosurgical ward.
- Bed rest +/– control of BP.

If aneurysm is confirmed, the bleed should be secured within the first few days, since about one-third of patients will have a second bleed within a few weeks. However, if the patient is very ill, the risks of intervention are increased and treatment may be delayed.

Once the aneurysm is secured, treat patient with 'triple H' (hypertension, hyperoxygenation, hypervolaemia) to prevent secondary damage, hence avoiding complications.

Surgical clipping vs. endovascular coiling

- Surgical clipping: the aneurysm is pinched at its base by a metal clip, and this is left in place permanently to prevent further haemorrhages.
- Coiling: this is a new technique based on angiography, and avoids surgery. Platinum coils are inserted into the inside of the aneurysm via arteries. The initial results are encouraging but the long-term effectiveness is uncertain.

Note
The International Subarachnoid Aneurysm Trial (ISAT) is the only multicentre, prospective, randomized trial conducted on patients with ruptured brain aneurysms, comparing the efficacy and safety of endovascular coiling with conventional surgical clipping. The primary results demonstrated a better 1-year outcome with endovascular coiling.

Complications

- Vasospasm: occurs in the first few days following SAH. The arteries of the brain may narrow, reducing blood flow and starving the brain of oxygen. It can be avoided with drugs and by maintaining a good BP, can be treated with angiography.

- Hydrocephalus: can occur immediately or months later. The presence of blood in CSF can lead to build-up of the fluid and pressure within the brain. Treated with LP, EVD or VP shunt.
- Epilepsy: can occur either at the time of the bleed or some time afterwards and may require treatment with drugs. Epilepsy is unlikely to develop if no fits have occurred within 2 years.

Rule of thirds

- One-third die before getting to hospital.
- One-third die within the first 6 months.
- One-third survive but many left with physical or cognitive deficits.

Helpful mnemonic for causes of SAH

BATS (*b*erry aneurysm, *a*rteriovenous malformations/*a*dult polycystic kidney disease, *t*rauma, *s*troke).

Cerebrospinal fluid

D : The CSF is produced from arterial blood by the choroid plexuses (70%) and secreted by the brain parenchyma (30%), and is absorbed by arachnoid graulations in venous sinuses. Total CSF volume in adults is 150 mL and total CSF turnover is 450–500 mL per 24 hours.

Functions

- Protection: provides a cushioning effect on the CNS and dampens the effects of trauma.
- Metabolite removal: serves as a vehicle for removal of metabolites from the CNS.
- Stable environment: provides a stable ionic environment for the CNS.

Composition of serum and CSF

Constituent	Serum	CSF
Protein (g/L)	60–78	0.15–0.45
Glucose (mmol/L)	3.9–5.8	2.2–3.9
Ca^{2+} (mmol/L)	2.1–2.5	1–1.35
K^+ (mmol/L)	4–5	2.8–3.2
Na^+ (mmol/L)	136–146	147–151
Cl^- (mmol/L)	98–106	118–132
Mg^{2+} (mmol/L)	0.65–1.05	0.78–1.26

I & S : depends on the CSF pathology.

A & P : The composition of CSF can alter in pathological conditions such as bacterial meningitis and SAH.

Alterations in CSF composition in some pathological conditions

Pathological condition	Protein	Glucose	Cells
Subarachnoid haemorrhage	Increased	Normal	Presence of RBCs
Viral meningitis	Increased	Normal	Presence of excessive number of WBCs (lymphocytes)
Bacterial meningitis	Increased	Decreased	Presence of increased number of WBCs (polymorphonuclear leukocytes)

D : CSF can be obtained by LP (puncturing the L5/L4 subarachnoid space) and sent for analysis to diagnose infection and neurological disorders (oligoclonal bands in multiple sclerosis). Most importantly, the CSF can be sent for urgent Gram staining to look for microorganisms +/− culture.

T & M : The CSF can be drained to reduce increased ICP or obtained for diagnosis (as above).

P : Depends on the initial pathology.

Hydrocephalus

D : Hydrocephalus denotes an excessive accumulation of CSF, which considerably enlarges the ventricles.

I & S : Not known. However, 1 in 500 children are affected.

A & P : Not known.

Classification

• Obstruction to CSF circulation.
• Over-production of CSF.
• Failure of CSF absorption at the arachnoid granulations.

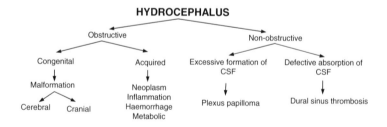

CF&D: The patients have symptoms of raised ICP: nausea, vomiting, headache. They will also have incontinence, dementia, gait changes, upgaze palsy.

T & M : Can be medical or surgical:
- Medical: acetazolamide may be helpful for temporizing, LP in non-obstructive hydrocephalus only.
- Surgery: the mainstay of treatment. CSF diversion with VP shunt or third ventriculostomy (hole in floor of third ventricle endoscopically).

P : Early diagnosis and treatment improves the chances of good recovery. The outcome varies from person to person depending on associated comorbidities and success of interventions.

> The Hounsfield unit (HU) is a measure of the X-ray beam on CT scan. Typically, dense bone is +600 HU (hyperdense) and air is –1000 HU (hypodense); brain has a value 20–40 HU and blood clot 75–80 HU.

Cauda equina syndrome

D : compression of the cauda equina (nerve roots below termination of spinal cord at L1).

I & S : uncommon; M = F.

A & P : trauma, HLD (usually central), spondylolisthesis, spondylosis, tumour, spinal epidural haematoma.

C F & D : may include some or all of symptoms/signs.

- Sphincter disturbance (retention 90% sensitivity > incontinence) +/– faecal incontinence: check post-micturition residual.
- Saddle anaesthesia (sensitivity 75%).
- Motor weakness.
- LBP.
- +/– Sexual dysfunction.

T & M : urinary catheter (measure residual), immobilize spine if traumatic, urgent MRI lumbosacral spine. Surgery: laminectomy; timing of surgery is controversial but early neurosurgical opinion essential (delay may result in negligence claim because of morbidity), normal practice to operate <24 hours may reduce long-term complications.

P : prognosis is worse in those who develop symptoms suddenly (especially for bladder function) as opposed to slowly progressive symptoms. Pain > sensation > motor > bladder > bowel > sexual function; improve in this order.

MCQs

Head injury (Answers, see p. 226)

1 A 30-year-old cyclist wearing no helmet was hit by a car travelling at 20 mph; he was taken to the local A&E department. On examination, he was confused, localizing to pain, and eye opening to speech. Which of the following are true and which are false?

    a His GCS is 11.
    b His GCS is 12.
    c He has a mild head injury by definition.
    d He should receive in-line traction of his cervical spine until cleared radiologically and clinically.
    e He should have a skull X-ray to exclude a linear fracture.

2 An 18-year-old driver is found unconscious after being ejected from his vehicle following a collision. He does not vocalize at all, he does not open his eyes to painful stimuli, and he has decerebrate posturing to supraorbital pressure. His BP is 90/65 mmHg and his pulse is 150 bpm. His left pupil is sluggishly reacting and larger than the right. Which of the following are true and which are false?
    a His GCS is 5.
    b The hypotension is likely to be related to the head injury.
    c He has Cushing's disease.
    d He has a right-sided expanding intracranial lesion.
    e He should receive a stat dose of steroids.

3 A 28-year-old man was assaulted with a baseball bat on the right side of his head. He suffered momentary loss of consciousness and was noted to have a boggy swelling over the right temporal–parietal region with an overlying laceration. He has a clear discharge emanating from the right ear and bruising behind the ear. Head CT showed a depressed parietal skull fracture and a base of skull fracture through the right petrous temporal bone. Which of the following are true and which are false?
    a Treatment for the base of skull fracture should include antibiotics.
    b He has Battle's sign and CSF rhinorrhoea.
    c The parietal fracture should be operated on.
    d His level of consciousness falls further in the A&E department. A repeat head CT shows a biconvex lens-shaped fluid collection. This collection is likely to be an acute SDH.

4 Regarding mannitol, which of the following are true and which are false?
    a It elevates BP and thus elevates CPP.
    b It reduces ICP by reducing oedema.
    c It provides glucose for the injured brain parenchyma.
    d It increases cerebral metabolism.
    e It increases the level of CO_2.

5 Regarding the main complication of ICP monitoring, which of the following are true and which are false?
    a Raised ICP.
    b Infection.
    c Leakage of CSF.
    d Seizures.

6 In head injuries, which of the following are true and which are false?
    a CPP = MAP + ICP.
    b The adult skull can accommodate an expanding volume of 50 mL without a significant rise in ICP.

c Lowering $PaCO_2$ causes cerebral vasoconstriction so should be avoided.

d Lowering PaO_2 should be encouraged.

e A high ICP reading in a patient with a closed head injury may be an indication for surgery.

EDH (Answers, see p. 227)

1 A 24-year-old man was hit on the right side of his head with a golf club 24 hours ago associated with a brief period of unconsciousness. He has now presented with persistent headache associated with vomiting and his GCS is 14/15. Why do you need to be cautious when taking this patient to the radiology department for imaging?

a Projectile vomiting will make scanning difficult.

b The patient's observation needs to be continuously monitored.

c The patient may become uncooperative and abusive.

d The patient may start fitting.

e The patient's GCS may drop.

2 Patients with EDH present with which of the following?

a Otorrhoea.

b GCS of 0.

c Urinary and faecal incontinence.

d Decrease in ICP.

e Fixed and dilated pupils.

3 An 8-year-old girl fell out of her second floor bedroom window, hitting her head on the roof the conservatory. On arrival at A&E her GCS is 15/15 and there is an obvious large haematoma under her laceration which is still oozing blood. Within minutes her GCS drops. What is your management?

a Insert two large-bore cannulas in the antecubital fossa.

b Call the trauma team.

c Fast bleep the anaesthetists to intubate the patient.

d Ask for 4 units of whole blood.

e Take her to the CT scanner.

4 Regarding secondary brain injury in a patient with a large EDH, which of the following are true and which are false?

a Brain atrophy.

b Haemorrhage.

c Infarction.

d Herniation.

e Diffuse axonal injury.

SDH (Answers, see p. 228)

1 Which of the following statements are true and which are false?

a Acute SDH and chronic SDH result from an acceleration/deceleration mechanism that results in tearing of the bridging veins.

b Chronic SDH results from rupture of the MMA.

c The precipitating event is unclear in almost half of patients with chronic SDH.

d In younger patients, the presentation is more commonly that of mass effect with symptoms and signs of raised ICP.

2 Regarding risk factors for developing acute SDH, which of the following are true and which are false?

a Subdural hygromas.

b Being female.

c Young age.

d Severe head injury.

e Dural tumour.

3 In chronic SDH, which of the following are true and which are false?

a MRI scan is the study of choice to demonstrate a chronic SDH.

b Diabetics have a lower recurrence rate than non-diabetics.

c Subdural hygromas can develop into chronic SDH.

d There is evidence of good clot formation within the chronic SDH.

4 Predispositions to the development of chronic SDH include which of the following?

a Being male.

b Older than 70 years of age.

c Alcoholism.

d Intracranial hypertension (i.e. raised ICP).

e Thrombophilia.

5 A 67-year-old man on warfarin for atrial fibrillation hit the top of his head while closing his garage door 1 week ago. He has not been himself since the accident, with continuous headache and nausea, episodes of confusion and unsteadiness on his feet. On his CT scan there is a large SDH that needs evacuation. What must you ensure before operating on this gentleman?

a An MRI scan to look for soft tissue changes.

b Echocardiogram to assess his heart function.

c Speak to his relatives.

d Check his INR.

e Give him antibiotics.

6 A retired GP on warfarin for prosthetic heart valve has presented with change in personality, decreased level of consciousness and 'off legs'. He undergoes evacuation of haematoma of his right chronic SDH. Post procedure, the nurses are concerned about the wet dressings on the patient's head. What do you do?

a Call the neurosurgical registrar immediately.

b Assess the patient's GCS and examine his pupils.

c Ask the nurses to apply a new dressing and repeat his observations.

d Undo the dressing to examine the operation site.

e Organize a head CT scan.

SAH (Answers, see p. 229)

1 Cerebral ischaemia in SAH can be prevented by which of the following?

a Introducing calcium channel antagonists such as nimodipine.

b Introducing antihypertensive agents.

c Hypertension.

d Haemoconcentration.

2 In SAH, which of the following are true and which are false?

a A non-uniform blood-stained CSF sample taken less than 6 hours after the onset of SAH can confirm the diagnosis.

b Pyrexia is a common finding.

c MI or cardiac arrythmias can occur.

d Bed rest reduces the risk of rebleed from aneurysmal SAH.

3 In a patient with a known unsecured aneurysmal SAH, a sudden deterioration in consciousness can be due to which of the following?

a Rebleed from the aneurysm.

b Hydrocephalus.

c Vasospasm.

d Epilepsy.

e Electrolyte imbalance.

4 Regarding SAH, which of the following are true and which are false?

a Patients may have ocular haemorrhages.

b Hydrocephalus may be obstructive in nature.

c Hydrocephalus may be communicating in nature.

d Approximately 30% of patients with aneurysmal SAH have more than one aneurysm identified on angiography.

e Giant aneurysms (>2.5 cm) are more likely to rupture.

5 Symptoms and signs of SAH include which of the following?

a Headache.

b Loss of consciousness.

c Whiplash.

d Anxiety attacks.

e Widespread maculopapular rash.

6 A 43-year-old woman collapsed in the high street and regained consciousness on arrival at A&E. There were classic signs and symptoms suggesting SAH, which was confirmed on CT of the head. Two days after cerebral angiogram and coiling, the patient complains of worsening headache associated with slurred speech. What is your management for this patient?

a Resuscitate the patient with blood.

b Start phenytoin infusion.

c Intubate and ventilate the patient.

d Ensure patient is hypertensive and hypervolaemic, and given hyperoxygenation.

e Repeat CT head.

CSF (Answers, see p. 230)

1 Regarding normal CSF, which of the following are true and which are false?

a Normal CSF pressure is $30\,cmH_2O$.

b CSF contains 3 mmol/L glucose.

c The presence of glucose in nasal secretions confirms CSF rhinorrhoea.

d Normal CSF contains HCO_3^-.

e CSF protein content >2 g/L is normal.

2 In the diagnosis of CSF leaks, which of the following are required?

a Radioisotope cisternography.

b CT head with reconstruction of skull base.

c CSF assay.

d Ultrasound.

e MRI myelography.

3 Regarding traumatic (non-surgical) CSF leak, which of the following are true and which are false?

a Most acute post-traumatic leaks stop within 10 days of injury.

b Conservative management involves stool softners and lumbar drainage.

c Persistent leaks after 10 days warrant surgical repair.

d Antibiotics have proven effective in reducing the incidence of meningitis in post-traumatic CSF leaks.

e The preferred elevation for patients with cranial leaks is flat bed rest.

4 Which of the following are indications for surgical intervention in CSF leak?

a A bout of meningitis is an indication for surgical intervention.

b Pneumocephalus (air within the cranium).

c Persisting leak.

d Patients with significant cardiovascular comorbidities require immediate repair.

Hydrocephalus and lumbar puncture (Answers, see p. 231)

1 Regarding lumbar puncture, which of the following are true and which are false?

a It is contraindicated in coagulopathy.

b It can be performed in communicating hydrocephalus.

c It should not be performed in meningitis.

d It is contraindicated in the presence of a suspected intracranial mass.

e It is useful for diagnosing cauda equina syndrome.

2 In a healthy individual, which of the following accurately describes the constituents of CSF?

a Has a higher concentration of glucose than plasma.

b Has the same osmolarity as plasma.

c Has the same concentration of sodium as plasma.

d Has the same pH as plasma.

e Is produced at a rate of 0.3 mL per 24 hours.

f Has a total circulating volume of 150 mL.

3 A 74-year-old man believed to have normal pressure hydrocephalus typically has which of the following?

a Gradual deterioration in mental state.

b Recurrent falls.

c Incontinence.

d Nystagmus.

e Dysphagia.

4 Symptoms of hydrocephalus include which of the following?
a Photophobia.
b Headache.
c Unsteady gait.
d Hallucinations.
e Nausea and vomiting.

5 Regarding types of hydrocephalus, which of the following are true and which are false?
a Acute hydrocephalus occurs over weeks.
b Obstructive hydrocephalus is the commonest type of hydrocephalus.
c Obstruction to the flow of CSF between the ventricles and subarachnoid space is a communicating hydrocephalus.
d Obstructive hydrocephalus is typically caused by a space-occupying lesion.
e SAH is a cause of communicating hydrocephalus.

6 Causes of hydrocephalus include which of the following?
a Migraines.
b Parkinson's disease.
c Metastatic tumours.
d Subarachnoid haemorrhage.
e Bacterial meningitis.

EMQs (Answers, see p. 232)

1 A 46-year-old driver is involved in a multi-vehicle collision. He is brought into A&E on a spinal board; the paramedics inform you that he was not wearing a seatbelt, at the scene, and that he was unable to move his legs. On examination, he has no sensation from below the umbilicus. He has a blood pressure of 70/40 mmHg, is bradycardic and agitated. Place in order of priority the treatment he should receive. Note that there may be one or more correct answers.
a His GCS should be calculated.
b He should be catheterized.
c He should be given inotropic support only if hypotension is not responding to fluid management.
d His airway should be assessed.
e His cervical spine should be immobilized.
f A blood glucose measurement should be done.

2 Link the patients with the location of their lesions.
a Temporal: memory disturbance.
b Frontal: personality change.
c Occipital: homonymous hemianopia.
d Parietal: motor deficit.
e Cerebellum: nystagmus.
For each case below, suggest the best diagnosis from the above list of options. Each option may be used once, more than once or not at all.

(i) A 67-year-old woman with previous breast cancer, who underwent a mastectomy and radiotherapy 2 years ago, presents with a 2-month history of receptive dysphasia. She is found to have nystagmus and papilloedema on examination.

(ii) A 28-year-old right-hand-dominant man presents with headaches, nausea and right upper limb weakness.

(iii) A 76-year-old hypertensive smoker presents with sudden headache and loss of vision as he looks to the right. On examination he is found to have a right-sided homonymous hemianopia with macular involvement.

(iv) A 32-year-old woman presents with headaches associated with pyrexia, dizziness and problems with balance.

(v) A 66-year-old gentleman bilingual in Spanish and English presents with progressive loss of inhibition and inability to speak Spanish.

3 Match the patients to the location of spinal pathology.
a C6/7 foraminal stensosis.
b Central disc prolapse L5/S1.
c Cervical canal stenosis.
d L3/4 disc prolapse.
e L4/5 disc prolapse.
For each case below, suggest the best diagnosis from the above list of options. Each option may be used once, more than once or not at all.

(i) A 43-year-old diabetic presents with progressive pins and needles, loss of fine hand movements and urgency micturating. Examination reveals brisk reflexes and increased tone more in the upper limbs than the lower limbs.

(ii) A 20-year-old builder presents with acute sensory loss in his perineum associated with right leg pain and difficulty passing urine.

(iii) Leg pain and paraesthesia in medial shin, weakness of plantar flexion.

(iv) Weakness in dorsiflexion and paraesthesia over knee.

(v) Weak elbow extension and numbness over the lateral forearm and the thumb and index finger.

4 Options:
a CT.
b Hyperdense.
c Hypodense.
d T1-weighted MRI scan, CSF dark.
e T2-weighted MRI scan, CSF white.
For each appearance below, suggest the best match from the above list of options. Each option may be used once, more than once or not at all.

(i) What is the appearance of an acute haemorrhage on head CT?

(ii) What is the appearance of air in head CT?

(iii) What is the appearance of an abscess on head CT?

(iv) Which scan is better to assess spinal fractures?

(v) Which imaging modality is best for looking at soft tissue injuries?

3 Ear, nose and throat

ENT conditions are common, constituting 10–15% of problems dealt with in primary care. It is also the largest surgical speciality within paediatrics.

Epistaxis

D: This is an acute bleed from the nostril (including nasal cavity and nasopharynx).
I & S : Common. Incidence 60%, M = F, peaks at ages 2–10 years and 50–80 years.
A & P : Bleeding can be from anterior nasal cavity (anastomotic network known as Little's area) or posterior and nasopharynx.

Predisposing factors

- Trauma: picking nose, fracture
- URTI: sinusitis
- Foreign body: peanut (child)
- Vascular: Little's areas (child), posterior arterial degeneration (elderly)
- Systemic disorders
- Neoplasm: nasopharyngeal carcinoma
- Disordered coagulation: warfarin, bleeding diatheses, DIC
- Others: postoperative, drugs (cocaine, heroin, tobacco, snuff)

C F & D : May present with haemoptysis (expectoration of blood) or haematemesis (vomiting blood); haemodynamic instability; visible bleeding in anterior nasal cavity. Nasal source confirmed when blood dripping from posterior nasopharynx.
T & M : ABC assessment; insert IV line; bloods for FBC, coagulation, G&S. Significant uncontrolled bleeding may require interventional embolization of the involved arteries or surgical ligation (tying with a ligature).
P : Excellent, if proper treatment given.

Haemodynamically stable patient

Apply pressure to the ala nasi for at least 15 min +/– apply ice to forehead to cause vasoconstriction of supplying arteries.

Haemodynamically unstable patient

- IV fluids for resuscitation with cardiac and BP monitoring.
- Prepare for theatre: arterial ligation of anterior ethmoidal or even external carotid.
- Embolization if stable enough.

EMQs and MCQs for Surgical Finals, 1st edition. © Hye-Chung Kwak, Imran Bhatti, Jaskarn Rai, Farhan Rashid, Bachittar Singh Jassar, Murthy Nyasavajjala, Viren Asher, Jon Lund and Mike Larvin. Published 2011 by Blackwell Publishing Ltd.

Initial management

1 Position patient comfortably, seated and ask to gently blow nose to remove blood clots to aid visualization.
2 Soak cotton-wool ball with lidocaine and adrenaline, insert into affected nostril to numb, use nasal speculum to visualize anterior bleed.
3 Use silver nitrate stick or bipolar suction diathermy to cauterize visible bleeding.
4 Persistent bleeding requires anterior nasal packing with ribbon gauze; posterior bleeding requires a posterior balloon, e.g. 14Fr Foley catheter filled with 6–10 mL saline, often with anterior packing.

French gauge: a tip

French gauge (FG) is simply the outer diameter of any cylindrical medical instrument in millimetres. Divide FG by π (roughly 3) to give the diameter in millimetres.

Earache (otalgia)

- Earache is a very common problem, with many different causes. We will concentrate on the common problems: otitis externa and otitis media.

Otitis externa

D: This is a skin condition of the external ear canal.

I & S: More common in children/teenagers, diabetics, up to 10% of population affected in their lifetime, M = F.

A & P: The external ear is self-cleansing, with skin squames migrating outwards from the centre of the eardrum. Earwax is acidic, hairs trap debris. Infection caused by trapped moisture (alters acidic environment), trauma breaking the skin lining (e.g. vigorous cleaning with cotton bud), infection in hair follicles.

CF & D: Pain especially on touching/pulling ear +/− itch, red and swollen canal +/− purulent discharge, tinnitus and dizziness. Examination with otoscope: erythema, swollen canal and exudates, but pain may hinder examination. Rule out tympanic membrane perforation associated with otitis media. Mastoiditis can be difficult to exclude (mainly headache, no ear pain/tenderness); seek ENT opinion.

T & M: Treated with topical antibiotics, cotton wick inserted superficially to keep canal patent, and aural toilet.

P: With appropriate treatment, should be pain-free after 24 hours and infection resolved within a week.

Acute otitis media

D: Acute middle ear bacterial infection associated with inflammatory fluid exudate which bulges drum.

I & S: Predominantly in children, M = F.

A & P: Risk factors as for URTIs, e.g. playgroups, contact with other children; tobacco smoke.

CF & D: Severe earache, temporary hearing loss (dampened vibrations). Examination with otoscope: bulging eardrum, perforated eardrum with copious discharge.

Complications include: Perforated eardrum, mastoiditis, meningitis, brain abscess.

T&M: Oral antibiotics (some controversy) or topical antibiotics with steroid drops for discharging ear. Treat surgically with grommet (typanostomy) tube to drain fluid from middle ear, or myringotomy to release the pus.

P: Good with antibiotics, most resolve without any treatment. Perforated eardrum usually heals spontaneously.

Other causes of ear pain

	Characteristics	Complications
Pinna haematoma (haematoma auris)	A haematoma develops below the perichondrium and compromises the blood supply to the cartilage of the ear. Immediate drainage and firm dressing required	Cauliflower ear Abscess formation
Necrotizing otitis externa	A potentially life-threatening form of osteomyelitis of the ear canal and skull base. Most common pathogen is *Pseudomonas aeruginosa*	CN VII (facial) nerve involvement, CN VI (abducens) and CN IX–XII neuropathy
Chronic otitis media with effusion (glue ear)	Middle ear effusion (1 month) without perforation/signs of infection. Usually resolves. A unilateral effusion in adults should raise suspicion of nasopharyngeal tumour	
Tympanic membrane perforation	The eardrum perforates due to infection, trauma and iatrogenic causes	Uncomplicated cases do not require intervention
Mastoiditis Cholesteatoma*	Abscess in the temporal bone Squamous keratinized epithelium invades the middle ear space. Treat with mastoidectomy	Sigmoid sinus thrombosis Hearing loss Chronic discharge Brain abscess

* Cholesteatoma is a cystic condition which develops in the middle ear and which may extend to the mastoid air cells. It is characterized by growth of a keratinizing, stratified, squamous epithelium. It has potential to grow and impair hearing and balance, erode bony structures, the ossicles and even the facial nerve unless it is removed surgically.

Definitions

- *Cerumen* is the medical terminology for earwax.
- Surgical incision of the eardrum is termed *myringotomy*.

Foreign bodies

D : Foreign bodies found in the ear, nose or throat can include anything from insects to sweets and small coins.

I & S : Common. Usually aged 1–9 years. Adults: fish bone, dentures.

A & P : Toddlers and children pick up objects and place in the ear, nose or mouth out of curiosity; trauma (e.g. falling onto an object).

C F & D : Depends on the foreign object, the number, type of FB and time of event.

Symptoms and signs

Ears
• Pain
• Impaired hearing
• Nausea and vomiting
• Bleeding

Nose
• No symptom
• Pain
• Difficulty breathing
• Nasal discharge
• Bleeding
• Vomiting blood

Throat/airways
• Pain
• Impaired swallowing
• Stridor
• Choking
• Wheezing
• Surgical emphysema in neck (oesophageal perforation)

Immediate attention needed if chemicals are involved (e.g. battery). Diagnosis may be obvious or may require fibreoptic scope/X-ray/CT imaging.

Complications

Ears
• May push FB further into the ear canal
• Infection

Nose
• May push FB further into the nose
• Sinusitis

Throat/airways
• May push FB further into airway, perforate oesophagus
• Pneumonia
• Lung abscess
• Death/hypoxic brain injury

T & M :

> *Ears*
> • For insects, place mineral oil into the ear to kill it prior to removal
> • Suction
> • Forceps, hooks
> • Remove under GA (epithelium too sensitive for LA)
>
> *Nose*
> • Blow nose with unaffected nostril closed
> • Suction if small
> • Wax hook or probe
> • Remove under GA (epithelium too sensitive for LA)
>
> *Throat/airways*
> • Heimlich manoeuvre in complete airways obstruction
> • Endoscopic removal

P : Once FB removed, prognosis usually good, i.e. no long-term damage. However, oesophageal perforation is possible as a result of fishbone and/or retrieval. Plain X-ray or CT may show free air.

Tonsillitis

D : Inflammation of pharyngeal tonsils (lymphoid tissues at back of throat).

I & S : Viral form common, bacterial form more common in children and young adults (5–15 years).

A & P :

> **Common causes**
>
> • *Streptococcus* group A bacteria (β haemolytic)
> • Epstein–Barr virus (EBV): causes glandular fever with ↑ nodes, splenomegaly
> • Coxsackievirus (may present like common cold in children)
> • Coryza (common cold)
> • Influenza virus

C F & D :

> **Symptoms and signs**
>
> • Swollen, red, inflamed tonsils +/– white pus spots
> • Fever
> • Throat fullness
> • Dysphagia, odynophagia
> • Otalgia, altered speech, headache, limb and back pain, regional node swelling
>
> **Characteristics**
>
> • Coated/white pus spots seen on tonsils
> • Infectious mononucleosis: the patient develops a rash on taking amoxicillin
> • Milder symptoms. Blisters on tonsils and top of mouth which scab and become painful

Complications of acute tonsillitis arise from infection spreading: cervical lymphadenitis, otitis media, laryngitis, peritonsillar abscess (quinsy), bronchitis, rarely septicaemia.

T & M : Usually requires no treatment. Admit patient if unable to swallow, take blood for EBV (Paul–Bunnell) and FBC; IV fluids, analgesia and antibiotics for 7 days if bacterial infection suspected; symptomatic management if considered likely to be viral. IV steroids if tonsils are hugely enlarged, infectious mononucleosis suspected, and signs of airways obstruction. Surgery: tonsillectomy for recurrent tonsillitis (more than five per year).

P : Good prognosis after surgery, but tonsillectomy does not guarantee freedom from further infections.

> EBV causes infectious mononucleosis; 90% of patients develop IM heterophil antibodies which are detected using the Paul–Bunnell test (sheep red cell agglutination in presence of heterophil antibodies). Monospot is an alternative which uses equine red cells.

Quinsy

D : Peritonsillar abscess, with pus in between the tonsillar capsule and lateral pharyngeal wall. Majority arise from untreated β-haemolytic streptococcal tonsillitis.

I & S : Common in teenagers and young adults.

A & P : May show mixed organisms:

- *Streptococcus* group A (β haemolytic)
- *Staphylococcus aureus*
- *Haemophilus influenzae*
- Anaerobic organisms.

C F & D : Examples of clinical features

Symptoms

- Throat pain
- Fever
- Drooling saliva
- Trismus
- 'Hot potato' voice

Signs

- Fetid breath
- Torticollis
- Drooling saliva
- Enlarged cervical nodes
- Uvula displaced away from lesion

Diagnosis is clinical (as above). Constitutional upset often present.

T & M : IV fluids, IV antibiotics (usually a penicillin derivative plus metronidazole), aspiration and drainage under LA (GA in children). Pus is sent for urgent Gram stain.

P: May rupture into parapharyngeal space. Recurrence ≈10% patientss within 1 year.

Parotid swelling

D: The parotid gland is the largest salivary gland, and produces watery (serous) saliva. It is located anterior and inferior to external auditory meatus, between mandible and mastoid process. Two lobes, superficial and deep, facial nerve runs between them. Deeper to facial nerve lies retromandibular vein, external carotid artery. Opening of duct is opposite the upper second molar.

I & S: Dependent on cause.

A & P: Surgical sieve: congenital, infective, inflammatory, neoplastic.

Causes	Clinical features	Diagnosis
Mumps (viral parotitis) Bacterial parotitis and chronic bacterial parotitis	Bilateral parotid swelling Pain on eating Purulent discharge from duct Systemically unwell	History and examination Blood tests including viral serology Pus: MC&S Sialography USS CT/MRI
Ductal stenosis, sialolithiasis (stone)	On/off pain and swelling around meal times	History and examination X-ray Sialography USS
Tumours	Various (see pleomorphic adenoma, below)	
Sjögren's disease (autoimmune)	Swelling and symptoms associated with Sjögren's disease	History and examination Autoantibodies Sialography Fine needle aspiration

CF & D: History and bimanual examination (gloved finger inside mouth) essential in all salivary gland swellings.

T & M: Combination management: symptomatic relief; I & D for abscess; parotidectomy for tumour, duct stenosis or stones; antibiotics for acute bacterial infections.

P: Dependent on cause. Mumps is self-limiting; acute bacterial parotitis is associated with a significant mortality risk; stones usually pass spontaneously (surgical dilatation or superficial parotidectomy is curative).

Parotid pleomorphic adenoma

D: Benign tumour of parotid, accounting for three-quarters of parotid tumours.

I & S: Most common in middle-aged females. M/F ratio 2 : 3.

A & P: Pleomorphic adenoma most common salivary tumour, consists of mesothelial and epithelial cells.

CF&D:

> **Symptoms and signs (few)**
> • Slow-growing firm parotid mass
> • Incidental finding on examination
>
> **Diagnosis**
> • Clinical assessment essential
> • USS with FNA
> • CT/MRI

T&M: Surgical removal recommended, as untreated may progress.
P: Postoperative recurrence rate 5%. If untreated, 5% become malignant.

MCQs

Epistaxis (Answers, see p. 234)

1 Where does Little's area receive its blood supply from?
   a Internal carotid artery only.
   b External carotid artery only.
   c Both internal and external arteries.
   d Subclavian artery.
   e Aorta.

2 In the management of epistaxis, which of the following are true and which are false?
   a Asking the patient to blow the nose worsens the effects of local fibrinolysis.
   b The application of lidocaine with adrenaline prior to the examination may reduce haemorrhage.
   c A posterior source of bleeding is more likely if there is drainage of blood in the posterior pharynx and failure to visualize an anterior source.
   d Posterior haemorrhage originates from branches of the sphenopalatine artery.
   e Cautery can be used to control bleeding from both nostrils simultaneously.

3 Which of the following general risk factors for epistaxis are true and which are false?
   a Fractured nose.
   b Sinusitis.
   c Hypertension.
   d Anticoagulation.
   e Tumour.

4 A 70-year-old man who has recently been started on warfarin for pulmonary embolism has presented with a 12-hour history of epistaxis. A posterior and

anterior nasal packing has been placed in both nostrils for posterior nasal bleeding. Why do you need to prescribe antibiotics for him?

a Sinusitis.

b Cerebrovascular accident.

c Septal haematoma.

d Septal mucosal necrosis.

e Aspiration.

5 A hypertensive 80-year-old woman has walked into A&E with epistaxis with haematemesis. On examination, she is pale, tachycardic, tachypnoeic and drowsy. What would you do next?

a Take a thorough history and examination.

b Call the anaesthetist to protect the airway.

c Take bloods for G&S and cross-match 4 units of blood.

d Insert two large-bore cannulas in the antecubital fossa and administer IV fluids.

e Ask the patient to pinch her nose.

6 Nasal packing increases the risk of which of the following?

a Mucosal pressure necrosis.

b Aspiration.

c Bleeding.

d Sinusitis.

e Hypoxia.

7 Epistaxis in the elderly may arise as a result of taking which of the following drugs?

a Antihypertensives.

b Aspirin.

c Warfarin.

d Aciclovir.

e Diuretics.

Earache (otalgia) (Answers, see p. 235)

1 Acute otitis media is a common problem in children, and as a junior doctor you may be asked to assess a child with a painful ear. With regard to glue ear, which of the following are true and which are false.

a Commonly follows URTI.

b Can lead on to chronic suppurative otitis media.

c Is associated with a family history of ear infections.

d Children are at increased risk of glue ear.

e Is associated with malformations of the head and neck area, such as cleft palate.

2 Symptoms of otitis externa include which of the following?

a Itching and earache.

b Swelling of the ear.

c Discharge from the ear.

d Ringing sounds in the ear.
e Touching the ear worsens the pain.

3 Which of the following statements about tympanic membrane perforations are true and which are false.
  a The commonest cause of tympanic membrane perforations is otitis externa.
  b The commonest cause of tympanic membrane perforations is otitis media.
  c Iatrogenic perforations heal better than perforations caused by infections.
  d Tympanic membrane perforation is an absolute contraindication to irrigation for earwax.
  e Purulent ear discharge is an indication of tympanic membrane perforations associated with infection.

4 With regard to glue ear (chronic otitis media with fluid), which of the following are true and which are false.
  a It is usually a self-limiting condition.
  b It is usually associated with hearing loss.
  c It is most common in adolescents.
  d It is common in the summer time.
  e Adenoidectomy and insertion of grommets are surgical management options.

5 Which of the following statements about cholesteatoma are true and which are false?
  a Surgical removal of cholesteatoma is recommended.
  b Cholesteatoma is a benign tumour.
  c Cholesteatoma is not associated with hearing loss.
  d Cholesteatoma is associated with dizziness and imbalance.
  e CT is required to assess cholesteatoma.

6 Which of the following statements about pinna haematoma are true and which are false?
  a It is usually caused by direct trauma.
  b This condition is managed conservatively.
  c A complication of pinna haematoma is cauliflower ear.
  d The patient requires no follow-up after treatment.
  e Needle drainage is the preferred treatment.

Foreign bodies (Answers, see p. 237)

1 With regard to foreign body in the nose, which of the following are true and which are false?
  a A 1-year-old toddler presents with a sweetcorn stuck in the right nostril. Treatment involves asking the toddler to blow her nose whilst blocking the left nostril.
  b A 7-year-old boy has a cotton bud stuck in his nose. The advice is to try to remove it at home.
  c In a 9-year-old with marshmallows stuck in both nostrils, inducing sneezing can push them out.

    d Choking is a serious complication of an FB in the nostril.

    e One of the symptoms of a nasal FB is bleeding.

2 With respect to foreign bodies in the throat and airway, which of the following are true and which are false?

    a Patients may present with a foreign body sensation in the throat, or pain on swallowing.

    b An FB in the airway should be suspected in a child with a noise from the upper airway.

    c X-ray is the main diagnostic tool.

    d Treatment can be carried out in the emergency department cubicle.

    e Foreign bodies in the throat can be managed conservatively.

3 Concerning foreign bodies in the ear, which of the following are true and which are false?:

    a They may affect hearing.

    b Water can be used to flush a dried pea from the ear.

    c They can be associated with pain the ear.

    d Infection caused by an FB may be treated with antibiotic ear drops.

    e Mineral oil can be used to kill an insect within the ear canal.

Tonsillitis and quinsy (Answers, see p. 237)

1 With regard to tonsillitis, which of the following are true and which are false?

    a It is usually a self-limiting condition.

    b Can be caused by bacteria or viruses.

    c The incubation period for *Streptococcus* infection is 1–2 hours.

    d Streptococcal infection is associated with small blisters on the tonsils.

    e Streptococcal infection is associated with milder symptoms.

2 Which of the following are complications of tonsillitis?

    a Quinsy.

    b Otitis externa.

    c Renal colic.

    d Lemierre's syndrome.

    e Airway compromise.

3 Regarding peritonsillar abscess, which of the following are true and which are false?

    a It is always caused by *Haemophilus influenzae*.

    b It is a complication of infectious mononucleosis.

    c Examination is difficult as the patient is usually uncooperative.

    d Patients have a 'hot potato' voice due to pharyngeal oedema.

    e The uvula is deviated towards the lesion.

4 Which of the following are complications of peritonsillar abscess?

    a Necrotizing fasciitis.

    b Pericarditis.

c Airway compromise.
d Mediastinitis.
e Spontaneous rupture resolves the problem.

5 In the management of peritonsillar abscess, which of the following are true and which are false?
a Peritonsillar abscess is treated successfully with antibiotics.
b Gram staining of pus is required.
c Tonsillectomy is never required.
d Steroids are contraindicated in the management of peritonsillar abscess.
e Analgesia should be offered as soon as possible.

6 Treatment for tonsillitis includes which of the following?
a The 'cold steel' method.
b Antibiotics.
c Using diathermy to operate on the tonsils.
d Coblation to surgically remove the tonsils.
e Laser treatment to remove the tonsils.

Parotid and parotid swellings (Answers, see p. 239)

1 In parotid gland obstruction, which of the following are true and which are false?
a Symptoms become apparent during fasting.
b Stones near the duct opening are removed by excision of the duct.
c Obstruction is common in young boys.
d The cause can be stenosis of the duct.
e The cause can be stones composed of mucus and cellular material.

2 Which of the following are complications of parotidectomy?
a Salivary fistula.
b Facial drooping.
c Facial fullness on the operated side.
d Skin numbness over the outer ear.
e Frey's syndrome.

3 Regarding salivary gland tumours, which of the following are true and which are false?
a They are most common in the smaller salivary glands.
b Benign salivary gland tumours are tender and hard.
c Acinic cell carcinomas of the salivary gland are classified as low-grade malignancies.
d Salivary gland tumours in the larger salivary glands are usually malignant.
e Mucoepidermoid tumours are the commonest salivary gland malignancy.

4 Regarding Sjögren's syndrome, which of the following are true and which are false?
a It is an autoimmune condition affecting smooth muscle.
b It is rare and mainly affects men.
c It can be diagnosed with Rose Bengal dye.

d Surgery is a treatment option.

e It decreases the risk of lymphoma.

5 With regard to sialadenitis, which of the following are true and which are false?

a It is caused by viral infection.

b It is due to underlying poor oral hygiene.

c It is usually asymptomatic.

d Should be treated with antibiotics.

e Affects young and healthy people.

6 Concerning parotid malignancy, which of the following are true and which are false?

a The commonest malignancy is acinic cell carcinoma.

b Facial nerve paralysis is a poor prognostic sign.

c More men are affected than women.

d FNA is the main diagnostic work-up.

e Pain is a poor prognostic sign.

EMQs (Answers, see p. 240)

ENT

1 Options

a Tonsillitis.

b Infectious mononucleosis.

c Viral laryngitis.

d Quinsy.

e Gastro-oesophageal reflux.

f Epiglottitis.

g Croup.

For each case below choose the single most likely diagnosis or investigation from the above list of options. Each option may be used once, more than once or not at all.

(i) A 3-year-old boy has been complaining of sore throat for 1 day and has been brought to A&E by his mother. On examination, he is pyrexial, there is drooling and he has difficulty speaking.

(ii) A 20-year-old man presents with fever and malaise for 1 week associated with a sore throat and cervical lymphadenopathy. On examination, his tonsils are red and swollen; there are generalized tender neck nodes, and tenderness in the left side of the abdomen.

(iii) A 50-year-old smoker with a BMI of 48 complains of a 1-year history of waking with a sore throat.

(iv) A 9-year-old girl is brought into A&E with a 5-day history of a sore throat, now associated with fever and difficulty swallowing. On examination, both tonsils are swollen and red with white pus spots.

(v) A 9-year-old girl has had 2 days of antibiotics for a sore throat but has come back to A&E with worsening symptoms, including increasing difficulty swallowing and limited opening of the mouth associated with fever. On examination, there is deviation of the uvula to the right side.

2 Options:
  a Pharyngitis.
  b Ulcerative tonsillitis.
  c Candidiasis.
  d Acute laryngotracheitis.
  e Ludwig's angina.
  f Lingual tonsillitis.
  g Foreign body.

For each case below choose the single most likely diagnosis or investigation from the above list of options. Each option may be used once, more than once or not at all.

  (i) An elderly diabetic patient receiving radiotherapy for oesophageal adenocarcinoma complains of a sore throat associated with difficulty swallowing. Endoscopic examination reveals white patches over inflamed pharyngeal and oesophageal mucosa.

  (ii) A 27-year-old woman complains of 3 days of right-sided throat pain radiating to the right ear, associated with bad breath and a foul taste in the mouth. On examination, there is an ulcer on the right tonsil.

  (iii) A 30-year-old man has had flu-like symptoms for 3 days and presents with a sore throat and rhinorrhoea. On examination, the nasopharyngeal mucosa is erythematous and oedmatous.

  (iv) A 51-year-old man presents with 1 day of a constant sore throat that is worse when trying to swallow saliva. He says that it feels as if there is something sharp stuck on the right side of his throat. On examination there are no signs of infection or inflammation.

  (v) A 42-year-old man is brought to A&E with fever and dehydration associated with a swollen neck and mouth. On examination, the mouth cannot be fully opened, but you can see that the tongue is pushed up against the roof of the mouth.

Parotid

1 Options:
  a Sarcoidosis.
  b Mucoepidermoid tumour.
  c Mumps.
  d Parotitis.
  e Pleomorphic adenoma of parotid.
  f Sialadenosis.
  g Sjögren's syndrome.
  h Warthin's tumour.

For each case below choose the single most likely diagnosis from the above list of options. Each option may be used once, more than once or not at all.

  (i) An 82-year-old woman has received 6 weeks of nasogastric feeding after a right-sided CVA. She has bilateral fullness in both cheeks, which are tender and she has a fever. What is the most likely diagnosis?

(ii) A 13-year-old boy is complaining of bilateral jaw tenderness associated with severe central abdominal pains associated with nausea and vomiting.

(iii) A 50-year-old smoker presents to his GP after his wife noticed a lump below his right ear. On examination it is soft and non-tender.

(iv) A 40-year-old woman who underwent a previous right-sided partial parotidectomy 2 years ago presents with a small parotid lump close to the previous scar. On examination, it is firm, non-tender and not tethered to the overlying skin. What is the most likely diagnosis?

2 Options:
  a Damaged facial nerve.
  b Facial asymmetry.
  c Frey's syndrome.
  d Greater auricular nerve trauma.
  e Haematoma.
  f Salivary fistula.
  g Wound infection.
  h All the above.

For each case below choose the single most likely diagnosis or complication from the above list of options. Each option may be used once, more than once or not at all.

  (i) In a surgical outpatient clinic, you see a 55-year-old man who complains of excessive sweating on eating. You notice that he has a scar on his right cheek close to the ear, suggestive of previous parotid surgery.

 (ii) A 47-year-old woman is 5 days post partial parotidectomy for pleomorphic adenoma, and is complaining of numbness over the scar and ear on the same side.

(iii) You are asked to assess a wound on the ENT ward. A frail 70-year-old woman has had a partial parotidectomy for mucoepidermoid carcinoma. The wound drain has been removed by accident and the nursing staff are worried about the continuous fluid leaking from the wound.

(iv) The same 70-year-old woman has now developed an erythematous wound which is tender and warm to the touch.

 (v) You receive a call from the surgical ward; a relative is concerned about facial drooping in her mother after parotid surgery.

(vi) You have been asked to explain superficial parotidectomy to a patient prior to consent being obtained. Which complications should you mention and explain?

4 Endocrine

Thyroid swellings

D : Diffuse thyroid swelling or discrete lumps (nodules) in the gland. In the UK, enlargements (goitres) affecting the entire thyroid are usually multinodular colloid goitres, as those from iodine deficiency are rare. Diffuse goitres may occur during puberty, pregnancy and lactation, in Hashimoto's disease and in thyrotoxicosis.

I & S : Common, 3000 cases annually, more common with increasing age; F > M; majority benign.

A & P : Some 10–20% of clinically solitary thyroid nodules prove to be malignant.

Differential diagnosis

- Adenoma/cacinoma/lymphoma
- Cyst: solitary or multiple
- Goitre: diffuse swelling with or without active functioning nodules

---

C F & D : Usually no symptoms, perhaps pain or difficulty swallowing. Patient, relative or friend may notice lump, sometimes an incidental finding. Take history and examine.

- Blood thyroid function tests: thyroid-stimulating hormone (TSH) and free T_4 (usually euthyroid), thyroid antibodies.
- Imaging: USS and thyroid isotope scans to assess characteristics.
- FNA essential for diagnosis, and ideally the first diagnostic test performed.

Isotope scan

Radioactive iodine is taken up by thyroid cells and scintigraphic images taken. Note that the test cannot differentiate benign and malignant nodules.

- Hot: dark spot. Much iodine is taken up, indicating increased TSH production.
- Warm: grey spot. Moderate amount of iodine taken up by the cells.
- Cold: light spot. Cells not taking up iodine, not making TSH.

T & M : Depends on cause. Surgery indicated in proven malignancy, atypical cytology, airway compromise, recurrent cysts, cosmetic reasons, failed medical management of hyperthyroidism.

P : Also depends on cause. For thyroid cancers, see below.

EMQs and MCQs for Surgical Finals, 1st edition.   © Hye-Chung Kwak, Imran Bhatti, Jaskarn Rai, Farhan Rashid, Bachittar Singh Jassar, Murthy Nyasavajjala, Viren Asher, Jon Lund and Mike Larvin. Published 2011 by Blackwell Publishing Ltd.

Thyroid cancers

I & S : In the UK around 3 per 100 000 are diagnosed with thyroid cancer. Approximately half are aged <50 years. M/F ratio 1 : 3.

A & P : There are risk factors for developing thyroid cancers.

Risk factors

- Benign thyroid disease: adenomas, goitre, thyroiditis.
- Radiation: history of exposure to radiation.
- Low iodine levels: leads to goitre.
- FAP: inherited bowel condition.
- Family history: medullary thyroid cancer may be inherited (MEN II syndrome).

C F & D : Symptoms include (i) neck lump; (ii) hoarse voice or sore throat >3 weeks; and (iii) rarely, loose motions and facial flushing. FNA and examination of cells under microscope required for diagnosis.

Thyroid cancer	Prevalence	Characteristics	Prognosis
Papillary	Up to 80%	Usually multifocal, slow-growing	90% 5-year survival
		Metastasize via lymphatics	
		Distinct histological appearance	
		Related to exposure to radiation	
		Best treated surgically	
		Seen in younger patients	
Follicular	15%	Metastasize via bloodstream to lung/bones	70% 5-year survival
		Diagnosis based on capsular invasion by tumour cells	
		Treated surgically, responds to radioiodine	
		Diagnosed in young/middle-aged patients	
Medullary	5–10%	Derived from calcitonin-producing C cells	90% 5-year survival
	Rare	Metastasize to lymph node and bone marrow	
		Associated with MEN II (thus familial)	
		Best treated surgically	
		Associated with *RET* proto-oncogene; thyroidectomy advised if positive for *RET*	
		Screening offered if positive family history	
Anaplastic (aggressive)	2%	In iodine-deficient areas or on background of existing thyroid disease, e.g. multinodular goitre	Zero 5-year survival
		May metastasize via blood or lymphatics	

(cont'd)

Thyroid cancer	Prevalence	Characteristics	Prognosis
Anaplastic (aggressive)	2%	Rarely treated surgically, unresponsive to radioiodine About 1 in 6 thyroid cancers, seen in older females	
Lymphoma	NHL: 2%	More common in women	85% 5-year survival
	HL: rare	Autoimmune thyroiditis is a risk factor	

T & M : Partial thyroidectomy for papillary/follicular cancers. Thyroidectomy and nodal dissection for medullary cancers. Many treated with radioiodine afterwards, most on lifelong thyroxine (blocks TSH growth effect).

> • Patients given radiotherapy should be advised to stay away from others for 2 days to prevent radiation exposure. Further information at www.cancerresearch.org.uk

Parathyroid gland and hyperparathyroidism

D: The parathyroid glands are four small endocrine glands located behind the thyroid gland in the neck, regulating calcium levels through parathyroid hormone (PTH). The commonest problem is over-production of PTH leading to hyperparathyroidism and hypercalcaemia. Primary hyperparathyroidism is the commonest form of hyperparathyroidism.

I & S : Approximately 42 cases per 100 000 (third commonest endocrine problem). M/F ratio 1 : 3.

A & P : Cause unknown for parathyroid adenoma, hyperplasia and carcinoma. Some association with ionizing radiation and MEN I and MEN II. The gland senses blood calcium levels and produces PTH in response to low calcium levels, but stops when calcium levels rise. In most cases of primary hyperparathyroidism, a parathyroid cell replicates to form a parathyroid adenoma (benign).

C F & D : Signs of hypercalcaemia are few.

Symptoms

- Lethargy
- Inability to concentrate
- Depression
- Headaches
- Bone pain
- Muscle weakness
- Osteoporosis
- GORD
- Renal stones
- Nausea
- Hypertension

- Atrial arrhythmias
- Constipation
- Abdominal pains

Diagnosis

- Raised blood and urinary calcium levels
- Raised or normal PTH: controls calcium and phosphate levels in the blood
- Hypophosphataemia
- DEXA scan: skeletal involvement
- Sestamibi scans: sestamibi is a protein labelled with technetium-99, taken up by active parathyroid cells

T & M : Excision of pararthyroid gland is the main option in primary hyperparathyroidism.

P : Excellent after surgery. Few develop hypoparathyroidism requiring calcium and vitamin D.

MCQs

Thyroid swellings (Answers, see p. 243)

1 A 30-year-old teacher presents with a lump on the right side of her neck. Which features favour a benign thyroid nodule?
   a Tenderness.
   b Mobile nodule.
   c New-onset hoarseness.
   d Lots of nodules.
   e Multiple swollen lymph nodes in the neck.

2 Which of the following are indications for thyroid surgery?
   a Atypical cytology and suspicion of cancer.
   b Airway compromise.
   c Large noticeable goitre without obstructive symptoms.
   d Failed medical therapy for hyperthyroidism.
   e Metastatic thyroid cancer with airway compromise.

3 Which of the following are advantages of FNA?
   a It provides tissue for cytology.
   b Safety.
   c It looks at iodine uptake in thyroid cells.
   d Its value in treating thyroid lumps.
   e The ability to assess the number of nodules.

4 A 60-year-old man has noticed a lump in his neck. You take a history and examine the patient. Which of the following features suggest malignancy?
   a Multiple nodules with a large dominant nodule on the left side of neck.
   b Frequent and loose motions.
   c Rapidly growing lump.

  d Engorged neck veins on the left side.
  e Enlarged lymph nodes in the neck.

5 Regarding investigations for thyroid lumps, which of the following are true and which are false?
  a Ultrasound scan will diagnose malignant lumps.
  b FNA is a final investigation.
  c Isotope scanning excludes benign lumps.
  d CT scan will be required to assess malignant lumps.
  e Most patients will have high TSH levels.

6 Regarding thyroid nodules, which of the following are true and which are false?
  a A 4-cm nodule containing follicular cells has a greater chance of malignancy than a 1-cm nodule.
  b Recurrent cystic nodules require aspiration only.
  c A 2-cm nodule can be observed.
  d A sudden change in size in thyroid nodule indicates infection.
  e Investigation for thyroid nodules includes haematology, radiology and FNAC.

Thyroid cancers (Answers, see p. 244)

1 With regard to papillary cell thyroid cancer, which of the following are true and which are false?
  a It is related to radiation exposure.
  b Total thyroidectomy with removal of all parathyroid glands is required.
  c Metastasizes via lymphatics.
  d Thyroxine is required after surgery.
  e Lymph node metastasis is associated with higher mortality.

2 With regard to follicular cell thyroid cancers, which of the following are true and which are false?
  a Vascular invasion is characteristic of follicular cancers.
  b More common in males.
  c Peak incidence is age 40–60 years.
  d Prognosis is unrelated to tumour size.
  e Lifelong thyroxine after surgery and radiotherapy does not influence mortality.

3 Regarding medullary thyroid cancer, which of the following are true and which are false?
  a Regional metastasis occurs early in the disease.
  b Inherited medullary thyroid cancer is the most aggressive form.
  c It is associated with radiation exposure.
  d Calcitonin is measured during follow-up.
  e Good prognosis when associated with MEN II.

4 With regard to anaplastic cancers, which of the following are true and which are false?
  a Affect more males than females.
  b Are slow-growing.

c Often arise within a more differentiated cancer.

d The presence of lymph node metastasis is associated with lower mortality rate.

e Patients may require tracheostomy.

5 Urgent investigation for thyroid lump is recommended in which of the following cases?

a History of radiation.

b Rapidly growing neck lump.

c Family history of thyroid cancers.

d Elderly gentleman with a cervical lymphadenopathy.

e Sore throat associated with high fever.

6 Radiotherapy can be used in which of the following thyroid cancers?

a Anaplastic thyroid cancer.

b Immediately after thyroid surgery.

c Recurrent thyroid cancer.

d Follicular thyroid cancer.

e Papillary thyroid cancer.

Parathyroid gland and hyperparathyroidism
(Answers, see p. 245)

1 Hypercalcaemia causes which of the following?

a GORD.

b Increased thirst as the patient loses ability to swallow.

c Brisk reflexes.

d Constipation due to dehydration.

e Renal stones.

2 With regard to primary hyperparathyroidism, which of the following are true and which are false?

a High blood PTH and calcium levels are diagnostic of primary hyperparathyroidism.

b Measuring 24-hour urine is one means of diagnosing hyperparathyroidism.

c Medical management is recommended.

d Normal calcium levels with low PTH is an indication for parathyroidectomy.

e Normal PTH and high calcium levels is secondary hyperparathyroidism.

3 With regard to sestamibi scan, which of the following are true and which are false?

a The radiolabelled sestamibi protein is taken up by all the parathyroid cells.

b High radiation levels are required.

c The radiolabelled sestamibi protein is injected into the vein.

d Best used in combination with radio-guided parathyroid surgery in the operating room.

e A negative scan excludes parathyroid tumour.

4 Regarding secondary hyperparathyroidism, which of the following are true and which are false?

a It is caused by chronic hypocalcaemia.

b It is usually seen in acute renal failure.

c May be associated with vitamin D deficiency.

d It is associated with very high levels of calcium.

e Surgery is the main treatment option.

5 Regarding tertiary hyperparathyroidism, which of the following are true and which are false?

a It is associated with hypocalcaemia.

b It is associated with low phosphate levels.

c Treated with medications.

d It is associated with acute renal failure.

e Patients with this condition have no symptoms.

6 The symptoms of hypocalcaemia include which of the following?

a Shortness of breath.

b Muscle cramps.

c Numbness and tingling in the extremities.

d Congestive cardiac failure.

e Oily skin.

EMQs (Answers, see p. 246)

1 Options:

a Radioactive iodine.

b Lifelong thyroxine.

c Vocal cord assessment.

d Endocrine tests.

e Total thyroidectomy and neck dissection.

For each case below choose the single most likely management or investigation from the above list of options. Each option may be used once, more than once or not at all.

  (i) A 55-year-old woman with a diagnosis of medullary thyroid cancer.

 (ii) A 25-year-old pregnant woman has noticed goitre.

(iii) After a total thyroidectomy and neck dissection for medullary tumour.

(iv) For complete treatment after a total thyroidectomy for a large aggressive follicular tumour.

 (v) After partial thyroidectomy for papillary tumour.

(vi) A 46-year-old woman is complaining of weakness in voice 2 days post total thyroidectomy.

2 Options:

a De Quervain's thyroiditis.

b Graves' disease.

c Hashimoto's thyroiditis.

d Postpartum thyroiditis.

e Subacute thyroiditis.

f Thyroid adenoma.

g Thyrotoxic crisis.

For each case below choose the single most likely diagnosis or investigation from the above list of options. Each option may be used once, more than once or not at all.

(i) A 46-year-old woman has been unwell with flu-like symptoms for 5 days, and now presents with a swollen painful neck associated with racing pulse and tremor. On examination there is generalized tenderness over her thyroid and tachycardia. Blood tests reveal elevated T_4/T_3 and decreased TSH, high ESR and negative thyroid antibodies.

(ii) A 28-year-old woman has presented with fatigue and irritability 1 month after giving birth to a full-term baby girl.

(iii) A 40-year-old woman presents to the ENT clinic with noisy breathing associated with a large neck lump. On examination, she has dry skin and there is exophthalmus and chemosis of the eyes.

(iv) A 42-year-old woman with a known history of hyperthyroidism presents with pyrexia of 40°C and tachycardia, vomiting and confusion.

3 Options:

a Central hypothyroidism.

b De Quervain's thyroiditis.

c Hashimoto's thyroiditis.

d Iatrogenic hypothyroidism.

e Postpartum thyroiditis.

For each case below choose the single most likely diagnosis or investigation from the above list of options. Each option may be used once, more than once or not at all.

(i) A 45-year-old woman presents with lethargy and irregular menstruation. On examination, there is a palpable goitre and thyroid function tests reveal high TSH and low T_4.

(ii) A 37-year-old woman has had radioiodine therapy for Graves' disease, and has come back to the outpatient clinic for a 1-year follow-up. She complains of tiredness and depression.

(iii) A 30-year-old woman who gave birth 4 months ago has been brought in by her sister with symptoms of depression and a neck swelling.

(iv) A 51-year-old woman has been feeling under the weather for a couple of weeks with flu-like symptoms associated with neck pain, fever and lethargy. Thyroid function tests reveal high TSH and low T_4.

4 Options:

a Paget's disease of bone.

b Primary hyperparathyroidism.

c Tertiary hyperparathyroidism.

d Post-surgical hypocalcaemia.

e Secondary hyperparathyroidism.

For each case below choose the single most likely diagnosis or investigation from the above list of options. Each option may be used once, more than once or not at all.

(i) A 28-year-old diabetic patient presents to the renal dialysis unit with the following symptoms: nausea, vomiting, confusion and weakness.

(ii) A 30-year-old woman has a routine blood test 4 hours after a total thyroidectomy. Calcium is 1 mmol/L and PTH is low.

(iii) A 22-year-old man with no surgical history presents with recurrent renal stones of unknown cause. The blood test reveals mildly raised calcium and further tests reveal raised PTH levels.

Part 3   Chest
5   Thorax

Penetrating thoracic trauma

D :   An object penetrates the chest wall creating a hole in the thoracic cavity, often incompatible with life.

I & S :   This type of injury is becoming increasingly frequent and the majority of victims are in the most productive years of their lives.

A & P :   The common modalities are stab injuries (low velocity), gunshot (medium to high velocity) and missiles (high velocity) due to explosions (low- vs. high-energy wounds): Potential injury to heart, lung, aorta, oesophagus, major vessels, trachea and bronchi.

C F & D :

Investigations/imaging

- Tension pneumothorax: clinical diagnosis.
- Cardiac tamponade: plain CXR (adjunct to primary survey).
- Open pneumothorax: spiral CT scan (gold standard).
- Airway obstruction: clinical diagnosis.

Other investigations like echocardiography, oesophagoscopy, bronchoscopy, aortogram are used to ascertain integrity of respective organs.

T & M :   The majority of these injuries are managed non-operatively. After initial resuscitation (following ABC), a symptomatic approach to the trauma helps delineate the organ systems. ATLS protocols recommend thoracostomy for any suspected penetrating injury. A collection of >200 mL/hour or 1500–2000 mL at initial thoracostomy (insertion of chest drain) is an indication for emergency thoracotomy/mediastinotomy. Cardiac tamponade (associated with Beck's triad: low mean arterial pressure, distension of neck veins, distant muffled heart sounds) and acute haemodynamic deterioration are the commonest indications for thoracotomy.

Management

- Tension pneumothorax: large-bore cannula in second ICS.
- Cardiac tamponade: thoracotomy.
- Open pneumothorax: sterile occlusive dressing taped on three sides.
- Airway obstruction: depends on the cause. Clear airway, intubate and ventilate.

EMQs and MCQs for Surgical Finals, 1st edition.   © Hye-Chung Kwak, Imran Bhatti, Jaskarn Rai, Farhan Rashid, Bachittar Singh Jassar, Murthy Nyasavajjala, Viren Asher, Jon Lund and Mike Larvin. Published 2011 by Blackwell Publishing Ltd.

A full admission history and examination, FBC, ABG and other blood tests are done after the patient is stabilized.

P : Patients who are clinically stable at presentation have better prognosis.

Blunt thoracic/cardiac trauma

D : A force propelled onto the chest wall that does not leave an open wound.

I & S : Blunt trauma to the chest wall and the heart is common in deceleration injuries.

C F & D : Clinical presentation depends on the injuries sustained. RuDusky classified this into five stages (0 to IV) according to severity and extent of trauma. These injuries are associated with severe dysrhythmias, coexisting vascular and pericardiac trauma.

Commonly diagnosed by abnormal ECG changes and elevated cardiac enzymes. Advanced investigations like transthoracic or transoesophageal echocardiogram may be useful in delineating areas of injury from healthy tissue.

T & M : Management of this type of trauma is supportive in intensive care and remains largely non-surgical. These patients may often need inotropic support and careful fluid balance. Any discontinuity of vascular integrity secondary to trauma/valvular damage may need immediate surgical intervention.

P : Various scoring systems predict outcomes of trauma using extensive algorithms (outside the scope of this book). Generally, most patients have good prognosis.

Rib fracture

D : One or more breaks in any of the rib bones making up the thoracic cage.

I & S : Approximately 10–15% of all blunt abdominal traumas will have at least one rib fracture. Flail chest is a clinical condition where ventilatory function of lungs is compromised because two or more fragments of ribs are dissociated from spine, resulting in paradoxical movements of the segment.

A & P : Usually caused by trauma.

C F & D : Fracture of posterior angle of ribs 4–9 most common site of injuries. Any other site will need enhanced work-up because forces required to cause such damage will be much more extensive. Sharp pain on inspiration or coughing, shortness of breath, local tenderness, paradoxical movement with respiration (in flail chest) are the immediate clinical features. Delayed presentation is often associated with focal or extensive consolidation due to reduced ability, or inability, to ventilate the lungs.

Diagnosis

- Often clinical crepitus is confirmed by a plain CXR (AP and lateral views).
- Rarely, much more extensive investigation is required to confirm a fracture (e.g. medicolegal purposes).
- However, if ribs 1, 2, 10, 11 and 12 are fractured, a CT scan with an angiogram is performed to ensure integrity of blood vessels in close proximity to them.

T & M : Assessment and management of rib fractures is part of primary pre-hospital care. Generally, rib fractures are managed on high-dependency unit with escalating levels of analgesia (as needed) and chest physiotherapy. Sometimes, they will need assistance such as CPAP or BiPAP.

P : If managed aggressively and early, outcomes are favourable. Younger patients with isolated fractures of ribs have better prognosis.

Tension pneumothorax

D : Pneumothorax is the presence of air in the pleural cavity compromising lung volume available for gas exchange. In tension pneumothorax, the increased intrapleural pressure displaces the mediastinal structures and causes cardiopulmonary compromise. This is an acute emergency.

I & S : Unknown.

A & P : Causes include iatrogenic and trauma. Lung parenchyma or bronchial injury acts as a one-way valve, trapping air in the pleual space.

CF & D : Chest pain and dyspnoea with tachycardia and distended neck veins. Deviation of trachea is also a frequent finding in these clinical situations. The diagnosis of tension pneumothorax is clinical. CXR is a good adjunct to clinical diagnosis.

T & M : Aim for full-blown lungs without any air in pleural cavity. British and American guidelines advise a risk stratification approach to management of asymptomatic/symptomatic pneumothorax. A wide-bore cannula placed in second ICS in mid-clavicular line relieves a tension pneumothorax. Further management is by a tube thoracostomy (chest drain).

P : Good prognosis with early diagnosis and immediate treatment.

Simple pneumothorax

In simple pneumothorax, the air in the pleural space does not build up significant pressure. It is managed with a chest drain if a significant (10–15%) portion of lung is collapsed, resulting in cardiopulmonary compromise. There is a role for expectant management if a stable patient with smaller pneumothorax is found on an incidental X-ray.

MCQs

Penetrating thoracic trauma (Answers, see p. 249)

1 A 26-year-old woman was found to be unconscious on a field trip after she accidentally tripped over onto a sharp object on left side of the anterior chest. She was transferred to hospital and was found to have a pneumothorax. On thoracostomy, she had 200 mL of blood in her chest in the first hour. Which of the following would be an indication for thoracotomy in this situation?

a Continuing traces of pneumothorax.

b More than 200 mL blood in next hour.

c Pain at chest drain site, 15 mL next hour.

d Inability to cough with thoracostomy *in situ*.

e More than 500 mL loss of serosanguineous fluid over next 48 hours.

2 In the investigation of penetrating trauma, which of the following should be considered?

a CXR.

b Chest CT.

c EUS.

d Bronchoscopy.

e ECG.

3 With regard to diaphragmatic injuries, which of the following are true and which are false?

a May result from stab injuries.

b Diagnosed with CXR.

c Previous injuries may present with visceral herniation.

d Always requires open repair.

e May be caused by blunt abdominal trauma.

Blunt thoracic trauma (Answers, see p. 249)

1 A 24-year-old man fell on a boulder and sustained bruising of his anterior chest. He took no notice of it, but later in the day noticed increasing shortness of breath and dizziness. He was rushed to A&E and found to have a haemothorax. He is haemodynamically stable, needing no further support. Which of the following would be the best approach to his condition ?

a Thoracotomy.

b CTA.

c Video-assisted thoracoscopy.

d Seldinger thoracostomy.

e Bronchoscopy.

2 A 28-year-old man was airlifted to a trauma centre following a car crash with no obvious injuries. After initial resuscitation and primary survey, he was found to have some bruising on anterior chest wall. Subsequently, over the next 3 hours he develops ECG findings suggestive of ischaemia. Further management of this patient would include which of the following?

a Immediate thoracotomy.

b Tube thoracostomy.

c Intensive/high-dependency care support.

d Discharge home with advice to return if he develops chest pain.

e Immediate coronary angiogram.

3 With regard to aortic injuries, which of the following are true and which are false?

a Caused by acceleration forces.

b Most common cause of mortality after blunt thoracic trauma.

c Results in increased radial pulses.

d Results in hypotension.

e May be associated with fractures of ribs 1 and 2 on the left-hand side.

4 With regard to cardiac tamponade, which of the following are true and which are false?

a Only occurs after blunt trauma.

b Blood leaks into the pericardial sac around the heart.

c Results in decreased venous pressure.

d Results in pulsus paradoxus.

e There is a 10% mortalilty rate.

5 With regard to haemothorax, which of the following are true and which are false?

  a Massive haemothorax is the accumulation of blood in the pleural space.

  b Caused by lung laceration.

  c There is increased tidal volume.

  d Results in signs and symptoms of shock.

  e There may be tracheal deviation.

6 In the management of pulmonary contusion, which of the following should be considered?

  a Oxygen.

  b Analgesia.

  c Thoracostomy.

  d Intubation and ventilation.

  e Pulmonary toilet.

Rib fractures (Answers, see p. 250)

1 With regard to flail chest, which of the following are true and which are false?

  a It is caused by a fracture on two ribs.

  b It is a segment of chest that does not have continuity with the rest of the chest.

  c There is paradoxical chest wall movement.

  d There is good air entry.

  e There may be crepitus of ribs with respiration.

2 A 30-year-old body-builder had acute focal chest pain in his right posterior chest wall, needing emergency admission to a surgical ward. He gives a history of anabolic steroid use and lifting heavy weights as part of his work-up. He was found to have a crepitus on the fifth rib, confirmed as a fracture on X-ray with no other findings. What would his management plan include?

  a Stopping anabolic steroids.

  b K-nailing the broken rib.

  c Analgesia and chest physiotherapy.

  d Immediate thoracotomy.

  e Reassurance and discharge to abstain from exercise for a week.

3 Which of the following would be appropriate in the management of rib fractures?

  a Nebulizers.

  b Patient-controlled nerve block.

  c Intercostal nerve blocks.

  d Lumbar punctures.

  e Regular physiotherapy.

4 The complications of rib fractures include which of the following?

  a Pneumonia.

  b Atelectasis.

c Cardiac arrest.
d Tracheobronchial fistula.
e Splenic haemorrhage.

Tension pneumothorax (Answers, see p. 250)

1 Regarding tension pneumothorax, which of the following are true and which are false?
a It is caused by an open chest wall injury.
b Air leaks from the pleural space into the lung.
c The remaining uninjured lung is compressed.
d There is an increase in heart size.
e Can result in death.

2 A 35-year-old man collapsed on a street and was wheeled into A&E with shortness of breath. He had a tube thoracostomy for tension pneumothorax. Which of the following methods is useful in diagnosing a tension pneumothorax?
a CXR.
b Clinical examination.
c CT scan of chest.
d Transoesophageal echocardiography.
e ECG.

3 Regarding open pneumothorax, which of the following are true and which are false?
a If the opening is one-third the diameter of the trachea, air passes through chest defect with respiratory effort.
b An open sucking chest wound allows free passage of air into and out of the pleural space.
c Results in lung collapse.
d Treat with 95% oxygen plus 5% carbon dioxide and occlusive dressing.
e Never develops into tension pneumothorax.

4 A 45-year-old man is admitted to the medical assessment unit by his GP with a pneumothorax, which was identified on plain X-ray during a routine examination for insurance purposes. A wide-bore cannula was inserted into the pleural space to treat the pneumothorax. Subsequent X-rays over the next few weeks showed recurrence of pneumothorax. This gentleman is keen on a solution for this problem. Which of the following would be the best advice in this situation?
a Wide-bore chest drain.
b Video-assisted thoracoscopic excision.
c Thoracotomy and excision.
d Seldinger chest drain.
e Conservative and recurrent aspirations.

5 Clinical features of tension pneumothorax include which of the following?
a Tachypnoea.
b Tachycardia.
c Hyporesonance on the affected side.

d Diminished breath sound on the unaffected side.

e Chest pain.

6 The treatment of tension pneumothorax shoud include which of the following?

a Non-invasive management.

b 100% oxygen.

c Needle decompression.

d Thoracostomy.

e Check CXR.

EMQs (Answers, see p. 251)

1 Options:

a Aortic rupture.

b Oesophageal rupture.

c Cardiac tamponade.

d Myocardial infarction.

e Tension pneumothorax.

f Pseudoaneurysm of aorta.

g Pericarditis.

h Sternal fracture.

i Thoracic outlet syndrome.

j Rib fractures.

For each case below suggest the likely diagnosis from the above list of options. Each option may be used once, more than once or not at all.

(i) A 34-year-old rock climber has had a slip off the rock face. In the emergency department, he is complaining of a choking sensation and tingling down his left arm. The patient required intubation due to rapid deterioration in his condition. During the secondary survey, there was a tense fluctuant lump on the left side of his neck and loss of bony prominences due to the increasing neck swelling. The CTA demonstrated injury to subclavian vessels.

(ii) An 88-year-old man was dragged into the bushes by his dog. The eyewitnesses who came to his aid found him clutching his chest and struggling to breathe. In the emergency department, there was ST elevation in the inferior leads of the ECG. He was admitted to the hospital for further management.

(iii) An 88-year-old woman had a fall onto her right chest 4 days ago. She presents to the surgical assessment unit with right-sided abdominal pain and difficulty breathing. The CXR suggests a right lobar pneumonia.

(iv) A 30-year-old man has been in a high-speed road traffic collision. In the emergency department, he is complaining of difficulty breathing and is becoming centrally cyanosed. There are no breath sounds in the left chest.

2 Options:

a Cardiac tamponade.

b Pericardial effusion.

c Endocarditis.

d Pneumothorax.
e Haemothorax.
f Pleuritis.
g Pneumonia.
h Mediastinitis.

For each case below suggest the likely diagnosis from the above list of options. Each option may be used once, more than once or not at all.

(i) A 32-year-old man has had a massive upper GI bleed after vomiting on a full stomach. He was managed in A&E and stabilized when the bleeding stopped. Subsequently, over the next 48 hours, he develops fever (39°C), malaise and shows signs of septicaemia. On plain CXR he was found to have gas in his mediastinum.

(ii) A 23-year-old woman presents to A&E with palpitations, malaise and fever. She gives a history of intravenous drug abuse and alcohol excess. She was stabilized and had a transthoracic echocardiography which shows vegetation on her mitral valve.

(iii) A 78-year-old woman has had a bypass graft earlier in the day and is being managed on the intensive care unit. She develops acute shortness of breath and reports tightness in her chest before losing consciousness. Her heart sounds are muffled and cardiac output is low.

(iv) A 53-year-old man has been treated for tuberculosis for 2 weeks. He develops occasional chest pain and tightness in his chest. His CXR shows a 'water-bottle-shaped heart'.

3 Options:
a Needle aspiration.
b Seldinger thoracostomy.
c Open thoracostomy.
d Pericardiectomy.
e Pericardiocentesis.
f Mediastinoscopy.

For each case below suggest the appropriate interventional procedure from the above list of options. Each option may be used once, more than once or not at all.

(i) A 45-year-old woman with cardiac tamponade.
(ii) A 32-year-old man with transudative pleural effusion.
(iii) A 75-year-old man with constrictive pericarditis.
(iv) A 16-year-old man with pneumothorax.

4 Options:
a Aortic rupture.
b Oesophageal rupture.
c Cardiac tamponade.
d Myocardial infarction.
e Tension pneumothorax.
f Pseudoaneurysm of aorta.
g Pericarditis.
h Sternal fracture.
i Thoracic outlet syndrome.

For each case below suggest the likely diagnosis from the above list of options. Each option may be used once, more than once or not at all.

(i) A 26-year-old woman was thrown against her car windscreen while involved in a rapid deceleration into a wall. She was fluid resuscitated on the scene but continues to be tachycardic and hypotensive. The CXR in the emergency department showed a widened mediastinum with a clear aortic knob visualized on left half of the aortic arch.

(ii) A 65-year-old farmer has been trampled in a stampede. He was airlifted to the nearest hospital where he received active resuscitation with oxygen and fluids. His ECG and AP erect CXR were normal but he complains of chest pain when taking a deep breath in. On examination, subcutaneous emphysema was obviously palpable on medial anterior chest associated with an audible crepitus.

(iii) A 45-year-old man was a train passenger involved in a high-speed train derailment. He hit the side of his chest and is complaining of chest pain. Following stabilization in A&E, the patient has a CTA. He was found to have an aortic injury which could be managed conservatively.

6 Breast

This section covers the following breast conditions:
- mastitis
- fat necrosis
- benign breast lumps
- breast cancer.

Mastitis

Inflammation of breast tissue. There are two causes:
- acute mastitis (synonym: puerperal or lactation mastitis)
- mammary duct ectasia (synonym: periductal mastitis)

Acute mastitis

I & S : Commonly in breast-feeding mothers, up to 3 months post partum.

A & P : Caused by infectious agents, local reaction to a systemic disease, a localized antigen–antibody reaction, idiopathic. There is cellulitis of the interlobular connective tissue within the mammary gland, resulting in abscess formation.

Risk factors: improper breast-feeding technique, leading to milk stasis and cracks or fissures of the nipple.

C F & D : The affected breast is erythematous, warm and swollen. It is tender to touch +/– fever and rigors. Because lactation mastitis is a result of cellulitis in the subcutaneous tissue, culture results are often reported negative. Majority are diagnosed clinically.

T & M : Abscess is assessed by USS and treated by needle aspiration +/– antibiotics. Stop breast-feeding in the presence of breast abscess.

P : Good prognosis for complete recovery.

Mammary duct ectasia

I & S : Middle-aged to elderly parous women (age 40–50 years), often non-lactating.

A & P : The duct becomes dilated, thickened and blocked during involution (glandular breast tissue changes to fatty tissue). Smoking has been implicated.

C F & D : The most common presentation is microcalcification on mammogram. Other presentations include:
- nipple discharge (grey to green)
- erythema, palpable mass under the nipple
- non-cyclical mastalgia
- nipple inversion or retraction.

EMQs and MCQs for Surgical Finals, 1st edition.   © Hye-Chung Kwak, Imran Bhatti, Jaskarn Rai, Farhan Rashid, Bachittar Singh Jassar, Murthy Nyasavajjala, Viren Asher, Jon Lund and Mike Larvin. Published 2011 by Blackwell Publishing Ltd.

Investigate with mammogram (microcalcifications in older women) and USS (aids differentiation between benign and malignant). Caution: mimics invasive carcinoma clinically.

T&M: Usually improves on its own. Antibiotics (for infection) +/− excision of the duct.

P: Good prognosis.

Fat necrosis

D: Benign non-suppurative inflammatory process of the fat padding of the breast.

I&S: Incidence <1%. Females 40–50 years old.

A&P: Caused by trauma.

CF&D: Often presents as an ill-defined spiculated dense mass, associated with skin retraction, ecchymosis, erythema, and skin thickness. No distinctive test to distinguish fat necrosis from a malignant lesion except histopathology.

T&M: Analgesics for pain. Resolves within 1 month. Lump excision performed if carcinoma suspected.

P: Excellent prognosis.

Benign breast lumps

The following benign breast lumps are covered:
- fibrocystic breast disease
- simple cysts
- fibroadenomata
- intraductal papillomas.

Fibrocystic breast disease (lumpy breasts)

D: Bilateral, multifocal, painful lesions. Increased risk of breast cancer (twofold to sixfold) in fibrocystic breast disease with hyperplasia or atypical hyperplasia.

I&S: Affects more than 60% of premenopausal women.

A&P: Hormone sensitive, often cyclical.

CF&D: Symptoms vary: breast pain, nipple itching, fullness in breast. Mobile lumps vary from one woman to another. Some are round with smooth borders; others are rubbery with irregular edges.

Diagnosis involves physical examination +/− USS +/− biopsy (to exclude breast cancer).

T&M: Symptom relief with analgesia, establish regular menstrual cycle (oral contraceptives). Regular self-examination and breast cancer screening is essential.

P: Excellent prognosis in the absence of abnormal breast cells.

Simple cysts

D: Simple cysts are benign fluid-filled sacs that usually occur in both breasts. They can be single or multiple and can vary in size.

I&S: Affects women between 30 and 40 years old.

A&P: The cause is unknown. Fibrocystic changes block ducts, causing duct dilatation and fluid accumulation.

CF&D: Lumps are firm, round or oval-shaped with distinct edges. Tenderness and lump size are often cyclical. Core needle biopsy or rarely aspiration and cytology for diagnosis.

T & M : Drain large and painful cysts. Most usually disappear after menopause.

P : Excellent prognosis.

Fibroadenomata ('breast mice')

D : Benign breast tumour.

I & S : Most common benign lesion in the female breast, age groups <30.

A & P : Arising from the interlobular stroma. Sensitive to estrogen; comes and goes with menstrual cycle. Exact cause unknown.

C F & D : Clinically present as a highly mobile, firm, non-tender and often palpable breast mass with distinct borders. Largely unilateral and solitary; sometimes multiple lesions occur in the same breast or bilaterally. Investigations may involve mammogram, USS or MRI. Diagnosis with FNA or core needle biopsy.

T & M : None required if the lesions stop growing. Surgical removal for larger, painful or growing lesions.

P : Excellent prognosis.

Intraductal papillomas

D : Small wart-like growths in the lining of the mammary duct near the nipple.

I & S : Usual lesion among those 40–50 years of age.

A & P : Cause and risk factor is unknown.

C F & D : Clinically presents as a nipple bleed or nipple discharge. Triple assessment with breast examination, USS or ductogram investigation. Diagnosis with FNAC or core biopsy +/– duct excision.

T & M : Excision biopsy and follow-up.

P : Excellent prognosis if there is one tumour.

Breast cancer

I & S : Breast cancer is the most common cancer and the second most common cause of death from cancer in women. Nearly 1% of breast cancer occurs in men.

A & P : Invasive breast cancers are typically ductal (85%) or lobular (15%) adenocarcinomas.

- Heterogeneous disease: multiple risk factors identified including early menarche, regular ovulation, and late menopause (in premenopausal women); obesity and hormone replacement therapy (in postmenopausal women).
- Hereditary breast cancers form only 5–10% of all breast cancers.

AJCC classification

The following is a list of breast cancer histological classifications. Infiltrating or invasive ductal cancer is the most common breast cancer histological type and comprises 70–80% of all cases.

Carcinoma, NOS

Ductal
- Intraductal (*in situ*)
- Invasive with predominant intraductal component
- Invasive, NOS

- Comedo
- Inflammatory
- Medullary with lymphocytic infiltrate
- Mucinous (colloid)
- Papillary
- Scirrhous
- Tubular
- Other

Lobular
- *In situ*
- Invasive with predominant *in situ* component
- Invasive

Nipple
- Paget disease, NOS
- Paget disease with intraductal carcinoma
- Paget disease with invasive ductal carcinoma

Other
- Undifferentiated carcinoma

The following tumour subtypes occur in the breast but are not considered to be typical breast cancers
- Phyllodes tumour
- Angiosarcoma
- Primary lymphoma

CF&D:

- Most common presentation: painless lump.
- Other presentations: breast pain or deformity, nipple discharge, and erythema or skin ulceration.
- Paget's disease: eczematous rash of the nipple and areola, itching and tenderness.
- Skin dimpling: retraction of Cooper ligaments.
- Peau d'orange sign: invasion of the subdermal lymphatic plexus.
  Diagnosis is with triple assessment:
- Clinical assessment
- Imaging: mammogram and USS (diagnosis and guidance for biopsy)
- Cytology/histopathology.

Surgical procedures for non-palpable lesions

- Image-guided core-needle biopsy
- Open biopsy with needle localization

Surgical procedures for palpable lesions

- FNA (sensitivity 80–90%, specificity 100%)
- Core biopsy
- Excision biopsy

T & M : Can be surgical or medical:

Ductal carcinoma *in situ* (DCIS)

• 85% of DCIS is detected on a mammogram.
• Management: mastectomy cures 98–99% of all types of DCIS, with a recurrence rate of only 1–2%.

Lobular carcinoma *in situ* (LCIS)

• LCIS is not a cancer; but increased risk of breast cancer.
• Management: active follow-up.

Treatment of invasive disease involves a multidisciplinary approach (surgery, chemotherapy, hormone therapy and radiotherapy). Prognosticating factors include age, menopausal status, lymph node status, ER/PR status and HER2 status. These factors form the basis for offering a particular treatment.

The following surgical treatments can be offered.

Surgery	Breast tissue	Axillary nodes	Pectoral muscles	Skin
Lumpectomy	Tumour + 0.5–1 cm normal tissue	Sampling	–	–
Radical mastectomy	Removed	Removed	Removed	Removed
Modified radical mastectomy	Removed	Partially/ completely	Fascia of pectoralis major	–
Total mastectomy	Removed	–	–	–

Adjuvant therapy involves hormone therapy (HT). The goal of HT in breast cancer is to induce an estrogen-deprivation state at the tumour level.

1 Receptor blockade, e.g. tamoxifen.
2 Suppression of estrogen synthesis:
  (a) Postmenopausal: aromatase inhibitors (e.g. anastrozole, letrozole).
  (b) Premenopausal: luteinizing hormone-releasing hormone analogues (e.g. goserelin).
3 Surgical oophorectomy or external beam radiation therapy in premenopausal women.

P : The 5-year relative survival for breast cancer is 80%.

M C Q s (Answers, see p. 252)

1 A 42-year-old woman had triple assessment for bilateral painful breasts, and a lump in her left breast. She was reassured by the surgeon that her symptoms

were part of benign breast disease. Which of the following statements are true?

a Cyclical mastalgia is the commonest reason for referral to the breast clinic.

b About 10% of fibroadenomata will disappear per year in women who have them verified by fine-needle aspiration follow-up.

c Benign breast disease is an important risk factor for breast cancer.

d Phyllodes tumour is always a benign fibroepithelial tumour.

e Fibroadenosis and microcysts disappear after menopause.

2 A 23-year-old woman is alarmed because of an accidental finding in her right breast. She noticed a painless lump that moves freely, and has some colourless discharge from both her nipples. She underwent triple assessment and was reassured by her surgeon. Regarding these types of lumps, which of the following statements are true and which are false?

a They are benign monoclonal neoplasms.

b Usually found in women younger than 30 years.

c Are rounded in outline and easily movable.

d At least 30% reduce in size over a 2-year period.

e Always have to be excised and studied by histopathology.

3 During breast self-examination, a 48-year-old woman has noted a non-tender mobile lump in her breast growing in size over the last 3 months. On clinical assessment, a firm 2-cm mass was palpable in the upper outer quadrant of her right breast. She underwent lumpectomy with axillary node sampling. The breast lesion is found to be HER2 positive and ER/PR negative. Which of the following additional treatment options is most likely to be efficacious in this woman?

a Anastrozole.

b Radical mastectomy.

c Epirubicin.

d Tamoxifen.

e Trastuzumab.

4 A 55-year-old woman has a routine screening mammogram and has an abnormal mammogram with multiple small areas of increased density. FNAC of an abnormal density reveals cells suspicious for a malignancy. Local wire-guided excision biopsy confirms an LCIS of the breast. Which of the following is the most likely finding associated with this woman's carcinoma?

a It is easily detectable on mammogram.

b It is multicentric often involving contralateral breast.

c A family history of breast cancer is unlikely.

d Estrogen receptor assay of this neoplasm will be negative.

e Mastectomy is strongly recommended for this type of lesion.

5 A 68-year-old woman was diagnosed with a 9-mm comedo intraductal carcinoma on histopathology after wide local excision of a mobile lump in her left breast. Which of the following is most likely associated with this type of cancer?

a It usually metastasizes early to the regional lymph nodes.

b Intraductal lesions larger than 5 cm tend to be focally invasive.

c This type of neoplasm needs routine axillary dissection at an early stage.

d Radical mastectomy is always advised for this type of lesion.

e Preoperative radiotherapy improves outcomes in this type of lesion.

EMQs (Answers, see p. 252)

1 Options:
   a Paget's disease of breast.
   b Puerperal mastitis.
   c Breast abscess.
   d Ductal ectasia.
   e Fibroadenoma.
   f Breast carcinoma.
   g Galactorrhoea.
   h Phylloides tumour.

For each case below suggest the likely diagnosis from the above list of options. Each option may be used once, more than once or not at all.

   (i) A 48-year-old woman presents with eczema-like rash affecting a recently inverted right nipple. The skin over the nipple and areola is itchy, red and inflamed. Fluid discharge from the nipple demonstrated a clump of abnormal cells.

   (ii) A 27-year-old lactating mother presents with redness and diffuse swelling of her left breast. On examination there is tenderness, with yellow-white nipple discharge on expression. USS shows a cystic collection in her breast.

   (iii) A 36-year-old woman presents with distressing nipple discharge and nipple retraction. She is a smoker of 10 cigarettes a day and has never breast-fed. On examination, she has white nipple discharge from her nipple, and on USS scan there is a retro-areolar abscess.

   (iv) An 18-year-old woman has noticed a recent painless rubbery and mobile lump in her left breast. Mammogram of the lesion showed a smooth round mass with a clearly defined edge. USS reveals a well-defined hypoechoic homogeneous mass 2.5 cm in diameter.

2 Options:
   a Postpartum mastitis.
   b Breast abscess.
   c Galactocele.
   d Periductal mastitis.
   e Fungal mastitis.
   f Cellulitis of breast.
   g Mammary fistula.

For each case below suggest the likely diagnosis from the above list of options. Each option may be used once, more than once or not at all.

   (i) A 23-year-old woman who is 2 weeks post partum has a localized cellulitis and multiple fissures and cracks on her nipple. Her symptoms worsen when she stops feeding her baby. USS of the breast shows no abscesses.

(ii) A 26-year-old woman has plugging of her lactiferous duct due to keratin plugs, resulting in a lump. On examination she has a fluctuant swelling in her peri-areolar region in upper outer quadrant.

(iii) A 36-year-old smoker who is an insulin-dependent diabetic, not currently lactating, has active inflammation around non-dilated subareolar breast ducts.

(iv) A 32-year-old woman with a BMI of 36 has redness and pain in the skin over the lower half of the breast which is tender on examination.

Part 4 Abdomen
7 Acute abdomen

Overview

D : Half the surgical admissions are admitted as emergencies, and more than half of all surgical emergencies present with acute abdominal pain.

I & S : Depends on the type of acute abdomen.

C F & D : Features of a typical patient heading for surgery:

- acute pain
- septic and toxic
- board-like abdomen
- absent bowel sounds
- WCC > 25 × 10^9/L
- Free air under diaphragm.

Differential diagnoses

Non-emergencies
- Mesenteric adenitis
- Acute enteric infections
- Acute enteric poisonings
- IBD
- Pancreatitis

Other
- DKA
- Heavy metal poisoning
- Acute porphyria
- Tabes
- Sickle cell crisis

Signs and symptoms can be divided into type, site, duration, character and radiation of pain and aggravating/relieving factors.

Types of pain

- Visceral: dull poorly localized pain in midline epigastrium, periumbilical region or lower mid-abdomen, crampy, burning and gnawing.
- Referred: pain felt in areas remote to the disease organ (e.g. subphrenic abscess felt as shoulder pain).

EMQs and MCQs for Surgical Finals, 1st edition. © Hye-Chung Kwak, Imran Bhatti, Jaskarn Rai, Farhan Rashid, Bachittar Singh Jassar, Murthy Nyasavajjala, Viren Asher, Jon Lund and Mike Larvin. Published 2011 by Blackwell Publishing Ltd.

Progression of pain

- Appendicitis: increases
- Gastroenteritis: decreases if clinically improving
- Colic: crescendo/decrescendo

Pain: aggravating/relieving factors

	Relieving factors	Aggravating factors
Peritonitis	Lie motionless	Movement
Renal colic	No relieving factors	Worse after micturition. Patient writhes, unable to find comfortable position
Biliary colic	No relieving factors	Fatty foods
Cholecystitis	Being still	Movement
Duodenal ulcer	Pain improves with eating	NBM
Gastric ulcer	Antacid tablets	Worse with eating
Mesenteric ischaemia	No relieving factors	Worse with eating

Diagnostic studies

- Blood tests: FBC, amylase
- Urine: urinary amylase, UTI
- Radionuclide scans: Meckel's diverticulum
- X-ray: AXR (obstruction), CXR (perforation)
- USS: biliary colic/liver abscesses, cholecystitis
- TVU: pelvic free fluid, ovarian mass/rupture
- CT abdomen/pelvis: visceral perforation/ischaemia

T & M : Depends on the condition but usually an operation (laparotomy or laparoscopy) is required to remove the problem.

P : Depends on the initial condition of the patient and the type of operation required.

Necrotizing fasciitis

D : This is a rapidly progressing, inflammatory infection of the deep fascia with secondary necrosis of the subcutaneous tissues caused by gas-forming organisms.

I & S : M/F ratio 2–3 : 1. Mean age is 38–44 years. Incidence in the UK is 500 new cases annually.

A & P : Risk factors include skin biopsy, needle puncture in IVDU patients, open fractures and surgical wounds. Predisposing factors include age >60 years, malnutrition, type 2 diabetes, alcohol abuse, peripheral vascular disease, renal failure, malignancy. It is most commonly caused by polymicrobial infections with both anaerobic and aerobic bacteria.

C F & D : The diagnosis is mainly clinical. The patient appears moderately to severely toxic with high temperature, tachycardia, hypotension and altered conscious level. It can affect any part of the body but most commonly the extremities, perineum (known as Fournier's disease) and truncal areas. Patients are unwell and a disproportionate amount of pain is present with only minor skin changes. Bullae, oedema, crepitus, erythema and necrosis may develop at a later stage (2–3 days).

Serum blood tests show a high WCC, abnormal renal function, hypoalbuminaemia and abnormal clotting profile. ABG may show metabolic acidosis from severe sepsis. X-ray shows soft tissue gas. MRI delineates the extent of infection which may help direct the extent of surgical débridement.

T & M : Manage airways and breathing with high-flow oxygen. Resuscitate patient with IV fluids. Primary treatment is with early and aggressive surgical débridement with IV antibiotics. The use of hyperbaric oxygen is controversial but has been shown to improve limb salvage.

P : Amputation and mortality rates are as high as 22%. Mortality is associated with delayed diagnosis, poor surgical technique and the presence of comorbidities such as diabetes.

Sigmoid volvulus

D : The sigmoid colon rotates around its mesenteric pedicle (usually more than 180° counterclockwise) resulting in partial or complete intestinal obstruction. There is a risk of ischaemia from venous congestion.

I & S : The commonest form of volvulus in the GIT. Older patients, M > F.

A & P : Anatomic defect: (i) the root of the sigmoid mesentery has a narrow attachment to the posterior abdominal wall; (ii) A long mesenteric axis. The site of torsion is typically 15 cm above the anal verge.

C F & D : Abdominal pain, distended abdomen, absolute constipation, nausea and vomiting. On examination there is tympanic abdomen +/– palpable mass.

DRE shows an empty rectum. Bowel loop seen on plain AXR. Can perform barium enema to locate obstruction, CT scan to diagnose ischaemic bowel.

T & M : Treatment with rigid sigmoidoscopy (can confirm diagnosis) and flatus tube +/– endoscopy +/– fluoroscopy. Laparotomy required for ischaemic bowel.

P : Half of patients will recur in the next 2 years. Mortality associated with sigmoid volvulus can be as high as 20%.

Shock

Life-threatening medical condition accompanied by a severe injury or illness in which the body suffers with insufficient blood flow causing hypoxia. There are five types of shock:

- septic
- anaphylactic
- cardiogenic
- hypovolaemic
- neurogenic.

Septic shock

D : Caused by bacteria multiplying in the blood causing release of toxins.

I & S : The incidence is on the rise, M ≈ F.

A & P : Cause is infective: pneumonia, appendicitis, meningitis, UTI, wound infection, etc.; 1.3% of all hospitalizations are from septicaemia and the incidence has increased threefold in the last two decades. The likely reasons for this increase include increasing elderly population, increased recognition of disease, organ transplantation, use of immunosuppressive and chemotherapeutic agents, increased use of indwelling lines, chronic disease and HIV.

The pathological process occurs from activation of host defence mechanisms through the influx of activated neutrophils and monocytes, release of inflammatory mediators, local vasodilatation, increased endothelial permeability and activation of coagulation pathways which results in end-organ dysfunction by formation of microthrombi.

CF&D: The symptoms and signs are variable. The American Society of Critical Care Medicine (www.sccm.org) defines systemic inflammatory response syndrome (SIRS) as meeting at least two of four criteria:

- temperature > 38°C or < 36°C
- tachycardia > 90 bpm
- tachypnoea > 20 breaths/min
- raised WCC > 12×10^9/L or < 4×10^9/L.

It is possible for a patient to have sepsis without meeting the SIRS criteria and furthermore SIRS may be present in the setting of many other illnesses. SIRS may lead to shock and then to multiorgan dysfunction syndrome (MODS).

General features

Fever is a common feature. The skin is usually warm in early septic shock due to peripheral vasodilatation and increased cardiac output. As septic shock progresses, depletion of intravascular volume and decreased cardiac output leads to cool clammy peripheries and delayed capillary refill. Petechiae or purpura can be associated with DIC.

Cardiovascular system

Tachycardia may occur as a physiological mechanism to increase cardiac output and oxygen delivery to tissues. It is an indication of hypovolaemia and the need for intravascular fluid replacement. Inotropic support should also be considered to counteract peripheral vasodilatation.

Respiratory system

Increased respiratory rate usually occurs from stimulation of respiratory centre in the medulla by endotoxins and also to compensate for metabolic acidosis from tissue hypoperfusion.

CNS

Altered mental status may be caused by cerebral hypoperfusion.

Investigations should include septic screen (FBC, CRP, microbiological cultures of blood, urine, wound, sputum, stool, CSF) and CXR. Further imaging includes USS and CT for intra-abdominal sepsis.

T&M: Early recognition and treatment is crucial. Administer appropriate antibiotics as soon as sepsis is noted together with volume replacement +/− inotropic support. It is also imperative to remove the source of sepsis as soon as possible (i.e. laparotomy for abdominal sepsis from stercoral perforation). Sequelae of septic shock include myocardial dysfunction, acute renal failure, DIC and liver failure. Specialist management is required.

P : Mortality rate is up to 50% depending on the severity of the sepsis.

Anaphylactic shock

D : Severe hypersensitivity reaction leading to shock.

I&S: Frequency of anaphylaxis has been explained by the increased exposure of subjects to allergens. The lifetime prevalence is up to 2% of the population as a whole.

A & P : Insect stings, medicines (especially antibiotics) or foods (nuts, berries, seafood). The effects of anaphylaxis are produced by release of mediators (including histamine, LTC_4, PGD_2 and tryptase) when the antigen binds to IgE antibody. This in turn results in increased secretion from mucous membranes, increased bronchial smooth muscle tone, decreased vascular smooth muscle tone and increased capillary permeability. Histamine release in the skin causes urticarial skin lesions.

C F & D :

- Skin/mucosa: urticaria, erythema, pruritis and angio-oedema with hypotension and bronchospasm.
- Eyes: itching and tearing with possible conjunctival injection.
- RS: cough, hoarseness, nasal congestion, sneezing, coryza, dyspnoea and hypoxia.
- GIT: nausea, vomiting, abdominal pain and diarrhoea are less common.

In general, investigations have no immediate role in the management of anaphylactic shock. Diagnosis is clinical. It is crucial to take a thorough history and exclude other causes of shock.

T & M : Treat in response to history and examination. Use the ABCDE approach and treat with IM or IV adrenaline, hydrocortisone and antihistamines.

P : Approximately 10–20 deaths/year in the UK occur from anaphylactic shock. Patients at high risk of shock should carry an adrenaline auto-injector.

Cardiogenic shock

D : Injury to the heart resulting in reduced cardiac output.

I & S : Cardiogenic shock occurs in approximately 7% of patients with acute MI.

A & P : The most common cause for cardiogenic shock is MI. A decrease in contractility results in reduced ejection fraction and cardiac output. These events lead to increased ventricular filling pressures, cardiac chamber dilatation, and eventually univentricular or biventricular failure that result in systemic hypotension and/or pulmonary oedema.

C F & D : Acute MI may present with chest/shoulder/jaw pain, shortness of breath, nausea and vomiting. Patients with cardiogenic shock may also present with noisy laboured breathing (due to pulmonary oedema) and pre/syncopal symptoms.

Careful cardiac examination is important. Cardiac murmurs may indicate valvular dysfunction whereas muffled heart sounds, raised JVP and pulsus paradoxus may indicate cardiac tamponade.

Differential diagnosis

- Differing BP from both arms may indicate a dissecting thoracic aneurysm.
- Distension of neck veins shows evidence of right ventricular failure or tamponade.

Investigations

- Blood tests: cardiac enzymes (troponin T), urea and electrolytes.
- Imaging: CXR will help assess heart size, pulmonary vascularity and mediastinal size to exclude aortic aetiology. Echocardiography when suspicion of valvular dysfunction or tamponade.
- 12-lead ECG: acute MI and old MI.

T & M : Follow the ABCDE approach. Anticoagulation and aspirin +/– inotropes +/– coronary angioplasty in acute MI.

P : Mortality in patients with acute MI and cardiogenic shock is 70% or more. Outcomes improve when rapid revascularization can be achieved.

Hypovolaemic shock

D : Severe blood/fluid loss reduces the preload of the heart resulting in reduced stroke volume.

I & S : Depends on the cause.

A & P : Ruptured abdominal aortic aneurysm (AAA), injury to a major blood vessel, severe diarrhoea and vomiting, and burns. Acute haemorrhage results in the activation of haematological, cardiovascular, renal and neuroendocrine systems.

Haematological system

Activation of the coagulation system and contracting blood vessels (releasing TxA_2). An immature blood clot is formed on the bleeding source by the activation of platelets. The damaged blood vessel exposes collagen, which causes fibrin deposition and formation of stable clot after 24 hours.

Cardiovascular system

Increase in heart rate, myocardial contractility and peripheral vasoconstriction. This occurs secondary to increased release of noradrenaline and decreased activation of baroreceptors (carotid arch, aortic arch, left atrium and pulmonary vessels).

Renal system

Activation of the renin–angiotensin system. Angiotensin II causes vasoconstriction and stimulation of aldosterone results in increased intravascular volume by retention of water and sodium.

Neuroendocrine system

Increase in antidiuretic hormone (ADH) from the posterior pituitary gland is released as a result of decreased firing of baroreceptors from hypotension and decrease in sodium concentration. ADH causes increased intravascular volume by resorption of NaCl and water at the distal tubule, collecting ducts and loop of Henle.

C F & D : BP alone should not be used as the main indicator for shock, especially in young people. Compensatory mechanisms prevent significant decrease in systolic BP until the patient has lost 30% of blood volume. More weight should be given to pulse, respiratory rate and skin perfusion. Patients taking beta-blockers may not present with tachycardia.

In suspected cases of hypovolaemic shock, investigate as follows:

- Blood tests: FBC, U&E, clotting profile, G&S or cross-match, ABG, β-HCG in females (ectopic pregnancy).
- Imaging: CXR for haemothorax/perforation of viscus, plain X-ray for long bone fractures, FAST for intra-abdominal bleeding, CT for stable patients with suspected bleeding.

Classes of haemorrhage have been defined, based on percentage of blood volume loss.

Class	Blood loss	Pulse rate (bpm)	BP	RR	UO	Conscious level
I	0–15%	Minimal tachycardia	↔ BP	↔	↔	Alert
II	15–30%	>100	↔BP, ↓PP	↑	↔	Alert
III	30–40%	>120	↓BP	↑	↓	Agitated, confused
IV	>40%	>120	↓↓BP, ↓PP	↑	↓/Anuric	Drowsy/LOC

Following trauma there are four areas in which haemorrhage may occur:

- Chest: auscultate for decreased breath sounds for a possible haemothorax.
- Abdomen: examine for abdominal tenderness or distension which may indicate intra-abdominal bleeding.
- Pelvis: examine for pelvic fractures.
- Thighs: examine for deformities or enlargement (signs of fracture and bleeding into thigh).

In trauma patients, the entire body should be examined for other external bleeding. In the patient without trauma, signs of AAA and perforated viscus should be identified.

T & M : Follow the ABCDE approach. Main goals: maximize oxygen delivery, fluid resuscitation, stop bleeding and fluid loss.

P : Dependent on the degree of blood loss.

Neurogenic shock

D : Spinal injury affecting sympathetic output and leading to hypotension, bradycardia, peripheral vasodilatation and hypothermia.

I & S : Approximately 20% in patients with isolated spinal cord injury.

A & P : Disrupted sympathetic outflow after spinal cord injury. It does not usually occur with spinal cord injury below T6.

C F & D : Hypotension (narrow PP), bradycardia (weak pulse), increased RR, cold clammy skin, dizziness or LOC, confusion/anxiety, low or no UO. Exclude all other causes of shock before diagnosing neurogenic shock.

T & M : Follow ABCDE approach. If patient is unable to maintain airway (i.e. GCS < 8, airway obstruction or hypoxia) emergency intubation may be required. Patients should be administered oxygen at 15 L/min through a non-rebreathing mask. Wide-bore cannulas should be inserted into the antecubital fossa, blood samples taken (FBC, U&E, LFT, coagulation profile, and G&S or cross-match depending on whether there is obvious blood loss), IV fluids infusion and catheterization (minimum UO of 0.5 mL/kg per hour). Inotropes may be given (with intensive monitoring) to increase BP to ensure good blood flow to vital organs.

Summary of treatments

Septic shock
Septic screen (CXR, urine, LP, stool sample, blood cultures, and possible USS or CT looking for intra-abdominal sepsis) and prompt administration of appropriate IV antibiotics.

Anaphylactic shock
Adrenaline, antihistamines and hydrocortisone. Salbutamol nebulizers maybe useful in bronchospasm.

Cardiogenic shock
Treat the underlying cause (i.e. MI, CCF). Cardiac inotropes maybe required in the intensive setting. Intra-aortic balloon pump (IABP) is recommended in situations where shock is resistant to pharmacological agents. IABP causes counterpulsation and reduces left ventricular afterload as well as improving coronary blood flow.

Hypovolaemic shock
Treat with IV colloids/blood. The underlying cause for bleeding must be stopped. Minimize further blood loss by splinting fractures, direct pressure over wounds, IV H_2 blockers and vasopressor for GI bleeds. Bleeding varices: first-line management is endoscopy, second-line management is lower oesophageal pressure using Sengstaken–Blakemore tube (lots of complications). Acute intra-abdominal bleed would require surgical intervention.

Neurogenic shock
IV fluids, immobilization and monitoring.

ATLS

The trauma team approach to managing seriously injured patients is crucial for improving patient management.

Primary survey

The first and key part of the assessment is primary survey, during which life-threatening injuries are identified and simultaneous resuscitation is initiated. ABCDE is a simple mnemonic for remembering in which order problems should be assessed.

A Maintain airway with C-spine protection
B Breathing and ventilation
C Circulation and haemorrhage control
D Disability (neurological assessment)
E Exposure and environment

A A talking patient is likely to have a clear airway. However, if the patient is unconscious, he or she may not be able to maintain the airway. With a GCS of 9–13 the airway can be opened using a chin lift or jaw thrust. Airway adjuncts (Guedel airway or nasopharyngeal airway; avoid in basal skull fracture) may be required; in an obstructed airway (blood or vomitus), suction instruments should be used to clear the blockage. A definitive airway should be instituted by an anaesthetist in patients who have GCS < 8 or severe maxillofacial and laryngeal injuries. The neck should be immobilized in a semi-rigid cervical collar, blocks and tape.

B The chest should be examined as routine (inspection, palpation, percussion and auscultation). Life-threatening injuries including tension pneumothorax, open pneumothorax, flail chest and massive haemothorax must be identified and treated immediately. Subcutaneous emphysema and tracheal deviation may suggest tension pneumothorax.

C Hypovolaemic shock is caused by significant blood loss. Two large-bore intravenous lines should be inserted, blood should be taken for FBC, U&E, cross-match and crystalloid solution is infused. If the patient does not respond, then type-specific or O-negative blood should be given. External bleeding is controlled by pressure although occult blood loss may be into chest, abdomen, pelvis or from long bones. Chest and pelvic bleeding can be identified on X-ray and bleeding into the peritoneum can be assessed by CT scan (stable) or laparotomy (unstable).

D Assess GCS. Pupils are examined for size, symmetry and reaction to light. A rapid neurological examination can be undertaken to check for lateralizing signs and signs of spinal cord injury.

E The clothes are removed and the patient is covered with a blanket to prevent hypothermia.

Secondary survey

Once the primary survey is completed, conduct a head-to-toe evaluation of the patient, including a complete history (AMPLE history) and examination.

AMPLE

A Allergies
M Medications currently used
P Past illnesses/pregnancy
L last meal
E Events/environment related to the injury

MCQs

Necrotizing fasciitis (Answers, see p. 253)

1 Treatment of necrotizing fasciitis mandates which of the following?
  a Emperical administration of antibiotics against Gram-positive, Gram-negative and anaerobic bacteria.
  b Hyperbaric oxygen has been proven to be useful.

   c Penicillins have not been indicated due to resistant species.

   d Operative intervention through the aggressive resection of tissues involved is mandatory.

   e Gram-positive organisms are treated with vancomycin.

2 Concerning necrotizing fasciitis, which of the following are true and which are false?

   a Impaired immune system is a common factor predisposing to this condition.

   b Mortality rates may be as high as 70%.

   c The infection only involves the superficial fascia alone.

   d It is likely to develop in the face of impaired fascial blood supply.

   e The infection is usually polymicrobial.

3 Necrotizing fasciitis can be a complication of which of the following?

   a Repair of rectal prolapse.

   b Oral antidiabetic medication.

   c Laparoscopy.

   d Breast-feeding.

   e Excision of skin lesion.

Sigmoid volvulus (Answers, see p. 253)

1 Risk factors for sigmoid volvulus include which of the following?

   a Mobile colon.

   b Hyperactive patients.

   c Diarrhoea.

   d Old age.

   e Irritable bowel syndrome.

2 A frail 70-year-old man is admitted from a residential home with chronic constipation, lower abdominal pains and abdominal distension. The AXR shows a large comma-shaped shadow in mid-abdomen. Both the clinical features and AXR indicate caecal volvulus. What is your management of this patient?

   a Consent the gentleman for a right hemicolectomy.

   b Resuscitate the patient.

   c Insert a flatus tube.

   d Request a double-contrast water enema.

   e Send urgent bloods for G&S.

3 The clinical features of colonic volvulus include which of the following?

   a Dull abdomen on percussion.

   b Distended abdomen.

   c Abdominal pain.

   d Shock.

   e Blood-stained stools.

4 A frail 77-year-old bed-bound man is admitted from a nursing home with a 7-day history of abdominal distension associated with absolute constipation.

The AXR shows a large coffee bean-shaped bowel loop arising from the pelvis and the observations indicate sepsis. What is your immediate management?
a CT abdomen.
b Immediate decompression with flatus tube.
c Send blood tests for U&E.
d Start the ABCDE sequence.
e Start IV antibiotics.

Shock (Answers, see p. 254)

1 Which of the following are criteria for diagnosing systemic inflammatory response syndrome (SIRS)?
a Abnormal haemoglobin level.
b Acidosis.
c Tachycardia.
d Raised WCC.
e Pyrexia above 38°C.

2 Which of the following statements best defines severe sepsis?
a Pyrexia alone with the presence of infection.
b SIRS with the presence of infection.
c SIRS with end-organ dysfunction.
d SIRS with hypotension despite fluid resuscitation.
e SIRS alone.

3 Which of the following is the most common initiating event for cardiogenic shock?
a MI.
b CCF.
c Penetrating injury to the myocardium.
d Cardiac contusion.
e Cardiac tamponade.

4 Haemorrhage initiates a series of compensatory responses. Regarding haemorrhagic shock, which of the following are true and which are false?
a Vasoconstriction associated with adrenergic response usually occurs at the arteriolar and precapillary sphincters.
b Immediate response is an increased sympathetic drive which causes tachycardia and vasoconstriction.
c Extracellular fluid becomes more hyperosmolar.
d Transcapillary refill occurs to restore circulating volume.
e Decreased activation of arterial baroreceptors leads to reduced pulse pressure and increased sympathetic response.

5 Regarding ATLS classification of haemorrhagic shock, which of the following statements are true and which are false?
a Class I shock is similar to a unit of blood donation.
b Class II shock will show signs of tachycardia, tachypnoea and significant BP drop.

c Class III can be managed with simple crystalloids.

d Class III shows a significant drop in BP.

e Class IV includes up to 40% blood loss and can be classified as life-threatening.

6 Regarding neurogenic shock, which of the following statements are true and which are false?

a Along with hypotension, both tachycardia and bradycardia may be observed.

b An alpha agonist is used for the mainstay of treatment.

c Severe head injury or spinal cord or high spinal injury may all cause neurogenic shock.

d There is loss of sympathetic tone.

e There is temporary loss of spinal reflex activity.

ATLS (Answers, see p. 255)

1 A 30-year-old male motorcyclist without a helmet was involved in an accident. On admission to the emergency department he was hypotensive (80/40 mmHg) with severe respiratory distress and appeared cyanotic. He was bleeding from his nose and had an open femur fracture. Breath sounds were decreased on the right side of his chest. What should be the initial management priorities?

a Tube thoracostomy of right hemithorax.

b Control of nose bleed with anterior and posterior packing.

c Obtain a C-spine and chest film.

d Obtain intravenous access and begin type O blood transfusions.

e Endotracheal intubation with in-line cervical traction.

2 Considering the diagnosis and treatment of cardiac tamponade, which of the following are true and which are false?

a Beck's classic triad of signs of cardiac tamponade includes distended neck veins, pulsus paradoxus and hypotension.

b Accumulation of more than 200 mL blood in the pericardial space will impair cardiac output.

c Cardiopulmonary bypass is required to repair most penetrating cardiac injuries.

d Approximately 15% of pericardiocenteses give a false-negative result.

e It is most frequently caused by blunt thoracic trauma.

3 The most common radiographic finding indicating a torn thoracic aorta includes which of the following?

a Presence of an apical 'pleural cap'.

b Deviation of the trachea.

c Left haemothorax.

d Widening of the mediastinum.

e Rib fractures.

4 Which of the following steps are part of the primary survey?

a Examining cervical spine.

b Measurement of BP and pulse.

c Evaluating the GCS.

d Protecting the airway and ensuring adequate ventilatory support.

5 What examination findings would you expect in a patient with a left-sided pneumothorax?

a Reduced breath sounds on the left.

b Reduced breath sounds on the right.

c Trachea deviated to the right.

d Trachea deviated to the left.

e Hyper-resonant percussion on the left with reduced expansion on the left.

6 During the secondary survey, the AMPLE history is taken. Which of the following are part of the AMPLE procedure?

a Previous anaesthesia.

b Medications.

c Pets in the home.

d Metal implants.

e Pregnancy.

EMQs (Answers, see p. 256)

1 Options:

a Colopexy.

b Barium enema.

c Urgent laparotomy.

d Elective surgery.

e Sigmoidoscopy and rectal tube.

f Resuscitation.

g Plain AXR.

h CT abdomen.

For each case below suggest the best intervention from the above list of options. Each option may be used once, more than once or not at all.

  (i) An 80-year-old bed-bound man has presented with a 5-day history of abdominal distension and tenderness. On rigid sigmoidoscopy for sigmoid volvulus, there is blood-stained fluid. What is your management?

 (ii) A 50-year-old has had a colonoscopic decompression of a sigmoid volvulus, but there are ongoing signs of sepsis associated with rebound tenderness in the right iliac fossa. What is your management?

(iii) A 40-year-old man with Down's syndrome presented with a 1-week history of abdominal bloating and constipation. On examination, he was dehydrated and his abdomen was soft and distended. What is your immediate management?

2 Options:

a Gastroenteritis.

b Pancreatic pseudocyst.

c Bowel obstruction.

d Incarcerated hernia.

e Toxic megacolon.
f Chorioamnionitis.
g Acute appendicitis.
h Uterine rupture.
i Acute pancreatitis.
j Strangulated hernia.
k Ovarian cyst rupture.
l Stercoral perforation.
m Hepatitis.
n Corpus luteal cyst.
o Placental abruption.
p Peptic ulcer perforation.
q Peptic ulcer.
r Inflamed Meckel's diverticulum.

For each case below suggest the best diagnosis from the above list of options. Each option may be used once, more than once or not at all.

(i) A 16-year-old adolescent male presents with a 1-day history of central abdominal pain radiating to right iliac fossa. He has fever (38°C) and tachycardia (110 bpm) on admission, and is peritonitic in the right iliac fossa.

(ii) A 42-year-old man with known gallstones presented to the emergency department with repeated bouts of projectile vomiting and severe pain in epigastric region and right hypochondrium. His blood tests showed WCC 15.5 × 10⁹/L, Hb 12 g/dL, platelets 240 × 10⁹/L, GGT 630 IU/L, bilirubin 12 µmol/L, ALT 246 IU/L, ALP 316 IU/L, amylase 1560 IU/L.

(iii) A 53-year-old woman presents to her GP surgery with recurrent bouts of severe epigastric pain around 2 hours after every meal. She also complains of bloating and abdominal fullness, water brash and occasional burning sensation in her chest. Her blood tests were unremarkable.

(iv) A 7-year-old boy has recurrent bouts of abdominal cramps and diarrhoea for the last 24 hours. His observations on admission were pulse 110 bpm, BP 110/78 mmHg, RR 16/min, temperature 37.1°C. On examination he has some mild generalized tenderness all over his abdomen.

(v) A 36-year-old man has noticed that he has developed yellowish discoloration of his sclera and high-coloured urine since his last foreign trip 8 days ago. Prior to this, he noticed he felt unwell, lost his appetite, had generalized body aches, fatigue and nausea. His liver profile is deranged and ALT in blood is much higher than normal.

(vi) A 76-year-old woman presents with a 5-day history of not passing faeces or flatus, gradual abdominal distension and vomiting. She has had two vaginal deliveries and was always fit and healthy before this episode of illness. The rest of her history was unremarkable. On examination, she has tenderness in left iliac fossa but no masses were felt. Rectal examination was unremarkable with an empty rectum.

(vii) An 82-year-old man is on aspirin and statin for his intermittent claudication, and takes regular paracetamol and ibuprofen for his arthritis. For the last 24 hours his family members noticed that he is drowsy, confused and almost crying out in pain when moved. On examination, he has a rigid abdomen with no audible bowel sounds.

(viii) A 29-year-old woman has been diagnosed with ulcerative colitis on histology from a biopsy taken at a recent colonoscopy. She was started on 5-ASA and steroids due to the severity of her symptoms, but has not improved clinically. On examination she is tender in her right iliac fossa and RUQ. A plain AXR showed grossly distended loops of bowel and her transverse colon has a diameter of 8 cm and the caecum measures 10 cm.

(ix) A 15-year-old boy presents with painless bleeding per rectum with central abdominal pain. He had his appendix removed 2 years ago. There is no family history of IBD. On examination he was noted to have tenderness in the right side of his abdomen with voluntary guarding in his right iliac fossa. A technetium-99 scan shows an active spot in his right iliac fossa.

(x) A 31-year-old sailor had a bout of acute epigastric pain while on a merchant trip to the Caribbean, which settled in 5 days. Since then he has noted that his upper abdomen is gradually increasing in size. His GP arranged for him to have USS, which showed a 5×6 cm collection of well-circumscribed fluid in the back of the stomach.

(xi) A 76-year-old woman has a long-standing history of chronic bronchitis. She developed sudden abdominal pain while lifting a chair. She was clinically stable. On examination, she had significant tenderness in her left upper quadrant and a firm and tender mass in left upper quadrant with discernible borders.

(xii) A 64-year-old man developed pain in the right side of his abdomen. He noticed a gradually increasing lump in his right groin which is now irreducible and tender on palpation. Over the next 4 hours, he develops peritonism in his right lower quadrant.

(xiii) A 45-year-old woman has a long-standing lump in her left groin that was reducible easily. Recently, she noticed that it was difficult to reduce and of late has been irreducible. It is tender to palpate with impulse on coughing.

(xiv) A 29-year-old woman developed sharp pain in her right iliac fossa, which gradually worsened over days. She was being treated for infertility with clomifene. Her periods have regularized since the start of treatment and her last menstrual period was 4 weeks ago. She had a negative ward pregnancy test.

(xv) An anxious 30-year-old woman is admitted to A&E with acute right iliac fossa pain. Her pain did not settle with analgesia, and she gave a history of her GP counselling her about an increased risk of endometrial cancer. On laparoscopy, she had free fluid in her abdomen.

(xvi) A 58-year-old man was admitted to A&E with a 2-day history of abdominal pain, constipation and altered sensorium. His carer gives a history of stroke 3 years ago. On examination, he is peritonitic in both the iliac fossae and suprapubic quadrants. A plain CXR shows no gas under diaphragm.

(xvii) A 21-year-old medical student presents repeatedly to A&E with bouts of copious vomiting, postprandial epigastric pain and weight loss. She has voluntarily lost a significant amount of weight in the last 12 months when she started developing these symptoms.

3 Options:
a Appendicitis.
b Biliary colic.
c Cholecystitis.
d Diverticulitis.
e Gastroenteritis.
f Meckel's diverticulitis.
g Mesenteric adenitis.
h Pancreatitis.
i Renal colic.

For each case below suggest the best diagnosis from the above list of options. Each option may be used once, more than once or not at all.

(i) A 12-year-old boy presents with a 4-day history of right-sided abdominal pain associated with a sore throat and fever. On examination, the abdomen is soft and minimally tender over the central region.

(ii) A 10-year-old boy who had his appendix removed 2 years ago presents with vague right-sided abdominal pains associated with 1 day of diarrhoea and fever.

(iii) A 38-year-old woman with known gallstones presents with a 1-week history of epigastric pain associated with nausea and vomiting. The abdomen is very tender and blood tests reveal a raised amylase level.

(iv) A 68-year-old obese man presents with central abdominal pain which has now settled in the right iliac fossa. On examination, he has rebound tenderness at McBurney's point and a temperature of 37.7°C. A CT abdomen with oral contrast reveals a thickened wall of the caecum and appendix.

(v) A 49-year-old man presents with a 1-day history of right iliac fossa and groin pain associated with nausea and vomiting. The abdomen is soft and non-tender. He is trying to get comfortable by pacing up and down the room. There are microscopic traces of blood and leucocytes in his urine.

8 Foregut

Dysphagia

D : Usually described as difficulty in swallowing and may or may not be associated with odynophagia (painful swallowing). A problem with any part of the swallowing process can lead to dysphagia.

I & S : Depends on the cause of dysphagia. Approximately one-third of elderly in nursing homes have some degree of dysphagia and half have dysphagia after a CVA.

A & P :

In the wall
- Diffuse oesophageal spasm or achalasia
- Inflammatory stricture or caustic stricture
- Tumour of oesophagus or GOJ
- Pharyngeal pouch
- Plummer–Vinson syndrome (anaemia, oesophageal web)
- Scleroderma
- Oesophageal web

Intraluminal
- Foreign body
- Locally advanced oesophageal tumour

C F & D : Duration and mode of onset of dysphagia are important in determining the diagnosis. It is important to determine if dysphagia is for solids or liquids or both, and whether a patient drools or chokes when eating. Malignancy usually presents with progressive dysphagia of sudden onset. The degree of dysphagia may progress from difficulty in swallowing solids, to liquids, then saliva.

Other symptoms

- Weight loss: suspicion of malignancy.
- Dyspepsia: due to GORD causing benign stricture.
- Haematemesis: from acid peptic disease or bleeding from a lesion of the oesophagus.
- Cough: secondary to aspiration of contents of pharyngeal pouch or mega-oesophagus.
- Lethargy: anaemia secondary to upper GI haemorrhage or chronic blood loss.
- SOB: as a result of anaemia or recurrent aspiration pneumonitis.

EMQs and MCQs for Surgical Finals, 1st edition. © Hye-Chung Kwak, Imran Bhatti,
Jaskarn Rai, Farhan Rashid, Bachittar Singh Jassar, Murthy Nyasavajjala, Viren Asher,
Jon Lund and Mike Larvin. Published 2011 by Blackwell Publishing Ltd.

Signs

Following the typical examination from hands to head, and down to the abdomen.
- Fingers/hand: pale, clubbing, +/– nicotine staining, koilonychia.
- Neck: supraclavicular lymphadenopathy, goitre +/– retrosternal extension.
- Chest: palpate for abnormal mass and auscultate for extra breath sounds.
- Abdomen: palpate for abdominal mass and auscultate for altered bowel sounds.

Investigations to exclude differential diagnosis

CXR
- Primary lung or mediastinal pathology
- Aspiration pneumonia
- Air–fluid level in dilated oesophagus (i.e. obstruction)

Barium swallow
- Narrowing at cardia ('rat tail') secondary to achalasia
- Oesophageal web or pharyngeal pouches
- Corkscrew oesophagus seen due to multiple simultaneous oesophageal contractions (diffuse oesophageal spasm)
- Benign stricture of oesophagus

Upper GI endoscopy
- Allows visualization of the tumour with biopsy and stenting

Bronchoscopy
- Bronchial carcinoma (causing extrinsic compression)

CT scan, CT/PET
- Structural abnormalities + stage of oesophageal tumour/cancer

EUS
- Staging of oesophageal cancer

Oesophageal manometry and pH monitoring
- Oesophago-gastric sphincter pressure
- Coordination and strength of peristaltic movement
- Underlying cause of the benign stricture such as acid reflux

T & M : Depends on the diagnosis. For oesophageal cancer, management depends on the stage of the tumour; it may involve neoadjuvant chemotherapy then surgery. Locally advanced cases are managed with chemotherapy, radiotherapy and usually a self-expanding metallic stent for dysphagia. Achalasia requires a Heller myotomy. GORD is treated medically with proton pump inhibitors (PPIs) or fundoplication. A pharyngeal pouch is dealt with by resection.

P : Depends on the cause of dysphagia.

Gastro-oesophageal reflux disease (heartburn)

D : The reflux of gastric contents into the oesophagus resulting in heartburn and sometimes oesophageal spasm. Heartburn is the most common digestive symptom. Regurgitation of gastric contents into the mouth (waterbrash) is termed 'volume reflux'. Patients with at least weekly heartburn and/or acid regurgitation have GORD.

I & S : This is a very common problem experienced by many people at some time in their lives. Prevalence in the Western world is 10–20%, whereas in Asia the prevalence is reportedly less than 5%. M > F.

A & P : See below.

C F & D : The majority of patients present with retrosternal pain with positional exacerbation, regurgitation into the mouth and occasionally with dysphagia if the patient develops stricture.

Common associations

- Loss of normal lower oesophageal sphincter pressure
- Hiatal hernia
- Abdominal obesity
- Smoking and strong alcohol

Common complications of GORD

- Oesophagitis
- Peptic stricture
- Barrett's ulcer
- Barrett's oesophagus (metaplasia, precancerous)
- Oesophageal adenocarcinoma

T & M : Endoscopy and biopsy allow inspection of inflamed mucosa. Barium swallow can also be used to assess reflux and the anatomy of hiatal hernia. The most definitive investigation is 24-hour pH monitoring, and manometry to exclude achalasia.

Medical treatment

- Changes in lifestyle: smoking cessation, weight reduction, decreased intake of alcohol, caffeine and spicy foods, raising head of bed.
- Pharmacological: simple antacids, alginates, H_2 antagonists, PPIs, prokinetics.

Surgical treatment

If the best medical therapy fails, then surgical intervention is indicated in the form of a hiatal hernia repair, and fundoplication (stomach wrapped around lower oesophagus).

P : Chronic recurring condition; lifetime risk of recurrence is about 80%.

Barrett's oesophagus

D : Barrett's oesophagus describes intestinal metaplasia of the normal oesophageal squamous epithelium, when it is replaced by gastric-type columnar epithelium. It is premalignant and may progress through the stages of dysplasia to cancer.

I & S : Barrett's oesophagus may be present in 5–15% of GORD patients in the Western population. The incidence of oesophageal adenocarcinoma is 0.4–0.5 % per year.

C F & D : Patients usually present with symptoms similar to GORD, including frequent long-standing heartburn, dysphagia and weight loss. Usually diagnosed with endoscopy and annual biopsy.

T & M : Treatment may consist of lifestyle changes and drugs as described above for reflux.

Surgical treatment

The American College of Gastroenterology (www.acg.gi.org) advocates surveillance endoscopy to detect high-grade intraepithelial neoplasia or cancer. The British Society of Gastroenterology (www.bsg.org.uk) advocates discussion with patients to decide whether surveillance is appropriate.

• Fundoplication to prevent reflux.
• Oesophageal resection only indicated for carcinoma or severe dysplasia.
• Endomucosal resection or ablation with argon plasma diathermy is sometimes offered.

P : Varies widely depending on the stage of the disease and the treatment available, but the current focus is on cancer prevention.

Malignant oesophageal tumours

D : Oesophageal cancer is a malignant tumour of the oesophagus, the two major types being squamous cell carcinoma (usually upper two-thirds) and adenocarcinoma (usually lower third).

I & S : 8000 cases per year in UK; more common in older males (60 years and above). M/F ratio 3 : 1. Adenocarcinoma is increasing in incidence and is related to reflux and Barrett's oesophagus.

A & P : Arises in the mucosa then invades submucosa and muscular layers.

Risk factors

• Barrett's oesophagus with dysplasia
• Environmental factors, e.g. smoking, alcohol and dietary nitrosamines
• Reflux oesophagitis (GORD)
• Achalasia

TNM staging for oesophageal adenocarcinoma

• Stage 0: carcinoma *in situ* (CIS), early stage of cancer
• Stage 1: T1–T2, N0, M0
• Stage 2 (A or B): T1–T3, N0–N1, M0
• Stage 3: T1–T4b, N1–N3, M0
• Stage 4 (A or B): any T, any N, M1

CF&D: Presentation with dysphagia, weight loss, acid reflux, hoarseness, sore throat and vomiting. Diagnosis involves investigation by endoscopy with biopsy (or barium meal) and staging of disease with CT chest and abdomen with EUS.

T&M: Treatment may consist of surgery, radiotherapy, chemotherapy or a combination. The type of resection will depend on the location of the tumour, with a combined abdomino-thoracic approach for distal lesions (the majority).

P: Overall 5-year survival in patients with oesophageal carcinoma is less than 25%.

Gastric cancer

D: Benign tumours include leiomyoma, haemangioma, neurofibroma and fibroma. Malignant tumours are more common and include adenocarcinoma (95%), GI stromal tumours (GIST), leiomyosarcoma, lymphoma (MALT) and carcinoids (neuroendocrine tumours). Benign tumours are rare and include adenomas, lipomas, leiomyomas and carcinoids. Adenocarcinoma spreads via lymphatics towards the nodes on the lesser and greater curvature of the stomach. From there it spreads to coeliac axis, hepatic nodes and then to the supraclavicular nodes via the thoracic duct. When it involves large areas creating a rigid thickened stomach it is referred to as linitus plastica.

I&S: In the UK stomach cancer is the eighth commonest cancer in adults, and the third most common GIT cancer, with an M/F ratio of 2 : 1. The peak age is 70–80 years. In Japan there is a very high incidence of gastric cancer and there are screening programmes in place for early detection.

A&P: Increasing age is a significant risk factor. Other risk factors associated with gastric cancer include:
- pernicious anaemia
- blood group A
- adenomatous polyps
- atrophic gastritis
- diet (excess nitrates, spicy and salty foods)
- smoking
- alcohol
- *Helicobacter pylori* infection.

CF&D: Patients may present with a variety of symptoms, including nausea, anorexia, weight loss, vomiting, epigastric pain, dysphagia, haematemesis and malaena. The following investigations are employed for diagnosis and staging.

- Gastroscopy: investigation of choice for confirming diagnosis with biopsy.
- Barium meal: can be used for diagnosis especially in linitis plastica.
- CT thorax and abdomen: for staging and planning further treatmen.
- FDG-PET: used to seek distant metastases.
- EUS: determines the extent of local disease, especially tumour T and nodal N stage.
- Laparoscopy: peritoneal seedings.

> **Gastric cancer stages and UICC equivalent**
>
> - Stage 0: CIS
> - Stage 1: T1, N0, M0 or T2, N0, M0
> - Stage 2: T2, N1, M0 or T3, N0, M0
> - Stage 3: T2, N2, M0 or T3, N1, M0
> - Stage 4: T1–T3, N3, M0 or any T or N, M1

T & M : Ideally curative, if not then palliative. Depending upon the stage of the disease, surgical resection with radical lymphadenectomy is the treatment of choice. The role of neoadjuvant (preoperative, 'downstaging') and adjuvant (postoperative) chemotherapy is debated. Palliative chemotherapy is often offered for inoperable tumour.

> - Partial gastrectomy: distal gastric cancer
> - Total gastrectomy with Roux-en-Y reconstruction: mid-gastric cancer
> - Distal oesophago-gastrectomy and Roux-en-Y reconstruction: proximal gastric cancer

P : The overall 5-year survival of stomach cancer is about 20%. However, there is great variability, depending on disease stage and treatment regimens.

MCQs

Dysphagia (Answers, see p. 258)

1 Which of the following describe the phases of swallowing?
   a Oral.
   b Orolaryngeal.
   c Deglutition.
   d Pharyngeal.
   e Oesophageal.

2 Which of the following are symptoms of dysphagia?
   a Sensation of food sticking in the chest.
   b Odynophagia.
   c Weight gain.
   d Sialorrhoea.
   e Choking while eating.

3 The causes of dysphagia include which of the following?
   a Achalasia.
   b Radiotherapy to the throat.
   c Radiotherapy to breast.
   d Parkinson's disease.
   e Alzheimer's disease.

4 Which of the following describe treatments for dysphagia?
 a Dysphagia caused by achalasia can be treated with botulinum toxin.
 b Dysphagia caused by oesophageal stricture can be treated with balloon dilatation.
 c Dysphagia caused by Parkinson's disease requires balloon dilatation.
 d Dysphagia caused by Plummer–Vinson syndrome is treated with surgery.
 e Dysphagia caused by pharyngeal pouch is treated with medications.

5 Which of the following are complications of dysphagia?
 a Aspiration.
 b Malnutrition.
 c Dehydration.
 d Atrophy of tongue.
 e Diminished taste.

6 Which of the following are investigations for dysphagia?
 a Barium swallow.
 b Endoscopy.
 c MR cholangiogram.
 d Manometry.
 e Abdominal USS.

GORD (Answers, see p. 259)

1 GORD usually presents with which of the following?
 a Heartburn.
 b Retrosternal pain with positional exacerbation.
 c Acid reflux into the back of the throat.
 d Dysphagia.
 e Fever.

2 Regarding GORD, which of the following statements are true and which are false?
 a It is cured by PPIs.
 b When mild may respond to simple lifestyle changes.
 c It is caused by *Helicobacter pylori* infection.
 d May result in a benign oesophageal structure.
 e Can often be treated successfully by fundoplication.

3 Which of the following are common complications of GORD?
 a Barrett's oesophagus.
 b Duodenal stricture.
 c Gastric ulcer.
 d Oesophagitis.
 e Oropharyngeal candidiasis.

4 Which of the following are risk factors for GORD?
 a *Helicobacter pylori* infection.
 b Heavy meals.
 c Oesophageal stricture.
 d Obesity.
 e Smoking.

5 Which of the following should be used in the investigation of GORD?
a Manometry.
b CT abdomen.
c OGD.
d Transthoracic echocardiogram.
e Barium swallow.

6 Which of the following should be used in the treatment of GORD?
a PPIs.
b Bisphosphonates.
c Lifestyle changes.
d Metronidazole.
e Fundoplication.

Barrett's oesophagus (Answers, see p. 260)

1 Regarding Barrett's oesophagus, which of the following are true and which are false?
a A change from columnar to squamous epithelium is termed 'Barrett's oesophagus'.
b GORD always leads to Barrett's oesophagus.
c The incidence of Barrett's oesophagus is rising in the Western world.
d 45% of oesophageal adenocarcinomas are associated with Barrett's oesophagus.
e All patients with Barrett's oesophagus need surgical resection.

2 Which of the following are risk factors for progression to adenocarcinoma?
a Female sex.
b GORD.
c Age > 45 years.
d Small area of Barrett's disease.
e Short reflux history.

3 Which of the following are symptoms of Barrett's disease?
a No symptoms.
b Dyspepsia.
c Heartburn.
d Hunger.
e Constipation.

4 How is Barrett's disease diagnosed?
a CT chest.
b OGD +/− biopsy.
c Barium meal.
d EUS.
e Manometry.

5 What is the management of symptomatic Barrett's disease?
a A course of PPI.
b Oesophagectomy.

c Endoscopic ablation.
d Fundoplication.
e Monthly surveillance.

Malignant oesophageal tumours (Answers, see p. 261)

1 Which of the following are risk factors for oesophageal cancer?
a Alcohol.
b Anaemia.
c Barrett's disease.
d Obesity.
e Male sex.

2 Which of the following are presentations of oesophageal cancer?
a Dysphagia.
b Weight loss.
c Diarrhoea.
d Headaches.
e Odynophagia.

3 Which of the following are used in the management of oesophageal cancer?
a Dilatation of oesophagus.
b Insertion of stent.
c Neoadjuvant chemotherapy.
d Endoscopic laser therapy.
e Radiotherapy.

4 Regarding oesophageal cancer, which of the following are true and which are false?
a The incidence of oesophageal cancer is increasing.
b Definitive diagnosis is by endoscopy and biopsy.
c When arising in Barrett's oesophagus is usually squamous cell carcinoma.
d The 5-year survival for node-negative resected oesophageal cancer is less than 25%.
e Is common in patients below 40 years of age.

Gastric cancer (Answers, see p. 261)

1 Which of the following are risk factors for gastric cancer?
a Cigarette smoking.
b Family history.
c Pernicious anaemia.
d Geographical location.
e Female sex.

2 Which of the following are presentations of gastric cancer?
a Dysphagia.
b Abdominal bloating.
c Pale stools.

d Weight gain.

e Anxiety.

3 How is gastric cancer diagnosed?
a Endoscopy with biopsy.
b Barium meal.
c EUS.
d Laparoscopy.
e CT scan.

4 Which of the following is the commonest type of malignant stomach cancer?
a Carcinoid.
b Lymphomas.
c Sarcoma.
d Adenocarcinoma.
e Fibroma.

5 Regarding linitis plastica, which of the following are true and which are false?
a It is associated with an improved prognosis.
b It is not linked with *Helicobacter pylori* infection.
c Can be missed or misdiagnosed at endoscopy.
d Is a common form of gastric cancer.
e May present with weight loss, poor appetite and vomiting.

6 What is the management of gastric cancer?
a Gastrectomy.
b Multidisciplinary approach to care.
c Chemoradiotherapy.
d Analgesia.
e PEG.

EMQs (Answers, see p. 262)

1 Options:
a Peptic oesophageal stricture.
b Globus hystericus.
c Boerhaave's syndrome (oesophageal perforation).
d Pharyngeal cancer.
e Oesophageal cancer.
f Cervical lympadenopathy.
g GORD.
h Achalasia (or diffuse oesophageal spasm).
For each case below suggest the single best diagnosis from the above list of options.
(i) A 32-year-old woman complains of difficulty in swallowing solids over the last 6 months, but has no problem when swallowing liquids. She was

diagnosed with GORD 3 years ago but has not been taking regular PPIs as advised. What is the most likely diagnosis?

(ii) A 75-year-old man presents with weight loss of 13 kg (2 stone) in the last few months associated with increasing difficulty in swallowing both solids and liquids.

(iii) A fit and healthy 32-year-old man has a problem initiating swallowing, and describes a sensation of food stuck in the back of his throat. After the food bolus passes down he feels fine, and there is no heartburn, indigestion, reflux or regurgitation. He has recently been made redundant and is being treated for anxiety.

(iv) An otherwise fit 35-year-old woman has experienced difficulty in swallowing for the past 3 years. She has not lost weight. She is able to swallow liquids easily but solids seem to stick in the distal gullet and this feels very painful. It is more likely if she 'bolts' her food.

(v) A 75-year-old woman presents with epigastric and lower chest pain of sudden onset. Over the last 6 hours she has experienced sudden onset of dysphagia whilst eating a roast chicken meal. On examination she is febrile, tachycardic, tachypnoeic and hypotensive. She has subcutaneous emphysema of the neck, and chest radiography shows bilateral pleural air–fluid levels and mediastinal emphysema. The ECG shows sinus tachycardia and troponin T is normal.

2 Options:
a Acute Crohn's disease.
b Acute appendicitis.
c Viral hepatitis.
d Perforated duodenal ulcer.
e Mesenteric embolus.
f Acute cholecystitis.
g Acute pancreatitis.
h Reflux oesophagitis.
i Duodenal ulceration.

For each case below suggest the single best diagnosis from the above list of options.

(i) A 38-year-old man complains of continuous epigastric pain. This becomes more severe if he does not eat for a while, regularly wakes him at 2 a.m. and is partly relieved by drinking milk or taking antacids. He denies any history of weight loss.

(ii) An obese 50-year-old man complains of burning retrosternal pain aggravated by drinking strong alcohol or hot drinks.

(iii) A 42-year-old man complains of weakness, depression and an inability to concentrate. He returned from a holiday in Thailand 18 days ago. On examination he is febrile, mildly jaundiced and vaguely tender in the RUQ and epigastric regions. He has a raised WCC and raised total bilirubin and transaminases.

(iv) A 46-year-old woman complains of localized RUQ pain radiating to the left shoulder, fever and nausea for 3 days. She has had similar milder episodes in the past but they have all settled within a few hours. On examination she is febrile, tachycardic and locally tender in the RUQ with a positive Murphy's sing. She has a raised WCC and CRP.

(v) A 60-year-old woman presents with sudden onset of severe epigastric pain, and the pain is worse when she moves or coughs. She consumes regular NSAIDs and steroids for long-standing rheumatoid arthritis. On examination she is febrile, tachycardic and diffusely tender, with generalized guarding. Serum amylase is normal.

3 Options:
   a Triple therapy.
   b Fundoplication.
   c PPIs.
   d H$_2$ receptor antagonists.
   e Simple antacids.
   f Long-term endoscopic surveillance.
   g Reassurance.
   h Upper GI endoscopy.
   i Heller's myotomy.

For each case below suggest the single best treatment from the above list of options.

   (i) A 77-year-old man, known to suffer from Barrett's oesophagus for 3 years, underwent endoscopy and multiple biopsies. The biopsy has shown no evidence of oesophageal cancer, nor any high-grade dysplasia. He takes high-dose PPI therapy.

   (ii) A 75-year-old woman suffering from osteoarthritis requiring regular NSAIDs for joint pain has developed dyspepsia. Endoscopy reveals gastric ulceration, from which multiple biopsies have confirmed inflammatory changes only, and are negative for *Helicobacter pylori* organisms.

   (iii) An anxious 29-year-old woman in her third trimester of pregnancy presents with occasional mild heartburn, which always improves with simple antacids.

   (iv) A 42-year-old man presents with several years of heartburn, which has been proven by endoscopy to be caused by reflux oesophagitis. His symptoms have not been controlled by high doses of PPI therapy for the last year, and 24-hour pH monitoring confirms significant acid reflux, with normal oesophageal manometry.

   (v) A 65-year-old woman presents with the recent onset of heartburn and indigestion.

9 Hepato-pancreato-biliary disease

Pancreatic cancer

D: Pancreatic cancer is a malignant tumour of the pancreas. The majority (95%) of pancreatic tumours are adenocarcinomas, with the remaining 5% consisting of other exocrine tumours of the pancreas, acinar cell and neuroendocrine tumours.

I & S: In the UK 7700 patients are diagnosed annually, mostly (80%) in patients aged over 60 years. M/F ratio 1.5 : 1.

A & P: The causes of pancreatic cancer are unknown but there are associated factors, with the strongest being smoking.

Risk factors

- Tobacco smoking: arcinogenic nitrosamines.
- Familial/hereditary: unknown genes, *BRCA1*, *BRCA2*, FAP, HNPCC.
- CP: prolonged inflammation.
- Type 2 DM: hyperinsulinaemia.
- Obesity: diet high in fat and sugars, lack of exercise and hyperinsulinaemia.

C F & D: Depending on the location of the cancer, 50% of patients present to the GP with painless jaundice.

Symptoms and signs

- Head of pancreas: progressive obstructive jaundice with steatorrhoea and dark urine.
- Body and tail of pancreas: early symptoms and signs are vague, including weight loss, nausea and back pain. Late symptoms and signs include diabetes, cachexia, vomiting (duodenal obstruction) and GI bleeding.

Elevated serum levels of tumour marker CA19-9 indicate the presence of pancreatic malignancy.

Investigations

- USS: dilated biliary tree with a pancreatic mass.
- ERCP: may demonstrate a periampullary tumour which could be biopsied. It may also show pancreatic or biliary stricture from which brushings may be acquired for cytology. Most importantly, this procedure can be used therapeutically to insert a stent and relieve biliary obstruction.
- CT: provides information about the extent of tumour and operability.

EMQs and MCQs for Surgical Finals, 1st edition. © Hye-Chung Kwak, Imran Bhatti, Jaskarn Rai, Farhan Rashid, Bachittar Singh Jassar, Murthy Nyasavajjala, Viren Asher, Jon Lund and Mike Larvin. Published 2011 by Blackwell Publishing Ltd.

USS and CT are appropriate for initial imaging in patients with suspected pancreatic cancer. If CT is indeterminate, EUS should be followed from which a diagnostic FNA biopsy can be taken. Histological diagnosis is necessary in patients who are not surgical candidates.

Furthermore, groups of patients with inoperable disease and obstructive jaundice should have biliary decompression by ERCP and may require relief of gastric outlet obstruction by duodenal stenting or bypass surgery.

Patients with resectable disease who are surgical candidates can undergo surgery without histology. Staging laparoscopy is reserved for patients with a high suspicion of metastasis who have not been identified by other means.

T & M : Either curative or palliative.

> • Curative: Whipple's procedure (pancreaticoduodenectomy); less than 15% of tumours are suitable for resection.
> • Palliative: biliary stent insertion for obstructive jaundice. Duodenal stent or gastroenterostomy for duodenal obstruction.

P : Pancreatic tumours have a poor prognosis due to late presentation (90% mortality within 1 year). However, if amenable to resection then the median survival is 18 months compared with 6 months in metastatic disease.

> **Useful hints and tips**
> • One may be able to palpate a distended gallbladder in the presence of jaundice (Courvoisier's law). In such cases the cause of jaundice is not likely to be gallstones but more likely a malignant cause.
> • Non-resectable disease is defined by distant metastasis, invasion of SMA, IVC, aorta or coeliac axis, or encasement of the portal venous complex.

Liver abscess

D : A collection of pus accumulated in a cavity within the liver.

I & S : Incidence 8–15 per 100 000 per year. M/F ratio 1 : 1.

A & P : Liver abscess may be of amoebic or bacterial origin. Bacterial infections are most common in the Western world.

> • Intrahepatic abscess: secondary to cholangitis or from spread of infection via portal circulation from infections such as diverticulitis or appendicitis.
> • Extrahepatic abscess: these develop secondary to intra-abdominal sepsis.

C F & D : Patients present with swinging pyrexia, rigors, malaise, anorexia, jaundice and right hypochondrial pain. Diagnosis is by USS. Serum blood tests show raised WCC and deranged LFTs.

T & M : Ultrasound-guided percutaneous drainage combined with systemic antibiotics/antihydatid agents.

P : Untreated pyogenic abscess is associated with 100% mortality. With early diagnosis, appropriate drainage and long-term antibiotics, the mortality rates fall to 15–20%.

Hepatocellular carcinoma

D : Hepatocellular carcinoma (HCC) is a primary malignancy of the hepatocyte frequently arising on a background of cirrhosis.

I & S : It is uncommon in the UK and accounts for only 2% of all cancers. The worldwide incidence is 1 million cases per year. M/F ratio 1.5–3 : 1.

A & P : Over 80% of HCC occurs in patients with cirrhotic livers. The major causes of cirrhosis remain alcohol consumption and hepatitis B and C infections. Other less common causes include inherited diseases such as haemochromatosis and α_1-antitrypsin deficiency.

C F & D : In patients with cirrhosis the diagnosis should be suspected when there is deterioration in liver function, development of upper abdominal pain and fever or an acute complication (ascites, encephalopathy, jaundice, variceal bleed).

USS will identify most tumours. The presence of a mass identified on USS within a cirrhotic liver together with a raised AFP (> 500 ng/mL) is diagnostic. Other forms of imaging such as CT or MRI may also be helpful. Biopsy should be avoided to prevent tumour seeding (1 in 1000).

T & M :

Surgical

- Resection and liver transplantation are the only treatments that offer cure.
- Resection is only feasible in 20% of patients mostly due to local spread of tumour and pre-existing cirrhosis.
- Liver transplantation has survival rates of 61.1% and can be offered in patients with cirrhosis.

Radiofrequency ablation

- Only used for small tumours less than 4 cm in size.

Chemotherapy

- Mainstay of treatment for patients with advanced disease who are not candidates for resection.

P : Patients able to undergo curative resection have a median survival of 4 years whereas patients who present with advanced disease have a median survival of 3 months.

Cholangiocarcinoma (advanced topic)

D : Malignancy of the bile duct system that may originate in the liver and extrahepatic ducts and terminate at the ampulla of Vater; 95% of the tumours are ductal adenocarcinomas and patients usually present with unresectable or metastatic disease.

I & S : The incidence is 1 per 100 000 patients per year. M/F ratio 1 : 2.5 in patients >60 years and 1 : 15 in patients <40 years.

A & P : Dysplasia is thought to be induced by chronic inflammation from conditions such as primary sclerosing cholangitis (PSC) or chronic parasitic infection.

C F & D : Patients present with jaundice, pale stools, dark urine, pruritis, weight loss and abdominal pain. If the cholangiocarcinoma is located distal to the cystic duct, patients may present with a distended gallbladder (Courvoisier's sign). Hepatomegaly may be noted in up to 25% of patients.

Tumour marker CA19-9 may be elevated greater than 100 U/mL. Essentially, USS or CT may reveal a mass lesion with dilated ducts. CT and MRI may be used for staging the disease. ERCP may be used for brushing cytology and stenting. If stenting is difficult with ERCP, then percutaneous transhepatic cholangiography (PTC) may be more helpful.

Treatment

- Surgical resection: the only therapy which offers a chance of cure, although only 10% of patients present at a stage where resection is possible.
- Medical: relieve jaundice by means of stenting using ERCP or PTC. Radiotherapy and chemotherapy have a limited role in the treatment of cholangiocarcinoma.

P: If complete surgical resection is achieved, then patients may experience a 5-year survival rate as high as 40%. A poor prognosis (<6 months) is expected for patients with irresectable disease.

Acute pancreatitis

D: Pancreatitis is an acute inflammatory condition of the exocrine pancreas.

I & S: This is a common disease affecting 10–20 per million every year. Sex distribution is dependent on the cause.

A & P: In up to one-third of cases the aetiology remains idiopathic and, until recently, studies have suggested that up to 70% of idiopathic cases are due to microlithiasis.

- Gallstones, 40%
- Alcohol, 35%
- ERCP, 4%
- Drugs (steroids, thiazides and statins), 2%
- Other causes: trauma (1.5%), infection (<1%) such as mumps, hypercalcaemia (<1%), pancreas divisum (<1%), hypertriglyceridaemia (<1%), vasculitis (<1%), autoimmune (<1%).

CF & D: Patients present with acute onset of epigastric pain radiating into the back. There is commonly an association of nausea and vomiting. Fever and tachycardia are the most common abnormal vital signs. Bruising of the abdominal wall (Grey Turner's sign: flank bruise; Cullen's sign: periumbilical bruise) may be present consequent to the tracking of blood-stained exudate.

Diagnosis is made by demonstrating an elevated serum amylase. Serum amylase rises from 2 hours and peaks at 12–72 hours from disease onset. Although it lacks sensitivity (75–92%) and specificity (20–60%), it is the most widely used method of diagnosing pancreatitis. Serum lipase is known to be more specific (50–99%) in identifying an acute episode.

In cases with elevated serum amylase it is important to rule out a perforated duodenal ulcer, which is confirmed by the presence of free subdiaphragmatic gas on erect CXR. Other causes of hyperamylasaemia which may require exclusion are discussed below.

Hyperamylasaemia

In the absence of clinical features of acute pancreatitis, an alternative diagnosis for high levels of amylase should be sought. There are many other organs which produce amylase, including pancreas, salivary glands, fallopian tubes, testes, lungs, thyroid and some malignant neoplasms.

- Salivary disease: parotitis caused by trauma, surgery, radiation or calculi within the duct of the parotid gland.
- Decreased clearance: renal impairment and liver disease including hepatitis and cirrhosis.
- Macroamylasaemia: amylase molecule binds with a large complex molecule, prolonging the half-life and decreasing clearance.
- Intestinal disease: obstruction, mesenteric infarction, IBD, appendicits and peritonitis.
- Female reproductive tract: ruptured ectopic, salpingitis, fallopian or ovarian cysts.
- Miscellaneous: ectopic secretion from lung, ovary, pancreas and colon malignancies, DKA, AAA.

The aetiology of the episode can be confirmed in 90% of cases. USS should be performed in all patients to confirm or exclude the presence of gallstone disease.

T&M: Initial treatment follows the ABC protocol: maintain the airway, support breathing, and fluid resuscitation to support the circulation. Pancreatitis is treated by supportive measures: oxygen delivery, analgesia, fluid resuscitation, monitoring of urine output, avoidance of oral intake and nasogastric tube insertion to rest the GIT. If possible enteral nutrition is preferred over parenteral nutrition in patients who are going to require long-term supportive treatment. There is some evidence for using antibiotics in patients with CT-proven pancreatic necrosis to prevent infection. Surgery is only indicated for draining infected collections, which are not amenable to percutaneous drainage.

P: Several scoring systems are available, mainly involving the Glasgow score which is applied 24 hours after admission.

Mortality rates according to Glasgow score

Glasgow Score	Mortality
0–2	2%
3–4	15%
4–6	40%
7–8	100%

Useful hints and tips

A common mnemonic for the causes of acute pancreatitis is 'I GET SMASHED', an allusion to the heavy drinking which is one of the main culprits.

I Idiopathic
G Gallstone
E Ethanol
T Trauma
S Steroids
M Mumps and other viruses (EBV, CMV)
A Autoimmune (polyarteritis nodosa, SLE)
S Scorpion bite
H Hypercalcaemia, hyperlipidaemia, hypertriglyceridaemia, hypothermia
E ERCP
D Drugs (steroids, sulfonamides, azathioprine, NSAIDs, diuretics)

Modified Glasgow Score

This score predicts the prognosis of patients with acute pancreatitis. Each parameter scores 1 point. A score of 3 or more predicts a severe episode. (An easy mnemonic to remember these parameters is PANCREAS.)

P $PO_2 < 8\,kPa$
A Age > 55 years
N Neutrophil (WCC) > 15 × 10^9/L
C Calcium (uncorrected) < 2 mmol/L
R Raised urea > 16 mmol/L
E Enzymes: ALT > 100 IU/dL, LDH > 600 IU/dL
A Albumin < 32 g/L
S Sugar (glucose) > 10 mmol/L

Chronic pancreatitis

D : Continuing chronic inflammatory process of the pancreas, characterized by irreversible morphological changes. This process can lead to chronic abdominal pain, impairment of endocrine and/or exocrine function.

I & S : Chronic pancreatitis has an annual incidence of 1 per 100 000 with a prevalence of 3 per 100 000. Males are more commonly affected than females (M/F ratio 2 : 1) and the mean age of diagnosis is 46 years.

A & P : The two most common causes of chronic pancreatitis are alcohol and gallstone disease (combined 60%), but up to 30% remain idiopathic.

C F & D : The most common presenting symptom of chronic pancreatitis is abdominal pain. The pain is often in the mid or left upper abdomen, occasionally radiating into the back. The pain may occur independent to meals and tends to be persistent, lasting several hours. Unfortunately, patients are undiagnosed for many years before a diagnosis is established. In most patients the severity either decreases or resolves over 5–25 years. In alcohol-induced pancreatitis, cessation of alcohol intake may reduce the severity of pain. Patient may suffer with steatorrhoea and weight loss due to pancreatic exocrine insufficiency.

A proportion will develop diabetes from endocrine insufficiency. Calcification seen on AXR is considered to be pathognomonic for chronic pancreatitis and is observed in around 30% of cases. CT scanning is indicated to look for complications of the disease. Recent studies have indicated that the best test for imaging the pancreas/pancreatic duct is EUS, especially when combined with FNA or Trucut biopsy.

T & M :

Medical treatment

- Pain control: advise patients to stop alcohol consumption and tobacco smoking. Strong analgesics in the form of opioids should be used to control pain.
- Restoration of digestion: use of supplemental pancreatic enzymes to compensate for pancreatic exocrine insufficiency thereby improving steatorrhea.
- Diabetic control: use of insulin to control blood sugars.

Surgical treatment

Procedures may be used to treat complications such as pseudocysts, abscess and fistula.

- Endoscopic: aimed at decompressing an obstructed pancreatic duct by passing a guidewire through the stricture and placing a stent after dilatation. This method of treatment can offer pain relief in 60% of well-selected patients after 5 years of follow-up.
- Open surgery: if the disease is limited to the head of the pancreas, then a Whipple's procedure can produce good results. In patients with intractable pain with diffuse disease, a subtotal or total pancreatectomy can be performed. However, quality of life and pancreatic function are impaired, with an operative mortality of 10%. Furthermore, symptomatic patients with a dilated pancreatic duct may require a pancreatojejunostomy (dilated pancreatic is divided and anastomosed to a loop of jejunum).

P : The overall survival is 70% at 10 years and 45% at 20 years. The risk of developing pancreatic cancer is 4% at 20 years.

Pancreatic pseudocyst (advanced topic)

D : These are the most common type of cystic lesions of the pancreas, containing amylase-rich, lipase-rich or enterokinase-rich fluid. After 4 weeks the pancreatic fluid causes an intense inflammatory response leading to the formation of a thick fibrous capsule (pseudocyst). It is most frequently located in the lesser sac in proximity to the pancreas.

A & P : The most common causes of pseudocyst include chronic pancreatitis, acute pancreatitis, pancreatic trauma and pancreatic cancer.

C F & D : Presentation with abdominal pain that persists for longer than 3 weeks after recovery from pancreatitis (80% of patients). Abdominal fullness, nausea, vomiting and weight loss may be seen in up to 50% of patients. Rarely, the cyst may also obstruct the CBD causing jaundice and pruritus. The most common acute complication of a pseudocyst is acute infection, which is heralded by fever, abdominal pain and systemic signs of sepsis.

CT is the preferred imaging modality required to diagnose and plan treatment.

T & M :

> • Ruptured pseudocyst: spontaneous rupture into the abdominal cavity causes an acute abdomen. This requires emergency drainage of fluid with cystic débridement.
> • Intact pseudocyst: endoscopic or surgical percutaneous drainage.
> • Pseudocyst eroding into a vessel: emergency angiogram with embolization of the blood vessel to control the severe bleed.

P : Most pseudocysts do not require treatment. The failure rate for drainage procedures is about 10%; recurrence is 20–25% and complication rates 15–20%.

Gallstones

D : Gallstones are concretions that are commonly formed in the gallbladder. Migration of the stones may lead to occlusion of the pancreatic or bile duct, cause pain (biliary colic) and produce acute complications such as acute cholecystitis, ascending cholangitis, or acute pancreatitis. Chronic gallstone disease may lead to fibrosis and loss of function of the gallbladder and predispose to gallbladder cancer.

I & S : The lifetime risk of developing gallstones in white people is 50% for women and 30% for men. Women are more likely to develop gallstones than men (M/F ratio 1 : 2–3).

A & P : Gallstone formation occurs as a result of certain constituents of bile becoming more concentrated such that they reach the limits of solubility. These constituents precipitate to form stones. Over 80% of gallstones are made from cholesterol and the rest (10–20%) are pigmented stones made up of calcium bilirubinate.

> **Cholesterol stones**
>
> Associated with:
> • female gender
> • European ancestry
> • increasing age
> • obesity
> • pregnancy
> • drugs (OCP, clofibrate).
>
> **Calcium bilirubinate stones**
>
> Associated with haemolytic disorders:
> • sickle cell anaemia
> • hereditary spherocytosis
> • β thalassaemia.

C F & D : Gallbladder disease may be thought of as having three stages: (1) asymptomatic gallstones; (2) biliary colic; and (3) complications of gallbladder stones.

Stage 1

No symptom for many years. Chance of developing symptoms is 1–2% per year.
Tests: usually detected incidentally on USS.

Stage 2

Gallstones impact the cystic duct during gallbladder contraction lasting 30–90 min. The pain is localized to the epigastrium or RUQ radiating to the right scapular tip. From onset, the pain increases steadily over 10 min and then persists over several hours before waning.

Tests: USS is the most sensitive, specific, non-invasive and inexpensive test for detection of gallstones.

Stage 3

Acute cholecystitis

Due to persistent impaction of the gallstone against the cystic duct, causing gallbladder distension and inflammation. The patient has worsening persistent pain and tenderness on palpation of gallbladder (Murphy's sign). Overgrowth of colonizing bacteria occurs and in severe cases there is an accumulation of pus known as gallbladder empyema. The gallbladder may become necrotic causing perforation and formation of a pericholecystic abscess.

Tests: neutrophilia +/– deranged LFTs from inflammatory injury. USS demonstrates oedema and pericholecystic fliud.

Gallbladder cancer

Uncommon, usually forms in the setting of gallstones and cholecystitis. Prognosis is poor unless localized to the gallbladder in which case cholecystectomy would be the curative procedure.

Cholecystoenteric fistula

A large stone erodes through the wall of the gallbladder into an adjacent viscus such as the small bowel, and causes gallstone ileus.

CBD stone

Due to gallstone migration from the gallbladder. May be asymptomatic although they can commonly obstruct by impacting distally at the ampulla of Vater, causing jaundice.

Tests: MRCP is imaging technique of choice. Initially, deranged liver ALT/AST and bilirubin, followed by ↓ALT/AST with ↑ALP and bilirubin.

Ascending cholangitis

Occurs from stagnation of bile above an impacted CBD stone producing purulent inflammation.

Acute pancreatitis

A stone may transiently obstruct the pancreatic duct causing activation of pancreatic proteases resulting in pancreatitis.

Causes of deranged LFT parameters

- Markers of function: albumin and bilirubin
- Markers of liver damage: ALT, ALP and GGT

- Hepatic process +/- duct stones: ↑ALT
- Intrahepatic cholestasis, cholangitis or extrahepatic obstruction: ↑ALP (found in epithelial cells lining the bile canaliculi)
- Cholestasis: ↑ALP +/- ↑GGT

USS is the standard for the diagnosis of gallstones and complications of gallstones associated with the gallbladder. The bile duct is often obscured by overlying bowel gas and therefore MRCP is best used to investigate for choledocholithiasis.

T & M:

Medical

- Ursodeoxycholic acid: this is a natural bile salt and a weak detergent, often requiring long-term compliance (6–18 months). Not very effective.

Surgical: cholecystectomy

- Laparoscopic/open: treatment of choice in symptomatic gallstones. CBD stone can be removed during surgery.
- ERCP +/- sphincterotomy: extraction of CBD stones. Can be used for patients not fit for surgery.

P: Following cholecystectomy 5–10% of patients develop diarrhoea, which is attributed to more bile salts reaching the colon. Also patients may develop pain resembling biliary colic, termed 'post-cholecystectomy syndrome'.

Useful hints and tips

Murphy's sign is elicited while the examiner maintains steady pressure over the RUQ and the patient inhales. This must be negative on the LUQ to be a true Murphy's sign.

MCQs

Pancreatic cancer (Answers, see p. 264)

1 Regarding pancreatic tumours, which of the following statements are true and which are false?

a The majority are malignant.

b All patients present with obstructive jaundice.

c Adenocarcinoma's strongest association is with diabetes.

d EUS can be used to relieve biliary obstruction.

e Curative treatment of adenocarcinomas is with radiotherapy.

2 Concerning the symptoms of pancreatic cancer, which of the following statements are true and which are false?

a Tumours involving the head commonly present with vague symptoms.
b Early symptoms of patients with tumours involving the body include cachexia and vomiting.
c Some of the late symptoms of tumours involving the body/tail of the pancreas include GI bleed, diabetes and vomiting.
d Steatorrhoea, dark urine and jaundice commonly occur in tumours involving the head of the pancreas.
e Depression

3 Which of the following are the signs of pancreatic cancer?
a Migratory thrombophlebitis (i.e. Trousseau's sign) more commonly occurs in pancreatic cancer.
b Presence of palpable gallbladder never occurs.
c Subcutaneous metastasis in the periumbilical area signifies advanced disease.
d A metastatic mass in the rectal pouch may be palpable on rectal examination.
e Ascites may be present in advanced intra-abdominal disease.

4 Regarding special investigations for pancreatic cancer, which of the following are true and which are false?
a 40% of patients with pancreatic cancer have elevated CA19-9.
b An elevated CA19-9 above 100 U/mL in the absence of biliary obstruction, benign pancreatic disease and intrinsic liver disease is highly diagnostic.
c 85% of patients with pancreatic cancer have elevated CEA.
d EUS has a detection rate of 99–100% including those tumours less than 3 cm in size.
e Using EUS-guided FNA, a cytological diagnosis can be made in 60% of patients.

5 Concerning the treatment of pancreatic cancer, which of the following are true and which are false?
a Surgery is the primary mode of treatment.
b The combination of gemcitabine and erlotinib leads to a higher median survival when used as adjuvant treatment.
c Radiation therapy can improve survival in pancreatic cancer.
d Patients with postprandial pain can have improvement following endoscopic decompression with stents.
e Approximately 50% of patients will present with duodenal obstruction which requires palliation with gastrojejunostomy.

6 Regarding the outcome of pancreatic cancer, which of the following are true and which are false?
a Mean survival for unresectable disease is 12 months.
b The 5-year survival rate is less than 3% in resectable disease.
c Median survival for patients undergoing resection is 24 months.
d The 5-year survival rate is 15–20% in resectable disease.
e Only 10% undergo curative surgical resection.

7 Regarding pancreatic carcinoma, which of the following are true and which are false?

a Adenocarcinoma of the pancreatic head has a better prognosis than cancer arising from the periampullary region.

b It is rare in young adults.

c Courvoisier's law is likely to be positive with a carcinoma at the head of the pancreas.

d Chronic pancreatitis is a predisposing factor.

e Most are acinar in histology.

8 Which of the following have been shown to be the strongest risk factors for development of pancreatic adenocarcinoma?

a Diabetes.

b Obesity.

c Gastrectomy.

d Chronic pancreatitis.

e Cigarette smoking.

Liver abscess (Answers, see p. 265)

1 Regarding hepatic abscess, which of the following are true and which are false?

a Hepatic abscesses are amoebic or bacterial in origin.

b *Entamoeba histolytica* is the most common cause for amoebic abscess.

c Bacterial abscesses are mostly caused by ascending cholangitis.

d Abscesses may rupture to cause peritonitis.

e Untreated abscesses are associated with a mortality of 50%.

Hepatocellular carcinoma (Answers, see p. 265)

1 Regarding hepatocellular carcinoma, which of the following are true and which are false?

a It is a primary malignancy of the biliary canaliculi.

b It commonly arises on a background of cirrhosis, 20–30 years after the initial insult.

c HCC is common and comprises 10% of all malignancies.

d Although cure is achieved through surgery, it is possible in fewer than 5% of all patients.

e Tumours are multifocal 75% of the time.

2 Which paraneoplastic syndromes are associated with HCC?

a Hypercalcaemia.

b Hypoglycaemia.

c Erythrocytosis.

d Thrombocytosis.

e Hyperglycaemia.

3 Which of the following has the weakest association with HCC?

a Hepatitis B.

b Hepatitis C.

   c Oral contraceptives.
   d Smoking.
   e Alcohol.

4 Concerning the treatment of HCC, which of the following are true and which are false?
   a 5% are suitable for transplantation.
   b The 5-year survival following transplantation is 75% with 5-year tumour recurrence rates at 15%.
   c Systemic chemotherapy, transplantation and tumour ablation are the mainstays of treatment in advanced disease.
   d Many surgeons use a cut-off of 5 cm as a criterion for surgery.
   e Intraoperative mortality in patients undergoing hepatectomy is doubled in patients with cirrhosis.

5 Regarding the investigation of HCC, which of the following are true and which are false?
   a AFP is elevated in 75% of cases with HCC.
   b The level of AFP inversely correlates with prognosis.
   c MRI has the best sensitivity and specificity in patients with nodular cirrhotic livers.
   d Biopsy is never omitted.
   e False-negative rates are as high as 30–40% in biopsies from tumours <2 cm.

6 Which of the following is the most common cause of cirrhosis in the UK?
   a Hepatitis B.
   b Autoimmune hepatitis.
   c Haemochromatosis.
   d Alcohol.
   e Primary biliary cirrhosis.

Cholangiocarcinoma (Answers, see p. 266)

1 Which of the following is the most common site for cholangiocarcinoma?
   a Lower one-third of CBD.
   b Intrahepatic.
   c End of CBD.
   d Cystic duct.
   e Heptic duct bifurcation.

2 Regarding cholangiocarcinoma, which of the following are true and which are false?
   a Radiation increases survival.
   b Transplantation is successful in patients with confined disease.
   c The more proximal the disease, the more likely it will be resectable.
   d Proximal disease is curable if resected.
   e None of the above is true.

3 Regarding the surgical treatment of cholangiocarcinoma, which of the following are true and which are false?

a Complete hepatic resection with transplantation has shown good results.
b Whipple is the best procedure for a resectable proximal tumour.
c Stenting of the biliary anastomosis is important prior to surgical resection of proximal biliary lesions.
d Klatskin tumours may require hepatic resection in attempt for cure.
e Transplantation is considered for patients with proximal disease who are not candidates for resection because of the extent of tumour spread.

4 Concerning cholangiocarcinoma, which of the following are true and which are false?
a Cholangiocarcinoma is more common than gallbladder cancer.
b Cholangiocarcinoma is more common in females.
c There is no association with gallstones.
d Ulcerative colitis is associated with cholangiocarcinoma.
e Choledochal cysts may be associated with the development of cholangiocarcinoma.

5 A 70-year-old man presents with obstructive jaundice. The patient's initial investigation begins with a CT scan. Which of the following is true regarding his diagnosis?
a A CT scan showing a non-distended gallbladder, intrahepatic duct dilatation and decompressed extrahepatic biliary tree is consistent with a hilar cholangiocarcinoma.
b Angiography is not required in the evaluation of a patient with cholangiocarcinoma.
c PTC would be preferred for visualizing the proximal extent of the tumour when dealing with proximal cholangiocarcinoma.
d Biliary obstruction on CT scan requires further investigation with percutaneous or endoscopic cholangiography.
e The use of a transhepatic biliary catheter can prove useful in surgical management of proximal bile duct cancers.

6 Regarding cholangiocarcinomas, which of the following are true and which are false?
a More than 90% are adenocarcinomas.
b The highest annual incidence is in Israel.
c Median survival is only 6 months.
d The parasite *Ascaris lumbricoides* has been implicated in cholangiocarcinoma.
e There is a strong relationship between PSC and cholangiocarcinoma.

Acute pancreatitis (Answers, see p. 267)

1 Regarding acute pancreatitis, which of the following are true and which are false?
a Hypercalcaemia is a common cause.
b It is associated with Grey Turner's sign (periumbilical bruising).
c A score of 2 on the Glasgow (Imrie) scale predicts a severe attack in most patients.
d Upper GI perforation can lead to a raised plasma amylase.
e Pseudocysts can occur as early as a week after the attack.

2 Which of the following statements are true regarding the BSG standards for managing pancreatitis?

a All patients should be managed in the high-dependency unit.

b Diagnosis should be made within 2 weeks.

c No more than 20% of cases should be attributed to an idiopathic aetiology.

d Patients with biliary pancreatitis should have definitive treatment within 2 days.

e Mortality should be above 30%.

3 Which of the following parameters are not included in Ranson's criteria?

a Elevated blood sugar.

b Amylase of greater than 1000.

c LDH > 600 IU/dL.

d ALT > 100 IU/dL.

e Leucocytosis.

4 Regarding standard supportive measures for patients with acute pancreatitis, which of the following is the best option for treatment?

a IV fluids and electrolyte therapy.

b Prophylactic antibiotics.

c Avoid the use of analgesia to allow for serial abdominal examinations.

d Nasogastric decompression.

e SC octreotide treatment.

5 Which of the following agents have been shown to demonstrate enhanced recovery from acute pancreatitis?

a H_2 receptor antagonists.

b Octreotide.

c Anticholinergic receptor antagonist.

d Beta blockers.

e None of the above.

6 Which of the following procedures increase the risk of acute pancreatitis?

a ERCP.

b CABG.

c Bile duct exploration.

d Distal gastrectomy.

Chronic pancreatitis (Answers, see p. 268)

1 Regarding chronic pancreatitis, which of the following are true and which are false?

a It is inevitable after recurrent acute episodes.

b For symptomatic patients with a dialated pancreatic duct caused by a stricture, longitudinal pancreaticojejunostomy (Peustow's procedure) is a sensible surgical option.

c Patients with chronic pancreatitis commonly present with jaundice, pruritis and fever.

d Total pancreatectomy is the best option in symptomatic patients.

    e Mesenteric angiography is useful in the evaluation of patients with chronic pancreatitis.

2 Which of the following investigations is best for confirming a clinical diagnosis of early chronic pancreatitis?
    a Urinary amylase clearance.
    b Serum CA19-9.
    c Serum amylase.
    d EUS.
    e ERCP.

3 Regarding chronic pancreatitis, which of the following are true?
    a In the UK the most common cause of pancreatitis is alcohol abuse.
    b The risk of alcohol-induced chronic pancreatitis can be reduced by consuming a high-protein diet.
    c Chronic pancreatitis usually develops 5 years after alcohol abuse.
    d Half of chronic alcoholics develop chronic pancreatitis.
    e In early-stage chronic pancreatitis, lasting pain relief can occur after abstinence from alcohol.

4 A 60-year-old male alcoholic presents to the clinic with chronic abdominal pain. ERCP findings include duct ectasia, ductal stones with alternating areas of stricture and dilatation. Which of the following would be the most appropriate operative procedure?
    a Total pancreatectomy.
    b Cholecystectomy and bile duct exploration.
    c Distal pancreatectomy with splenectomy.
    d Distal pancreatectomy with end panreaticojejunostomy.
    e Longitudinal pancreaticojejenostomy.

5 Which of the following is the most common cause of obstructive jaundice in patients with chronic pancreatitis?
    a Pancreatic pseudocyst formation.
    b Gallstones.
    c Head of pancreas tumour.
    d Stricture of bile duct.
    e Cholangiocarcinoma.

6 Which of the following is the most common clinical manifestation of chronic pancreatitis?
    a Jaundice.
    b Diabetes mellitus.
    c Steatorrhoea.
    d Epigastric pain.
    e Weight loss.

Pancreatitic pseudocyst (Answers, see p. 269)

1 A 49-year-old man presents with acute pancreatitis from acute alcohol abuse. By the ninth day in hospital the patient is noted to have a recurrent fever

(38.5°C), leucocytosis and tachypnoea. On imaging, there is a fluid collection around his pancreas. What is the next step in managing this patient?

a IV antibiotics.

b Laparotomy and pancreatic débridement.

c ERCP and stenting.

d CT/EUS-guided aspiration of peripancreatic collection.

e None of the above.

2 A 68-year-old man has a pancreatic collection. The medical team decides for conservative treatment for 10 weeks. A follow-up CT scan reveals a 6-cm pseudocyst in the region of the body of the pancreas. The pseudocyst is unilocular and the distal part of the stomach is displaced anteriorly; 300 mL of fluid is aspirated using CT-guided aspiration. What is the risk of pseudocyst recurrence after simple aspiration?

a 20–25%.

b 40–45%.

c 60–65%.

d 80–85%.

e 100%.

3 Which of the following classification systems are used for pancreatic pseudocysts?

a TNM staging.

b Glasgow score.

c Ranson criteria.

d Nealon's classification.

e Frey and Wardell classification.

4 In which of the following sites are pancreatic pseudocysts most frequently located?

a Greater sac.

b Paracolic gutters.

c Pelvis.

d Mediastinum.

e Lesser sac.

5 Which of the following is the most common acute complication of a pancreatic pseudocyst?

a Infection.

b Rupture.

c Bleeding.

d Obstruction.

e Pain.

6 What proportion of pancreatic pseudocysts become infected?

a 30%.

b 40%.

c 25%.

d 10%.

e 60%.

Gallstones (Answers, see p. 270)

1 Regarding gallstones, which of the following are true and which are false?
   a β-Glucuronidase-producing bacteria form pigmented stones.
   b Boas' sign results from cholecystitis.
   c They are the most common cause of jaundice.
   d Chenodeoxycholic acid can be used to treat uncomplicated cholesterol stones.
   e Conventional open cholecystectomy is performed with Kocher's incision.

2 Regarding jaundice, which of the following are true and which are false?
   a In haemolytic jaundice there is a fall in urobilin and urobilinogen within the urine.
   b May occur postoperatively.
   c Carotenaemia can be clinically confused with jaundice.
   d With the presence of Murphy's sign is associated with ascending cholangitis.
   e In obstructive jaundice preoperatively, phytomenadione may be used to correct clotting abnormalities within 6 hours.

3 Which of the following are typical biochemical features of obstructive jaundice?
   a Reduced ALP.
   b Reduced ALT.
   c Bilirubin < 20 μmol/L.
   d Raised AFP.
   e Raised amylase.

4 Regarding ascending cholangitis, which of the following are true and which are false?
   a Commonly occurs in a CBD partially obstructed by gallstones.
   b Causes a triad of signs and symptoms named after Charcot.
   c In late stages LFTs are deranged showing a hepatitic picture.
   d Anaerobes most commonly cause the infection.
   e Surgical exploration is the most common approach for definitive treatment.

5 A 70-year-old woman presented with pruritis, dark urine and epigastric pain. Physical examination reveals jaundice. LFTs reveal a bilirubin of 84 μmol/L, a mild rise in the transaminases and ALP three times above the upper limit. Which of the following is the most appropriate initial investigation?
   a USS of abdomen.
   b ERCP.
   c MRI of abdomen.
   d CT of addomen.
   e EUS.

6 Which of the following are indications for cholecystectomy?
   a The presence of asymptomatic gallstone disease in a patient with IDDM.
   b The presence of asymptomatic gallstones.
   c The presence of symptomatic gallstones in patients with uncontrolled angina.

d The presence of gallstones with intermittent episodes of RUQ abdominal pain radiating into the back.

e Following the confirmation of gallstones in a patient with jaundice.

7 Which of the following options is the initial treatment for acute cholangitis with sepsis?

a Remove an obstructing CBD gallstone.

b Alleviate jaundice and prevent liver damage.

c Prevent cholangiovenous reflux by decompressing the biliary system.

d Perform a laparoscopic cholecystectomy and CBD exploration.

e Perform a sphincterotomy with ERCP.

EMQs (Answers, see p. 272)

1 Options:

a CT scan.

b ERCP.

c PTC.

d ^{99}Tc iodide scan.

e Barium follow-through.

f MRCP.

g Endoscopy.

h Laparoscopy.

i Oral cholecystogram.

For each case below choose the single most likely investigation from the list above. Each option may be used once, more than once or not at all.

(i) A 76-year-old woman presents with obstructive jaundice and a palpable gallbladder. USS shows a dilated CBD and past history includes Pólya gastrectomy for a bleeding ulcer.

(ii) A 60-year-old man presents with obstructive jaundice. The USS revealed no gallstones, normal liver and a CBD measuring 12 mm. His past history includes a gastrectomy carried out 15 years ago.

(iii) A 55-year-old obese woman presents with acute upper abdominal pain. Examination demonstrates pyrexia and tenderness in RUQ. An erect CXR reveals no subdiaphragmatic free air. USS failed to confirm the diagnosis.

(iv) A 60-year-old woman presents with upper abdominal pain and obstructive jaundice. The gallbladder is not palpable clinically. USS shows gallstones and dialated common bile duct.

2 Options:

a Pancreatic carcinoma.

b Gallstones.

c Mumps.

d Cystic fibrosis.

e Alcohol.

f Hypothermia.

g Polyarteritis nodosa.

h Hypertriglyceridaemia.

i Iatrogenic.

j Thiazide diuretic.

k Hypercalcaemia.

For each case below choose the single most likely diagnosis from the list above. Each option may be used once, more than once or not at all.

(i) A 50-year-old woman with polyuria, haematuria, abdominal pain and bone ache.

(ii) A 55-year-old obese woman with recurrent episodes of RUQ abdominal pain.

(iii) A 70-year-old man with progressive jaundice, new-onset diabetes and weight loss.

(iv) A 13-year-old girl presents with fever, anorexia, headache, malaise and trismus.

(v) A 10-year-old girl with a history of recurrent chest infections and sinusitis with abdominal pain.

3 Options:

a Acute cholecystitis.

b Alcoholic liver disease.

c Carcinoma of the head of the pancreas.

d Choledocholithiasis.

e Haemolytic anaemia.

f Hepatic abscess.

g Metastatic hepatic disease.

h Pancreatitis.

i Portal vein thrombosis.

For each case below choose the single most likely diagnosis from the list above. Each option may be used once, more than once or not at all.

(i) A 40-year-old woman presents with progressive jaundice and severe discomfort in the epigastrium without pyrexia; 10 months previously she had undergone laparoscopic cholecystectomy.

(ii) A 25-year-old IVDU presents to hospital with suspected appendicitis and becomes acutely unwell with a high swinging pyrexia, jaundice, and palpable tender hepatomegaly.

(iii) A diabetic 47-year-old man presents with severe weight loss and painless progressive jaundice. His gallbladder is palpable on examination.

(iv) A 53-year-old hotel worker has a 10-day history of increasing jaundice and confusion. He also gives a history of loss of sensation in hands and feet. On examination he has spider naevi, palmar erythema and palpable enlarged liver.

(v) A 29-year-old woman has a 2-week history of mild jaundice and pallor, following an upper respiratory infection (pharyngitis). On examination the spleen is palpable. Urinalysis shows excess urobilinogen, but no bilirubin.

4 Options:

a Carcinoma of pancreas.

b Hepatocellular carcinoma.

c Gilbert's syndrome.

d Primary biliary cirrhosis.
e Sclerosing cholangitis.
f Chronic active hepatitis.
g Dubin–Johnson syndrome.
h CBD stones.
i Rotor's syndrome.
j Hepatitis A.
For each case below choose the single most likely diagnosis from the list above.
Each option may be used once, more than once or not at all.

(i) A 70-year-old woman presents with jaundice and backache. Clinical examination reveals mass in the RUQ, acanthosis nigricans and superficial thrombophlebitis.

(ii) A 30-year-old man presents with jaundice and a 6-month history of bloody diarrhoea. His Hb is 10 g/dL, bilirubin 75 µmol/L and elevated liver enzymes including AST, ALT (140 U/L) and ALP (450 U/L).

(iii) A 13-year-old boy presents with jaundice after an episode of tonsillitis. Serum bilirubin rises further on fasting. USS was normal.

(iv) A 45-year-old woman presents with obstructive jaundice 4 weeks after laparoscopic cholecystectomy. Blood test results include bilirubin 105 µmol/L, ALP 750 U/L, ALT 150 U/L.

(v) A 50-year-old woman presents with obstructive jaundice and hepatomegaly. She has a past history of Sjögren's syndrome and antibody blood tests reveal positivity for anti-mitochondrial antibody. Liver biopsy shows ductal destruction, proliferation and granulomas.

5 Options:
a ERCP and stenting.
b Cholecystectomy with T-tube in CBD.
c Laparoscopic cholecystectomy within 2 weeks.
d Elective laparoscopic cholecystectomy.
e Ursodeoxycholic acid.
f Whipple's procedure.
g Open cholecystectomy.
h Cholecystostomy.
For each case below choose the single most likely treatment from the list above.
Each option may be used once, more than once or not at all.

(i) An 80-year-old woman with multiple comorbidities and limited exercise tolerance presents with RUQ pain, jaundice and rigors. Blood tests show bilirubin 110 µmol/L, ALP 734 U/L and ALT 110 U/L. USS reveals CBD dilatation and presence of a stone.

(ii) A 44-year-old woman presents with RUQ abdominal colic lasting less than 24 hours. Blood tests are normal and USS reveals a gallbladder containing stones with no wall thickness.

(iii) A 66-year-old man presents with jaundice, weight loss and recent-onset diabetes. Abdominal examination reveals a palpable gallbladder.

(iv) A 52-year-old man presents with acute epigastric pain and vomiting. Serum amylase was > 1000 U/L and USS reveals multiple small gallstones.

(v) A 90-year-old woman with ischaemic heart disease presents RUQ pain and swinging fever. Blood tests reveal WCC 30×10^9/L, and LFTs within normal limits. USS shows a large distended gallbladder. Treatment with intravenous antibiotics does not improve her clinical condition.

6 Options:
   a Alcoholic liver disease.
   b Autoimmune hepatitis.
   c Chronic obstructive pulmonary disease.
   d Congestive cardiac failure.
   e Infective hepatitis.
   f Lymphoma.
   g Metastatic liver disease.
   h Polycystic liver.
   i Primary biliary cirrhosis.

For each case below choose the single most likely diagnosis from the list above. Each option may be used once, more than once or not at all.

   (i) A 76-year-old woman is admitted with dyspnoea 3 days post MI and found to have a palpable tender liver.
  (ii) A woman of 20 years of age with known IDDM is found to have hepatomegaly at routine follow-up.
 (iii) At an insurance medical examination a woman of 50 years of age is noted to have xanthelasma, skin pigmentation and a palpable liver.
  (iv) A 45-year-old publican, who attends the dermatology clinic with severe psoriasis, is noted to be jaundiced and have a large liver.
   (v) A 70-year-old woman with constant upper abdominal pain, anorexia and weight loss is found to have an enlarged irregular liver.

7 Options:
   a Haemochromatosis.
   b Wilson's disease.
   c Primary biliary cirrhosis.
   d Osler–Rendu–Weber syndrome.
   e Alcohol.
   f Methotrexate.
   g Cardiac cirrhosis.
   h Budd–Chiari syndrome.
   i α_1-Antitrypsin deficiency.
   j Cystic fibrosis.

For each of the signs described below, choose the single most likely cause of cirrhosis from the list above. Each option may be used once, more than once or not at all.

   (i) Parotid enlargement and Dupuytren's contracture.
  (ii) Clubbing, coarse crepitations at both lung bases.
 (iii) A middle-aged woman with xanthelasma.
  (iv) Breathlessness, ankle oedema and a raised JVP.
   (v) Multiple telangiectasiae around the lips.

8 Options:
  a Chronic active hepatitis.
  b Primary biliary cirrhosis.
  c Wilson's disease.
  d Hepatic adenoma.
  e Haemochromatosis.
  f Cholecystitis.
  g Gaucher's disease.
  h Galactosaemia.
  i Gilbert's syndrome.
  j Alcoholic liver cirrhosis.

For each case below choose the single most likely diagnosis from the list above. Each option may be used once, more than once or not at all.

  (i) A 30-year-old woman presented with anorexia, weight loss, lethargy and arthralgia for 3 weeks. On examination she was pale and jaundiced. The liver was palpable two finger-breadths below the costal margin as the tip of the spleen. Blood test results were as follows: ALP 150 U/L, AST 875 U/L, bilirubin 39 μmol/L, albumin 21 g/L, globulin 52 g/L.

  (ii) A 45-year-old man presented with worsening limb twitches and facial tics. He has been an inpatient in a psychiatric hospital for the last 5 years and has a family history of psychiatric illness.

  (iii) A 38-year-old woman presented with generalized pruritis for 5 months. On examination she was tanned and spider naevi were present on her chest. The patient also had hepatomegaly and splenomegaly.

  (iv) A 17-year-old boy presents with flu-like illness followed 3 days later by abdominal pain, nausea, vomiting and jaundice. All his blood tests were normal apart from increased unconjugated bilirubin.

  (v) A 30-year-old woman presents with acute abdominal pain. Her bowels were regular with normal stools. She was taking the OCP and on examination there were no features of chronic liver disease. She was tender over the RUQ and the right lobe of the liver was palpable.

10 Spleen

The spleen is a lymphoid organ that produces cells involved in immune responses, destroys old blood cells, removes debris from the bloodstream and acts as a reservoir of blood.

Anatomy

The spleen is present in the left hypochondrium and measures approximately 2.5 × 7.5 × 12.5 cm. It usually lies with its long axis along the line of the tenth rib. It occupies the space between the left ninth and the eleventh rib. The two important ligaments around the spleen are the lienorenal (from spleen to kidney) and the gastrosplenic (stomach to spleen).

Functions

The spleen helps to sequester and remove old red blood cells and platelets from the systemic circulation. It produces antibodies like IgM, which help to fight foreign antigens. It acts as a storage place for platelets; about 30% of the total platelets are within spleen. Spleen recycles iron and filters capsulated microorganisms, e.g. pneumococcus.

Causes of splenomegaly

Haematological disorders
- Myeloproliferative disorders (myelofibrosis)
- Haemolytic anaemia
- Leukaemia and lymphoma
- Thalassaemia
- Sickle cell disease

Infective
- Acute (infective endocarditis, HIV, CMV, EBV)
- Chronic (malaria, leishmaniasis, toxoplasmosis)

Portal hypertension
- Cirrhosis; portal, hepatic or splenic vein thrombosis

Systemic pathology
- Rheumatoid arthritis
- Felty's syndrome
- Sarcoidosis or amyloidosis

EMQs and MCQs for Surgical Finals, 1st edition.   © Hye-Chung Kwak, Imran Bhatti,
Jaskarn Rai, Farhan Rashid, Bachittar Singh Jassar, Murthy Nyasavajjala, Viren Asher,
Jon Lund and Mike Larvin. Published 2011 by Blackwell Publishing Ltd.

Indications for splenectomy

- Trauma: bleeding.
- Iatrogenic: during surgery (e.g. gastrectomy/bowel surgery).
- Hypersplenism: autoimmune thrombocytopenia, haemolytic anaemia, thrombotic thrombocytopenia, hereditary spherocytosis, sickle cell/thalassaemia, staging procedure in Hodgkin's lymphoma.

Vaccinations prior to splenectomy

- *Haemophilis influenzae* type B
- Meningococcus (*Neisseria meningitidis*)
- Pneumococcus (*Streptococcus pneumoniae*)
- In addition, lifelong penicillin and prophylaxis against malaria when required.

Mnemonic for the spleen: all the odd numbers

'1, 3, 5, 7, 9, 11': the dimensions of the spleen are 1 × 3 × 5 inches. It weighs 7 ounces and it underlies ribs 9–11.

MCQs (Answers, see p. 275)

1 Which of the following are indications for splenectomy?
 a Massive splenic injury.
 b Iatrogenic.
 c Idiopathic thrombocytopenic purpura.
 d Staging procedure in Hodgkin's lymphoma.
 e Total gastrectomy.
 f Splenic neoplasm.

2 Which of the following are the vaccinations required after splenectomy?
 a *Haemophilus influenzae* type B.
 b Pneumococcus.
 c Meningococcus.
 d Hepatitis C.
 e HIV.

3 Regarding splenic rupture, which of the following are true and which are false?
 a It is more common in patients with infectious mononucleosis.
 b It may be delayed up to 7 weeks following blunt abdominal trauma.
 c It can lead to raised hemidiaphragm.
 d It produces a negative Kehr's sign.
 e Left lower rib fracture can lead to splenic rupture.

EMQs (Answers, see p. 275)

1 Options:
  a Administer analgesia.
  b Call your senior.
  c Cross-match blood.
  d Establish IV access and administer fluids.
  e Group and save.
  f Insertion of chest drain.
  g Laparotomy.
  h Record the observations.
  i Ultrasound scan.
  j Urgent blood glucose check.
  k Urgent CT abdomen.
For each case below suggest the most appropriate management from the above list of options. Each option may be used once, more than once or not at all.
  (i) A 28-year-old man presents with LUQ pain after being assaulted. On erect CXR, there is a suspicion of posterior lower rib fractures and a raised left hemidiaphragm. There are no other associated injuries. What is your management?
  (ii) A 40-year-old man has had a fall, hitting his left lower ribs and lower back on the corner of the dining table. He had a tender LUQ on palpation, he is haemodynamically stable and haemoglobin level is normal.
  (iii) A 38-year-old woman presented with sudden onset of LUQ pain associated with persistent vomiting. There was guarding and rebound tenderness over the LUQ. Erect CXR revealed a displaced gastric bubble.
  (iv) A 45-year-old woman presented to A&E following a severe road traffic collision. Her abdomen was rigid, associated with tachycardia and hypotension. An urgent ultrasound of her abdomen revealed free fluid.
  (v) You have been asked to review the fluid requirements of a 60-year-old man who had a splenectomy for trauma 2 hours ago. The observations clearly indicate increasing pulse rate and decreasing blood pressure.

2 Options:
  a CT scan of abdomen and pelvis.
  b Laparotomy and splenectomy.
  c Long-term low-dose penicillin prophylaxis.
  d Mesenteric angiogram.
  e Overwhelming post-splenectomy infection.
  f Prophylactic immunization.
  g Splenectomy.
  h Ultrasound of the abdomen.
For each case below suggest the most appropriate treatment/investigation from the list above. Each option may be used once, more than once or not at all.
  (i) A 45-year-old man presents to the medical assessment unit. He looks very unwell. He is showing signs of sepsis including fever, hypotension and tachycardia. He gives a history of splenectomy about 2 years ago for trauma.

(ii) A 38-year-old man admitted to A&E has been involved in a road traffic accident 2 hours ago and is complaining of left upper abdominal pain. He is tachycardic, hypotensive and ultrasound of the abdomen has suggested a peri-splenic fluid collection. He has not responded to vigorous intravenous colloid and crystalloid infusions.

(iii) A previously fit and healthy 60-year-old man with a history of a fall from a flight of stairs presents to the surgical assessment unit. He is haemodynamically stable. The CXR has confirmed left lower rib fractures with no evidence of haemothorax/pneumothorax. He is now developing increasing left upper abdominal pain and tenderness. The repeat observations suggest stable pulse and blood pressure. What should be the next investigation?

(iv) A 40-year-old factory worker has been diagnosed with primary splenic tumour. He is awaiting an elective splenectomy in 2 weeks time. What should be done before the splenectomy?

(v) A 48-year-old man who underwent elective splenectomy 2 days ago is waiting to be discharged from the hospital today. He has already had prophylactic immunization against *Haemophilus influenzae*, *Streptococcus pneumoniae* and *Neisseria meningitidis*. What is the next step before discharging the patient?

11   Midgut

Acute appendicitis

D: Acute inflammation of the appendix.

I & S :   In the UK, around 10% of the population will develop acute appendicitis. Common in children and young adults. M/F ratio approximately 1.5 : 1.

A & P :   Obstruction of the appendiceal lumen.

C F & D :   Typical presentation is periumbilical pain (midgut origin) migrating to the right iliac fossa (peritoneal irritation by the inflamed appendix) +/− pyrexia, nausea and vomiting.

Diagnosis is clinical. Additional tests: WCC, urinalysis to exclude UTI (and pregnancy test), USS can aid in diagnosis, CT abdomen in difficult cases.

Symptoms

- Right lower quadrant pain
- Nausea and vomiting
- Anorexia

Signs

- Tenderness
- Rebound tenderness
- Guarding
- Rovsing sign
- Psoas irritation
- Fever and tachycardia

T & M :   Follow the ABCDE approach and keep patient NBM for laparoscopic or open appendicectomy.

P :   Greater mortality in perforated appendicitis (abscess formation and other complications), excellent prognosis after surgery.

Small bowel obstruction

D :   Obstruction of the small bowel causing strangulation is a surgical emergency.

I & S :   Approximately 5% of acute surgical admissions are due to SBO.

A & P :   Caused by adhesions, hernias, malignancy, volvulus, Crohn's disease. There is proximal bowel dilatation, fluid accumulation and increased peristalsis, and eventually venous flow is impaired followed by arterial flow.

EMQs and MCQs for Surgical Finals, 1st edition.   © Hye-Chung Kwak, Imran Bhatti, Jaskarn Rai, Farhan Rashid, Bachittar Singh Jassar, Murthy Nyasavajjala, Viren Asher, Jon Lund and Mike Larvin. Published 2011 by Blackwell Publishing Ltd.

CF&D: The patient may look very unwell and dehydrated with a distended abdomen.

Symptoms

- Colicky abdominal pain
- Nausea and vomiting
- Absolute constipation

Signs

- Abdominal tenderness
- Abdominal distension
- Tinkling bowel sounds
- Dehydration
- Fever
- Tachycardia

Following history and examination (look for any hernias), consider the following investigations:

- Blood: FBC (look at Hb and WBC), U&E (assess dehydration, correct any abnormal electrolytes), G&S (for surgical intervention).
- Plain AXR: look for distended small bowel with air–fluid level, prominent valvulae coniventes, absent gas in the large bowel. Cannot distinguish whether bowel is strangulated on AXR, therefore may need further imaging.
- CT scan: diagnose strangulated bowel, find aetiology of SBO.

T&M: Begin with **ABCDE approach, NGT for decompression, IV line for fluid resuscitation, catheter to monitor UO, continuous monitoring, consider antibiotic cover for Gram-negative and anaerobic microorganisms.** Contact the surgeons early.

In simple or partial SBO, a 3-day trial of conservative management can be considered. Most will resolve.

P: Early surgery has better outcomes.

Meckel's diverticulum

D: A remnant of the vitello-intestinal duct from embryonic life which lies on the antimesenteric border of the ileum. It is present 60 cm proximal to the ileocaecal valve, about 5 cm in length. It is a true diverticulum containing all three intestinal layers.

I&S: It is present in 2% of the population. No sex predilection but males are more likely to have symptomatic diverticula.

CF&D: Mostly asymptomatic but may present with the following complications:

- Acute inflammation: right-sided abdominal pain.
- Intussusception: right-sided abdominal pain and mass.
- Bleeding and perforation: the gastric mucosal lining of the diverticulum may bleed or perforate.

• Obstruction: band adhesional obstruction of the small bowel from the tip of the diverticulum to the umbilicus.

> **Investigations**
>
> • Ultrasound
> • Contrast studies of the bowel
> • Technetium-labelled red cell scan in the presence of active bleeding

T & M : Surgical excision (wedge resection or small bowel resection).

P : Mortality for surgery can be up to 5%.

MCQs

Appendicitis (Answers, see p. 277)

1 Regarding the anatomy and function of the appendix, which of the following are true and which are false?

a The appendix is a true diverticulum.

b It develops as an outgrowth from the terminal ileum.

c The position of the tip of the appendix remains constant.

d It functions as a major essential part of the GALT.

e It is approximately 4 inches (10 cm) in length.

2 Regarding the epidemiology of appendicitis, which of the following are true and which are false?

a It is the second most common acute surgical emergency in the UK.

b It is more common in cultures that have a higher intake of dietary fibre.

c It does not occur in patients over 60 years of age.

d Perforation rate is higher at the extremes of age.

e There is a higher incidence in females.

3 Regarding the symptoms associated with appendicitis, which of the following are true and which are false?

a Typically symptoms present with periumbilical pain radiating to left iliac fossa.

b The typical presentation was first described by Allen Whipple.

c Subcaecal appendix may present as diarrhoea and urinary frequency.

d Vomiting usually precedes the pain in appendicitis.

e Appendicitis can present with RUQ pain.

4 Regarding the signs associated with appendicitis, which of the following are true and which are false?

a In uncomplicated appendicitis the vital signs are mostly significantly changed.

b Rovsing's sign is the demonstration of pain upon flexion and internal rotation of the right hip.

c Point of maximal tenderness is over McBurney's point.

d Alvarado's score is a 9-point scoring system to assist the diagnosis of appendicitis.

e A positive right psoas sign suggests that the inflamed appendix is located under the liver.

5 Which of the following investigations are useful for appendicitis?
a AXR.
b Urinalysis.
c Inflammatory markers.
d USS is the most sensitive and specific imaging modality.
e CT abdomen.

6 Regarding the treatment of appendicitis, which of the following are true and which are false?
a One should withhold analgesia to prevent masking of symptoms and signs.
b Perioperative antibiotics help reduce faecal leak rates.
c Treatment with antibiotics can lead to spontaneous resolution.
d Delay in treatment results in a higher risk of morbidity and mortality.
e The operation is always a laparoscopic procedure.

7 Regarding the complications of appendicitis, which of the following are true and which are false?
a Appendicectomy is a safe procedure with a low mortality rate.
b Wound infection risk is highest in simple appendicitis.
c A pelvic abscess may be treated with high-dose intravenous antibiotics.
d Risk of perforation is higher only in the young patient.
e There is no risk of stump appendicitis.

Small bowel obstruction (Answers, see p. 278)

1 Which of the following are causes of small bowel obstruction?
a Hiatal hernia.
b Adhesions.
c Large abscesses.
d Irritable bowel syndrome.
e Intussusception.

2 Which of the following should be considered in the differential diagnosis of small bowel obstruction?
a Gastroenteritis.
b Pancreatitis.
c Acute appendicitis.
d DKA.
e Endometriosis.

3 Which of the following are investigations for small bowel obstruction?
a Barium enema.
b CT abdomen and pelvis.
c MRA.

d USS.

e AXR.

4 Which of the following are complications of small bowel obstruction?

a Intra-abdominal abscess.

b Wound dehiscence.

c Pulmonary oedema.

d Cerebrovascular accident.

e Short bowel syndrome.

Meckel's diverticulum (Answers, see p. 279)

1 Regarding Meckel's diverticulum, which of the following are true and which are false?

a It is present at the duodenojejunal flexure.

b It is present at the mesenteric border of the small bowel.

c It may contain heterotopic gastric, pancreatic or duodenal tissue.

d Consists of all intestinal layers.

e It is thought to be 10 cm in length.

2 Regarding the presentation of Meckel's diverticulum, which of the following are true and which are false?

a All are symptomatic.

b Children may present with bleeding per rectum.

c May include intestinal obstruction.

d May present as intussusception.

e May present like acute appendicitis.

3 Regarding the management of Meckel's diverticulum, which of the following are true and which are false?

a Can always be diagnosed with technetium-labelled red cell scan.

b Erect CXR can be helpful in the presence of perforated Meckel's diverticulum.

c Meckel's diverticulitis should be resected surgically.

d An inflamed diverticulum found during appendicectomy should be left alone.

e Acute Meckel's diverticulitis may be an intraoperative diagnosis.

4 Which of the following are indications for surgical resection of Meckel's diverticulum?

a Umbilico-ileal fistulae.

b Ileus.

c Intestinal obstruction.

d Haemorrhage.

e Asymptomatic healthy diverticula.

5 A 50-year-old fit and healthy man was admitted to the general surgical ward with generalized abdominal pain associated with feeling very unwell. His observations indicate sepsis and on examination there was localized peritonism over the right side of his abdomen. What is your management?

a Follow the ABCDE sequence to resuscitate the patient.

b CT abdomen and pelvis.
c Plain erect AXR.
d Take the patient to theatre for a laparotomy.
e Observe the patient overnight.

6 A 29-year-old woman presents with right-sided abdominal pain associated with nausea and vomiting. There is abdominal guarding and rebound tenderness. What is the most appropriate management?
a Pregnancy test.
b Urgent blood tests.
c Book an exploratory laparoscopy.
d AXR.
e Urgent CT scan.

EMQs (Answers, see p. 280)

1 Options:
    a Appendiceal mucocele.
    b Gangrenous appendix.
    c Perforated appendix.
    d Pelvic abscess.
    e Sepsis.
    f Ileus.
    g Carcinoma of the appendix.
    h Wound infection.
For each case below choose the single most likely diagnosis from the list above. Each option may be used once, more than once or not at all.

  (i) A 24-year-old woman has presented with urinary frequency and swinging fever 1 week after laparoscopic appendicectomy.
 (ii) A 19-year-old man presents with fever and tenesmus, 10 days after open appendicectomy.
(iii) A 29-year-old woman presents with a 4-day history of increasing right-sided abdominal pain associated with fever, nausea and anorexia. There is guarding and rebound tenderness over her lower abdomen associated with tachycardia and hypotension. Blood tests reveal neutrophilia and raised CRP.
 (iv) A 54-year-old man has developed nausea and projectile vomiting 3 days after appendicectomy.
  (v) A 20-year-old woman has had right-sided abdominal pains for 5 days. At exploratory laparoscopy, there is an enlarged appendix with black patches.

2 Options:
    a Laparotomy.
    b Laparoscopy.
    c Conservative.
    d CT-guided drainage.

e Barium meal.

f Laparostomy.

For each case below suggest the most appropriate management from the above list of options. Each option may be used once, more than once or not at all.

  (i) A 60-year-old man has had a right hemicolectomy for malignancy 36 hours ago. He is now complaining of generalized abdominal bloating and pain associated with nausea and vomiting. His AXR reveals dilated small bowel loops and his potassium levels are very low.

 (ii) An overweight 49-year-old woman presents with a 2-day history of severe abdominal pain. On examination, there is a large paraumbilical hernia (10 × 10 cm) which is tender and tense, with bowel sounds heard on auscultation. The skin overlying the paraumbilical hernia is red and hot.

(iii) A 61-year-old man had a laparotomy for gallstone ileus 2 weeks ago. He now presents with sepsis associated with vague abdominal discomfort. There is one large pelvic collection.

12   Colorectal

Diverticular disease

D :   There are terms and definitions:
- Diverticulosis: presence of diverticulae in colon without inflammation.
- Diverticular disease: presence of symptomatic diverticulae.
- Diverticulitis: colon with inflamed and infected diverticulae.

I & S :   Equal gender predisposition; one in two adults by the time they reach 60 years. Most elderly have diverticulae by 85 years of age.

A & P :   Perhaps resulting from lack of fibre in diet, hypertrophy of colonic muscle to overcome small stool volumes causes high pressure within lumen, with mucosa being pushed out next to weak points in colonic wall (where arteries perforate the circular muscle layer).

C F & D :   Majority (75%) asymptomatic. Often present as intermittent ache and tenderness in the left iliac fossa. One-quarter of all diverticulae are associated with inflammation that is often suppurative. Complications are abscess, phlegmon, perforation (often the presenting feature of previously unsuspected diverticular disease) bleeding, fistula and stricture.

Differential diagnosis

- Infectious colitis
- IBD
- Malignancy
- Ischaemic colitis, other causes of hollow viscus perforation

---

Investigations

- Routine bloods to confirm inflammatory process and to ensure adequate blood counts
- Plain X-ray to exclude perforation
- CT scan to stage the extent of inflammation (Hinchey scoring system)

Hinchey scoring of severity of acute diverticulitis

Grade 1   diverticulitis with phlegmon (1a)/pericolic or mesenteric abscess (1b)
Grade 2   diverticulitis with walled-off pelvic abscess
Grade 3   diverticulitis with generalized purulent peritonitis
Grade 4   diverticulitis with generalized faecal peritonitis

EMQs and MCQs for Surgical Finals, 1st edition.   © Hye-Chung Kwak, Imran Bhatti, Jaskarn Rai, Farhan Rashid, Bachittar Singh Jassar, Murthy Nyasavajjala, Viren Asher, Jon Lund and Mike Larvin. Published 2011 by Blackwell Publishing Ltd.

T & M : Most uncomplicated acute episodes are treated conservatively with antibiotics. Surgical option increasingly discouraged. Acute indications for surgery include overwhelming sepsis from extensive abscess/phlegmon, bleeding that cannot be controlled by less invasive methods. Abscesses can be adequately treated by percutaneous drainage. Lararoscopic washout has been shown to be beneficial in trials. Most common indications for elective surgery include chronic symptoms of pain with recurrent flare-ups, stricture causing obstruction and colovesical/colovaginal fistulae.

Hartmann's procedure

This is often an emergency procedure. Left-sided colonic resection is performed, the rectum closed, and the proximal colon brought to the skin as an end stoma.

P : Lifestyle and dietary advice with regular laxatives and stool softeners.

Colorectal cancer

D : Most common gastrointestinal cancer; around 37 500 new cases every year in the UK alone (100 every day).

I & S : Third most prevalent cancer in UK. Risk increases with age, peaking at 70 years of age (*Source*: Office of National Statistics).

A & P :

Risk factors

- Sedentary lifestyle
- Diet, obesity
- Family history of CRC
- Ulcerative colitis
- Hereditary syndromes (e.g. FAP, HNPCC)
- Juvenile polyposes

Polyps occur universally in FAP, but FAP accounts for only 1% of CRCs. The adenoma–carcinoma sequence proposed by Vogelstein and Kinzler states that CRCs arise from a series of histopathological and molecular changes that transform normal epithelial cells into dysplastic cells. Intermediate next step is the adenomatous polyp, dysplastic cells that do not breach the basement membrane. The majority of CRCs arise as adenomas and progress to carcinoma. Adenomatous polyps are common in general population (33% at age 50, 70% at age 70).

Diagnosis of HNPCC using Amsterdam criteria II

- Three or more family members with HNPCC-related cancers, one of whom is a first-degree relative of the other two.
- Two successive affected generations.

> • One or more of the HNPCC-related cancers diagnosed under age 50 years.
> • FAP has been excluded.
> • Two cases of colorectal cancer where families are small (one aged under 55).
> • Two cases of colorectal cancer and one case of endometrial cancer, other early-onset cancer.

CF&D:

- General examination of the patient: anaemia, weight loss.
- Abdominal examination: mass.
- DRE: manual palpation of the polyp/ulcer.
- Faecal occult blood test: screening tool, but not useful in diagnosis of an individual patient outside a screening programme.
- Sigmoidoscopy and colonoscopy: for complete visualization, identify potential synchronous lesions, tissue biopsy. Sigmoidoscopy with rigid or flexible scope.
- Double-contrast barium enema using air and barium contrast: good at identifying luminal and circumferential lesions. May miss up to 10% of significant lesions.
- CT pneumocolon: used in patients not fit for colonoscopy or where colonoscopy has technical difficulties.
- Staging CT scan: for staging and for determining status of metastases.
- MRI: preferred for rectal cancer along with CT scan staging.
- PET: used in detecting metastases/local recurrence of cancer.

Up to one-third of all colorectal cancers present as emergencies.

Right-sided lesions

- Iron-deficiency anaemia
- Abdominal pain
- Mass lesion
- Change in bowel habit
- Significant weight loss
- Rectal bleeding

Left-sided lesions

- Abdominal pain
- Abdominal mass
- Change in bowel habit
- Obstruction

Common constitutional symptoms include weight loss, loss of appetite, night sweats and fever. All tend to be late symptoms and signs.

Staging

Multiple systems are used to describe the tumour. However, national guidelines require minimum dataset comprising AJCC and Dukes classifications.

Dukes classification

A	Invasion into but not through the bowel wall
B	Invasion through the bowel wall but not involving lymph nodes
C1	Lymph node involvement, apical node not involved
C2	Lymph node involvement, apical node involved
D	Widespread metastases

AJCC (TNM) classification

Tis	Tumour confined to mucosa; cancer *in situ*
T1	Tumour invades submucosa
T2	Tumour invades muscularis propria
T3	Tumour invades subserosa or beyond (without other organs involved)
T4	Tumour invades adjacent organs or perforates the visceral peritoneum
N1	Metastasis to one to three regional lymph nodes
N2	Metastasis to four or more regional lymph nodes
M0	No distant spread seen
M1	Distant metastases present. Any T, any N

Stage grouping

0	Tis, N0, M0
I	T1, N0, M0 or T2, N0, M0
II-A	
II-B	
III-A	
III-B	
III-C	T N2 M0
IV	any T, any N, M1

P: More than 20 000 deaths annually from CRC. Patients with early-stage CRC have better prognosis than those who present with more advanced disease. Overall, 50% 5-year survival.

Dukes cancer staging: 5-year survival (*Source*: Cancer Research UK)

- Dukes A: 93%
- Dukes B: 77%
- Dukes C: 48%
- Dukes D: 6.6%

Inflammatory bowel disease

There are two main types: ulcerative colitis (UC) and Crohn's disease (CD).

Ulcerative colitis

D: Chronic inflammatory and ulcerative disease largely affecting colon and rectum.
I & S: Affects ≈ 120 000 people in the UK. Usually presents before 30 years of age, with another peak at 50–60 years of age.

A & P : Exact aetiology unknown. Mucosal and submucosal lesions normally begin in the rectum and spread proximally in a continuous pattern.

C F & D : Majority of the patients present with rectal bleeding associated with mucus, diarrhoea, urgency and frequency. Severe cases present with toxic features like fever, SIRS and rarely peritonitis. UC may display extraintestinal manifestations such as peripheral arthritis, episcleritis, aphthous stomatitis, erythema nodosum, pyoderma gangrenosum, ankylosing spondylitis and primary sclerosing cholangitis. Only the last does not resolve with improvement of the underlying UC.

Risk of developing colon cancer is dependent on length of symptoms, roughly around 7–8% per 10 years. It correlates with disease proximal to the splenic flexure and severity of the first attack in addition to duration of disease. Surveillance with biopsy should be employed for patients with long-standing disease.

Toxic/fulminant UC: the term 'toxic megacolon' is increasingly discouraged because all the 'toxic' features may be present without signs of colonic dilatation or impending perforation. This condition is normally refractory to usual escalating medical management. This condition is managed like any other surgical emergency using the ABC approach. Supportive management and detailed blood picture (FBC, U&E, clotting profile, G&S) should be initiated while arranging for further tests. Usually, endoscopy is avoided during an acute toxic episode and a surgical option is considered.

Routine bloods are not usually confirmatory but do contribute to management of a patient with UC. Definitive diagnosis is visualization of the area by endoscopy in non-acute situations and by taking a tissue biopsy that is examined under microscope (pathological diagnosis).

T & M : Medical treatment is administered to induce remission of the disease. Commonly used drugs include an escalating protocol comprising 5-ASA, corticosteroids, azathioprine/6-mercaptopurine, infliximab and ciclosporin. In addition, metronidazole is added to the treatment to reduce effects of superadded infections. Once the symptoms are controlled, remission is maintained using 5-ASA, tapering doses of corticosteroids, and azathioprine.

> A surgical option is indicated for steriod dependence, fulminant disease, haemorrhage and perforation. Proctocolectomy is curative. Reconstruction by ileoanal pouch is often performed.

Crohn's disease

D : A chronic inflammatory condition involving the full thickness of bowel (transmural) that can affect any part of the digestive tract, from mouth to anus.

I & S : Approximately 7 per 100000 per year in the UK, mostly diagnosed between ages 16 and 30 years. Slightly more women affected than men.

A & P : Most common site affected is distal ileum. Macroscopic features include bowel wall thickening and mesenteric fat wrapping of the affected part of the bowel, hence fistulation, stenosis and mesenteric abscess formation are typical of CD.

C F & D : CD presents as chronic diarrhoea associated with abdominal pain and lethargy. Presentation may also be with signs of bowel obstruction, fistulae and abscesses. Perianal complications are not uncommon (fistula and fissure).

CD is diagnosed by endoscopy and tissue biopsy. Barium studies, MRI of the small bowel and enteroscopy are some of the other diagnostic tools available.

T&M: Escalating treatments for CD are similar to those for UC, often only difficult to induce remission and maintain it. More than 60–70% of patients diagnosed with CD need surgical intervention for symptom relief or curative intent to improve quality of life.

P: Younger patients diagnosed with CD have worse prognosis than those diagnosed later in life. Overall life expectancy of CD patients is less than that of general population.

Lower gastrointestinal bleeding

D: Bleeding beyond ligament of Treitz. Often source unknown at presentation; around 15–20% are upper GI, small bowel causes.

I&S: Total incidence is unknown. Occurs most often in the elderly.

A&P: Depends on the cause:
- Diverticulitis/diverticular disease: bleed from vasa rectae in the submucosa
- Anorectal pathology
- Colitis
- Neoplastic lesions
- Ischaemia
- Meckel's diverticulum
- Angiodysplasia
- Aortoenteric fistula
- Medical causes (e.g. coagulopathy).

CF&D: Acute GI bleeding is an emergency. Presentation varies with severity of bleed. There may be malaena or bright red blood per rectum +/– abdominal pain +/– hypotension, tachycardia +/– diarrhoea. A thorough history (previous bleed and risk factors of upper GI bleeding) and examination (ensure it is bleeding per rectum by a DRE) is required to assess the origin and severity of bleed.

Investigations

- FBC, U&E, clotting screen, cross-match.
- Upper GI endoscopy to exclude upper GI bleed if patient unstable with ongoing active bleeding
- Colonoscopy (after bowel preparation in a patient where bleeding not settled after admission)
- CTA
- Mesenteric angiogram and selective embolization

T&M: ABCDE approach. Actively resuscitate using two large IV cannulas in the antecubital fossa and IV fluids; correct obvious haematological and clotting dysfunction. Often self-limiting (>95%) if all obvious haematological dysfunction corrected.

P: Precise localization of bleed is the key to treatment of a massive bleed. Acute resuscitative management may often be followed by a definitive management plan that needs a structured, systematic and detailed series of investigations.

> **Definitions**
>
> • *Haematochezia*: fresh/altered blood mixed with stool resulting in maroon-coloured stool (in brisk upper GI bleed or lower GI bleed).
> • *Melaena*: digested dark tarry black stool (upper GI bleed).

Haemorrhoids

D : Haemorrhoids are clusters of vascular and adventitious tissue in the anus, lined by normal anal epithelium. They are classified as follows:

• Internal haemorrhoids: haemorrhoids occurring above dentate line. Three primary sites at 3, 7 and 11 o'clock positions. They are in the insensate area of the anus, hence are rarely painful.

• External haemorrhoids: haemorrhoids occurring below dentate line, in the sensate area and hence often painful when engorged.

I & S : Up to one-third of all humans have some extent of haemorrhoids at some point in their lives. M = F. Most commonly treated in 40–60 year olds.

A & P : Exact aetiology is not clear, but increased incidence in patients with IBD and pregnancy. Small quantities of low-fibre stools have been associated with haemorrhoids (straining and chronic constipation).

> **Grading of internal haemorrhoids**
>
> Stage I   Do not prolapse
> Stage II   Prolapse with straining but return spontaneously
> Stage III Bleed and prolapse with straining and need manual effort for returning to anus
> Stage IV   Prolapse and stay outside, cannot be reduced manually

C F & D : Rectal bleeding associated with bowel movements, perianal itching, rectal lump/mass are common presentations of internal haemorrhoids. Perianal spasms, pain and irreducible tender rectal lump are features of strangulated or thrombosed haemorrhoids.

> **Differential diagnosis**
>
> • Perianal abscess
> • Fistula in ano, pruritus ani
> • Condylomata accuminatum
> • Viral or bacterial dermatitis

Haemorrhoids is often a diagnosis of exclusion, after detailed colonoscopy or barium enema or other investigations for rectal bleeding.

• Check for anaemia
• External haemorrhoids: seen on examination
• Internal haemorrhoids: proctoscopy.

T & M : Treatment depends on grade of haemorrhoids (prolapse). Medical management of haemorrhoids (laxatives and stool softeners) is the main approach for early haemorrhoids. Surgery for haemorrhoids is tailored to individual patient needs and extent of disease.

Surgery for haemorrhoids

For early grades
- Simple sclerotherapy
- Electrocoagulation/cryocoagulation
- Submucosal injection is often choice of treatment

For more progressed stages
- Simple measures like rubber-band ligation
- Formal haemorrhoidectomy (conventional or stapled) may be necessary

---

P : Complications and recurrence rates are often quoted at 5–8% even in the best centres.

Fissure in ano

D : Fissure in ano (anal fissure) is a breach in the lining of the anal canal distal to the dentate line. Most cases of fissure in ano are posterior (90%).

I & S : They are more common in women than men, aged 20–60 years, major preponderance in fertile women, particularly post partum. Other causes include anal trauma, abscesses, infections and rarely CD.

A & P : The precise aetiology is unknown, but ischaemia of the area involved in the process causes fissures. Contrary to popular belief, constipation and hard stools are only associated with fissures and only rarely a cause of fissures. It is hallmarked by three distinct features:
- enlarged anal papilla
- ulcer in the anal epithelium with induration
- sentinel pile/skin tag.

Anal fissures lasting longer than 6 weeks are termed chronic fissures.

C F & D : **Pain in ano often associated with defecation; painful rectal bleeding and pruritus ano are common presentations of fissures**. Diagnosis by history and detailed examination. Clinical examination should be thorough, sometimes needing EUA.

T & M : Medical management includes dietary advice, laxatives/stool softeners, analgesia, glycerine cream/calcium-channel blocker cream. Botulinum toxin injection helps in reversible surgical intervention, while more elaborate surgery is by lateral sphincterotomy with fissurectomy.

P : Anal fissures need to be followed up for the fear of continence (up to 5%).

Fistula in ano

D : A fistula is an abnormal connection between two epithelial surfaces. In fistula in ano, this abnormal connection is usually between anal canal and perineum.

I & S : Fistulae are more common in men than women (M/F ratio 2 : 1). They affect 20–50 year olds.

A & P : Cryptogenic abscess theory states that up to 30% of all perianal abscesses eventually give rise to fistulae. Other causes include chronic anorectal infections, CD, foreign bodies, diverticulitis and immunocompromise.

C F & D : Soiling of clothes, discharge (malodorous), difficulty in maintaining hygiene and pruritus are some of the common clinical presentations of anal fistulae. Extensive fistulae cause systemic illness.

Diagnosis of fistula in ano is by meticulous history and detailed examination. In complex cases, fistulogram/endorectal USS or MRI scan of pelvis and pelvic floor are useful adjuncts.

T & M : Depending on anatomy of fistula in relation to anal sphincter, they are classified as follows:

- Subsphincteric: below external anal sphincter.
- Trans-sphincteric : through the external sphincter.
- Intersphincteric: through superficial and deep components of external sphincter.
- Extrasphincteric: extending over and above the anal sphincter complex.

It is important to determine the type of fistula as management strategy differs for each of these fistulae.

- Simple fistulae can be managed with a fistulotomy (fistula is laid open over a probe) or fistulectomy (fistula tract is excised). Sometimes a seton stitch is used to help drain sepsis in long-standing fistulae.
- Complex fistulae need more extensive surgical management with repeat procedures to treat fistulae.

The main aim of acute treatment of any fistula is to treat the sepsis. A typical fistula treatment is easily remembered using the mnemonic SNAP.

S	Treat sepsis: antibiotics and surgical drainage
N	Nutrition
A	Determine anatomy
P	Perform the definitive procedure

P : Good outcome with treatment. Recurrence more likely in those with IBD.

Goodsall's rule of fistulae

- If the external opening of the fistula is anterior to an imaginary transverse line across the anus, the fistula tract is a straight line opening into the anal canal.
- If the anterior fistulae are more than 3 cm anterior to the line, the tract will curve posteriorly, terminating in the posterior midline.
- The tract of the posterior fistula will curve with its opening in the posterior wall of the anal canal.

MCQs

Diverticular disease (Answers, see p. 281)

1 A 76-year-old woman presents to A&E with left iliac fossa pain and temperature of 38.1°C. She has a long-standing history of constipation, requiring her to use laxatives daily. On examination, she was tender in her left iliac fossa with no guarding or rigidity. What should be the immediate management of this patient?
a Flexible sigmoidoscopy and biopsies.
b Active fluid resuscitation and analgesia.
c Emergency CT scan.
d Surgical exploration and bowel resection.
e Barium enema investigation.

2 A 68-year-old man was referred to the surgical clinic with recurrent general abdominal pain and passing of hard stools. He was found to have numerous diverticulae all over his colon at colonoscopy and no other anomalies. Other underlying causes of constipation had been excluded. What should be the further management of this patient?
a Follow-up colonoscopy every 2 years.
b Dietary and lifestyle advice.
c Parenteral nutrition.
d Referral for surgical resection.
e CT scan every year.

3 A 55-year-old man with known diverticular disease presents to the acute surgical admissions ward with tender abdomen and abdominal pain on deep inspiration and coughing. On examination, he had rebound tenderness in his left iliac fossa with guarding. He was actively fluid resuscitated and administered intravenous antibiotics. What would be the best modality for investigating this patient further?
a T1-weighted MRI of pelvis.
b Technetium-99 scan.
c CT abdomen and pelvis.
d Emergency barium enema.
e USS abdomen.

4 A 75-year-old otherwise fit woman was found to have a pelvic collection due to extensive sigmoid diverticular inflammation. She continues to require increasing organ system support. She was taken to theatre for surgery, which requires which of the following procedures?
a Ileostomy and segmental resection.
b Sigmoid colectomy and Hartmann's procedure.
c Sigmoid colectomy and end-to-end anastamosis.
d Abdomino-perineal excision of rectum.
e Total colectomy.

5 Which of the following are symptoms and signs of diverticulitis?
a Right lower quadrant pain.
b Hunger.

c Tachycardia.
d Abdominal mass.
e Rectal bleeding.

6 Which of the following are complications of diverticulitis?
a Fistula.
b Perforation.
c Pelvic abscess.
d Stricture.
e Obstruction.

Colorectal cancer (Answers, see p. 281)

1 A 68-year-old man was referred to colorectal clinic by his GP, who suspects colorectal cancer. He presents with a 6-week history of painless rectal bleeding and diarrhoea. Which of the following investigations would you arrange?
a Stool culture and faecal occult blood test.
b Colonoscopy.
c CT scan of abdomen and pelvis.
d PET scan.
e MRI pelvis.

2 A 75-year-old woman had rigid sigmoidoscopy and was found to have a circumferential tumour at 9 cm from the anal verge. Biopsies of this mass confirm it to be a rectal cancer. MRI of pelvis has confirmed radiologically T3 disease with obvious N1 nodal spread. This patient's further options would include which of the following?
a Multidisciplinary team discussion, neoadjuvant chemoradiotherapy, surgery.
b Multidisciplinary team discussion, surgical resection.
c Endomucosal resection of the tumour and watchful waiting.
d Surgical resection and adjuvant chemotherapy.
e Staging laparoscopy.

3 A 19-year-old woman suspects that due to a strongly positive family history she might have Lynch syndrome (HNPCC). Which of the following criteria would exclude HNPCC?
a Three first-degree relatives with colon cancer aged less than 50.
b Family history of FAP.
c Family history of ovarian and gastric cancer aged less than 50.
d Father and sister with colon cancer, brother with villous adenomata.
e Strong family history of renal cancer.

4 A GP receives a letter about his 75-year-old patient stating that he has had an anterior resection with primary anastamosis without stoma formation Based on the information available which of the following parts of the colon have been removed?
a Lower rectum and anal sphincter.
b Ascending colon and hepatic flexure.

c Rectosigmoid.
d Splenic flexure and descending colon.
e The whole colon and rectum.

5 Which of the following are the symptoms and signs of colorectal cancer?
a Constipation.
b Rectal bleeding.
c Weight loss.
d Anaemia.
e Perianal abscess.

6 Which of the following are risk factors for colorectal cancer?
a Old age.
b IBD.
c Colonic lipomas.
d FAP.
e Lynch syndrome.

IBD (Answers, see p. 282)

1 A 53-year-old man was diagnosed with ulcerative colitis from a biopsy at colonoscopy. He has mild symptoms that require the induction and maintenance of remission. This is best done by using which of the following first-line drugs?
a Mesalazine.
b Prednisolone.
c 5-ASA.
d Metronidazole.
e Methotrexate.

2 A 24-year-old woman recently had flexible sigmoidoscopy for lower GI bleeding and altered bowel habit and was diagnosed as having colonic Crohn's disease. Which of the following statements best describes her condition?
a Continuous lesions all over rectosigmoid is common.
b Pancolitis with crypt abscesses.
c She has a better prognosis than a newly diagnosed 60-year-old man.
d Should always be treated by excising the inflamed part of the bowel.
e Inflammation is confined to the distal duodenum.

3 A 40-year-old man was found to have large ulcerated areas that were biopsied from his rectosigmoid during an elective colonoscopy. He had diarrhoea, which settled with a 2-week course of 5-ASA. Which of the following statements best describes his clinical condition?
a He has an increased risk of developing colorectal cancer.
b His remission should always be maintained with steroids.
c He will need surgery to remove the ulcerated areas.
d His ulcerations will benefit from routine use of antibiotics.
e He needs a modified diet.

4 A 25-year-old man presented with change in bowel habit and abdominal pain. He has been diagnosed with a mild form of ulcerative colitis. With regard to the pathology of ulcerative colitis, which of the following is true?
a It shows full-thickness inflammation.
b The rectum is almost always spared.
c Enterocutaneous or intestinal fistulae are common.
d The serosa is usually normal.
e Fissuring ulcers are usually present.

5 A very unwell 32-year-old woman has pneumaturia and anterior wall fistula secondary to a 10-year history of Crohn's disease. Further management of this patient would include which of the following?
a Antibiotics, total parenteral nutrition, abdominal CT scan.
b USS of abdomen, nasogastric feeding, steroids.
c Regular diet, plain AXR, analgesia.
d Immediate surgical excision and ileostomy.
e Antispasmodics and analgesia.

6 With regard to ulcerative colitis, which of the following are true and which are false?
a Ulcerative colitis is a disease confined exclusively to the colon.
b Crohn's disease often involves left side of the colon.
c Gross rectal bleeding is a regular feature of ulcerative colitis.
d Perianal lesions differentiate Crohn's disease from ulcerative colitis.
e Asymmetric bowel involvement and skip lesions are characteristic of Crohn's disease.
f Crohn's disease lesions are well-demarcated ulcers with distinctive edges.
g Transmural fissuring and pancolitis are hallmarks of Crohn's disease.
h Transmural inflammation of ulcerative colitis depicts severity of disease.
i Masses and abscess in the abdomen are common with ulcerative colitis.
j Lymphoid granulomas are typical in Crohn's disease.

7 Which of the following is the most appropriate procedure for a patient with uncontrolled UC?
a Hartmann's procedure.
b Abdomino-perineal resection.
c Loop colostomy.
d Panproctocolectomy and end ileostomy.
e Loop ilestomy.

8 Panproctocolectomy is used for patients with which of the following conditions?
a Crohn's disease.
b Familial polyposis.
c Diverticular disease.
d Colorectal cancer.
e Ulcerative colitis.

9 Concerning stomas, which of the following are true and which are false?
a Right-sided stoma is invariably an ileostomy.
b A loop ileostomy is temporary.

c Ileostomy rarely has a spout.

d A stoma is performed to protect a proximal anastomosis.

e Hartmann's procedure is resection of colon with formation of ileostomy.

Lower gastrointestinal bleeding (Answers, see p. 283)

1 A 68-year-old man presents with a 3-week history of rectal bleeding mixed with stool, increased frequency of defecation and nausea. On examination, his rectum showed significant mucosal telangiectasia. He received radiotherapy for prostate cancer 2 years ago. Which of the following is the likely diagnosis of his condition?

a Diverticulitis.

b Radiation proctitis.

c Rectal carcinoma.

d Ischaemic colitis.

e Infective colitis.

2 An 83-year-old man presented to A&E with redcurrant jelly-like rectal bleeding and abdominal pain. He was tachycardic on arrival and needed resuscitation to maintain his blood pressure. He is currently on aspirin, clopidogrel, simvastatin, ACE inhibitors and bendroflumethiazide and uses GTN spray. Which of the following best describes his likely diagnosis?

a Rectal carcinoma.

b Ischaemic colitis.

c Infective colitis.

d Haemorrhoids.

e Intussusception.

3 A 78-year-old man presented to A&E with bright rectal bleeding and clots associated with diarrhoea. Prior to this admission, he was treated for recurrent chronic left lower quadrant pain and chronic constipation. He had low-grade fever (37.4°C) and tachycardia on arrival and was found to have an Hb of 6.8 g/ dL. Which of the following best describes his likely diagnosis?

a Crohn's disease.

b Wegener's granulomatosis.

c Diverticular abscess.

d Infective colitis.

e Diverticular bleed.

4 A 25-year-old woman has had an uneventful delivery 3 weeks ago. Since her childbirth, she has had difficulty and pain during defecation. On examination she was found to have a breach of the anal mucocutaneous junction with an indurated area around the breach and a tag distal to the breach. Which of the following best describes her likely diagnosis?

a Haemorrhoids.

b Fissure in ano.

c Fistula in ano.

d Anal warts.

e Solitary ulcer.

5 A 42-year-old man presents to his GP surgery with a 1-year history of fresh intermittent rectal bleeding. He has had no change in bowel habit or loss of weight or appetite. Which of the following best describes his likely diagnosis?
a Perianal haematoma.
b Solitary ulcer.
c Haemorrhoids.
d Fissure in ano.
e Colitis.

6 A 32-year-old man presented to his GP surgery with pruritus ani and inability to maintain hygiene after opening his bowels. On examination, he was found to have a cluster of papillomata surrounding the anal aperture. Which of the following best describes his likely diagnosis?
a Fistula in ano.
b Anal warts.
c Anal cancer.
d Perianal abscess.
e Perianal haematoma.

Haemorrhoids (Answers, see p. 284)

1 Regarding haemorrhoids, which of the following statements are true and which are false?
a Internal haemorrhoids originate above the dentate line.
b There are four major haemorrhoidal cushions.
c Haemorrhoids contain blood vessels.
d Botulinum toxin injection is a management option for haemorrhoids.
e Rectal bleeding is the commonest presenting symptom of haemorrhoids.

2 Which of the following are risk factors for haemorrhoids?
a Obesity.
b Pregnancy.
c Renal disease.
d Colonic malignancy.
e Prolonged sitting.

3 Regarding haemorrhoids, which of the following statements are true and which are false?
a Symptomatic prolapsed haemorrhoids are treated surgically.
b Haemorrhoids that prolapse with straining but which return spontaneously require haemorrhoidectomy.
c All patients presenting with rectal bleeding have haemorrhoids.
d Asymptomatic haemorrhoids do not require treatment.
e Haemorrhoids are more common in females.

4 A 30-year-old pregnant woman with a long-standing history of haemorrhoids presents to A&E with acute-onset pain in her anal canal. On examination,

there is a bluish discoloured firm tender tense lump. Further management of this patient would include which of the following options?

a Immediate haemorrhoidectomy.

b Delayed haemorrhoidectomy.

c Analgesia and stool softeners.

d Diltiazem anal cream.

e Incision and drainage under GA.

5 A 55-year-old man was referred to the surgical department by his GP for recurrent rectal bleeding. On examination, he has grade IV haemorrhoids. He has had a recent colonoscopy and barium enema which were both clear. The best treatment would include which of the following?

a Stapled haemorrhoidectomy.

b Rubber-band ligation.

c Emergency haemorrhoidectomy.

d Conservative management.

e Sclerotherapy.

6 Which of the following would help prevent haemorrhoids?

a Increase straining.

b Increase fibre in the diet.

c Exercise.

d Refrain from emptying bowels when the urge occurs.

e Keep well hydrated.

Fissure in ano (Answers, see p. 284)

1 Treatment of fissure in ano would include which of the following?

a Partial internal sphincterotomy.

b Topical calcium channel agonists.

c Nitroglycerin spray.

d Botulinum toxin injection.

e Antibiotics.

2 Which of the following are the complications of fissure in ano?

a Sentinel pile.

b Faecal impaction.

c Fistulae.

d Incontinence.

e Haemorrhoids.

3 A 23-year-old man presents to the surgical clinic with a 2-week history of painful defecation and residual bleeding on the toilet tissue. On examination, he was found to have fissure in ano. Which of the following is *not* a feature of anal fissures?

a Sentinel pile (skin tag).

b Hypertrophied anal papilla.

c Increased vascularity.

d Ulcer.

e Pain.

4 A 40-year-old man presents with a chronic anal fissure of 3 months' duration refractory to medical management. He is keen on some surgical intervention for this. Which of the following options is *not* part of modern surgical practice?
a Digital anal stretch.
b Anal botulinum injection.
c Internal sphincterotomy.
d Fissurectomy.
e Colostomy.

5 A woman presents with perineal discomfort. On examination, there is tenderness on posterior aspect of her anal canal. The pathological condition she has is likely a result of which of the following?
a Increased vascularity to anal mucosa.
b Ischaemia of lining of anal canal.
c Cervical effacement during labour.
d Chronic constipation.
e Chronic diarrhoea.

6 A 16-year-old boy with a history of chronic anal ulcer for 4 months is seen in the surgical clinic. On examination there are two ulcers at the 4 and 7 o'clock positions with inflamed surrounding skin and a right lateral fistula opening into his right buttock. The surgeon treating him takes a biopsy of the tissue under anaesthetic. Which of the following is the likely diagnosis?
a Bowen's disease.
b Anal cancer.
c Crohn's disease.
d Ulcerative colitis.
e Diverticulitis.

Fistula in ano (Answers, see p. 285)

1 Which of the following conditions is *not* associated with fistula in ano?
a Diverticulitis.
b Crohn's disease.
c Pelvic inflammatory disease.
d Diabetes.
e Irritable bowel syndrome.

2 Which of the following are the presentations of fistula in ano?
a Rectal pain.
b Mucoid discharge.
c Pruritis.
d Rectal bleeding.
e Early satiety.

3 Which of the following are the treatments for fistula in ano?
a Seton.
b Fistulectomy.
c Sphincterotomy.

d Fistulotomy.

e Fibrin glue.

4 A 35-year-old man with known Crohn's disease presents to the acute surgery department with a perianal fistula pouring copious amounts of pus on expression. The next appropriate surgical option for this patient would include which of the following?

a Incision and drainage of perianal abscess.

b MRI scan of pelvis.

c Total parenteral nutrition with ileostomy.

d IV antibiotics and expectant management.

e Fistulotomy.

5 A 17-year-old college student has had a perianal abscess that drained itself spontaneously 6 weeks ago. He has a residual tender area with a small induration that seeps clear fluid when expressed. His further surgical management would include which of the following?

a Immediate CT abdomen and pelvis.

b EUA and fistulotomy.

c MRI pelvis and fistulogram.

d Defunctioning ileostomy with flap reconstruction of the floor.

e Repeat incision and drainage.

6 Regarding fistula in ano, which of the following statements are true and which are false?

a A trans-sphincteric fistula is more difficult to treat than a subsphincteric fistula.

b While applying seton suture, the patient needs to be informed about incontinence.

c All anal fistulae need parenteral nutrition to help healing.

d According to Goodsall's rule, anterior fistulae are complex to treat.

e All patients with perianal abscess should be warned of the possibility of fistula prior to surgical drainage.

13 Nutrition in surgical patients

D: The provision of fuel substances to maintain life.

I & S: In the UK 2 million people are affected by malnutrition and up to 40% of inpatients are malnourished. Those left NBM for greater than 72 hours and critically ill surgical patients who generally have impaired utilization of fuel substrates will need special attention.

Sources of energy	Energy content	Recommended daily intake
Carbohydrates	4 kcal/g	Minimum 47% total daily calories
Amino acids	4 kcal/g	0.6–0.75 g/kg daily
Lipids	4 kcal/g	11% total daily intake

A & P: Patients at risk are those who have chronic diseases (e.g. IBD) and the elderly population. These fuels are regulated by insulin and glucagon.

C F & D: Assess the history and overall appearance of the patient including dentition, and mucosa for hydration. When you ask the patient to be NBM, the following should be considered.

	Liver	Muscle	Fat
12 hours	Glycogenolysis provides glucose	Glycogen converted to lactate Protein breakdown to amino acids Both transported to the liver and converted to glucose	Lipolysis, to provide energy to muscle tissue
48 hours	Gluconeogenesis from amino acids	Each day, 75 g protein broken down to amino acids for conversion to glucose	Start of glycerol and triglyceride use, fatty acids become main fuel for tissues
Prolonged fasting	Ketogenesis from fatty acids	Reduced protein breakdown as ketones are used as fuel	

EMQs and MCQs for Surgical Finals, 1st edition. © Hye-Chung Kwak, Imran Bhatti, Jaskarn Rai, Farhan Rashid, Bachittar Singh Jassar, Murthy Nyasavajjala, Viren Asher, Jon Lund and Mike Larvin. Published 2011 by Blackwell Publishing Ltd.

Nutritional status and requirements should be assessed in all patients depending on age, sex, weight, activity and presence of disease, and referred to the dieticians for review.

T & M : Methods of feeding are described below.

Route	Description		Provides
Enteral	Oral *In patients unable to maintain adequate oral intake*	Preferred method	Calories, nitrogen, essential fluids, vitamins, minerals, trace elements
	NGT/NJT	Nutritional support for up to 6 weeks	
	PEG/RIG	Long-term feeding in patients with upper GI obstruction	
	Percutaneous jejunostomy	Patients with GOO, recurrent aspirations, pancreatic disease	
Parenteral	TPN through large vein	Concentrated hypertonic nutrient solution. For patients unable to absorb from GIT for >10 days. Supplement for patients with high caloric and nutritional needs *Advantages*: bypasses the gut, reduces activity in gallbladder, pancreas and small bowel *Disadvantages*: morbidity from line sepsis	Can tailor the diet/feed/formula according to patient needs

Patients also require fluids. The daily fluid requirement for a healthy individual is 2–2.5 L.

Electrolyte	RDI	
Sodium	100 mmol (2 mg/kg daily)	Consider GI losses, insensible losses from wounds, third space losses (up to 20 L due to increased capillary permeability, hypoalbuminaemia and impaired renal homeostasis). Adults should get 30 mL/kg daily of fluids
Potassium	60 mmol (1 mg/kg daily)	
Magnesium	300–350 mg/day	
Calcium	800–1200 mg/day	
Phosphorus	800–1200 mg/day	

> **P:** Improving nutrition before and after surgery enhances recovery and results in shorter hospital stays.

MCQs (Answers, see p. 286)

1 Regarding electrolytes, which of the following are true and which are false?
 a Hypophosphataemia is associated with muscular weakness.
 b Hypomagnesaemia can lead to tetany.
 c Hypokalaemia leads to myocardial infarction and death.
 d Hyponatraemia leads to loss of consciousness.
 e Hypercalcaemia causes nausea and vomiting.

2 Regarding malnutrition, which of the following are true and which are false?
 a It is associated with longer hospital stays.
 b Approximately 40% of patients admitted to hospital are malnourished.
 c Is associated with inadequate diet in the UK.
 d Is associated with alcoholism.
 e Malnutrition Universal Screening Tool (MUST) is used to diagnose malnutrition.

3 Regarding TPN, which of the following are true and which are false?
 a Emergency bowel cancer surgery is the only indication for TPN.
 b TPN has limited value for well-nourished patients with a healthy GIT likely to resume normal function within 10 days.
 c TPN is indicated in a terminal oesophageal cancer patient on the Liverpool care pathway.
 d Consists of carbohydrates, lipids and proteins.
 e Reduces activity in the gallbladder, pancreas and small intestine.

4 Regarding nasogastric feeding, which of the following are true and which are false?
 a Can be commenced as soon as the NGT is inserted.
 b Is appropriate for a stroke patient.
 c The NGT is in the right place if there is acidic aspirate.
 d A large-bore Ryle's tube can be used for nasogastric feeding.
 e Requires dietetic input.

5 Which of the following are the complications of TPN?
 a Infection.
 b Electrolyte abnormalities.
 c Distended neck veins, swollen face and ipsilateral arm swelling.
 d Hypoglycaemia.
 e Hiccups.

6 Regarding refeeding syndrome, which of the following are true and which are false?

a Occurs in severely malnourished patients when you introduce high-carbohydrate feeds.

b Occurs only when feed is introduced enterally.

c Is characterized by hyperkalaemia, hypermagnesaemia and hyperphosphataemia.

d Can precipitate acute cardiac failure.

e Surgical patients kept NBM for more than 10 days are at high risk of refeeding syndrome.

EMQ (Answers, see p. 288)

1 Options:

a Oral intake.

b NGT feeding.

c Jejunostomy.

d Keep NBM.

e PEG feeding.

f TPN.

For each case below choose the single most likely form of nutrition from the list above. Each option may be used once, more than once or not at all.

(i) A chronically malnourished alcoholic man with GOO due to acute pancreatitis has been kept NBM for 8 days, and there is a need to start some sort of nutrition.

(ii) A 60-year-old woman has had a high anterior resection 2 days ago for a malignant polyp in the rectosigmoid junction.

(iii) A 45-year-old man has had a pylorus-preserving pancreaticoduodenectomy for pancreatic tumour.

(iv) A 20-year-old man who has survived a decompression craniectomy for severe head injury now has residual right-sided weakness and communication difficulties.

(v) A 34-year-old woman with Crohn's disease has been admitted with severe flare-up of her inflammatory bowel condition. She is unable to eat and drink enough to meet her nutritional needs.

14 Hernias

Overview

A hernia is a protrusion of a viscus or part of a viscus beyond its normal confines. Abdominal hernias occur at natural points of weakness (e.g. umbilicus, inguinal canal, femoral canal) but may be caused by nerve damage causing weakness (e.g. post appendicectomy). Also iatrogenic weakness (incisions) can predispose to hernia formation. These weaknesses can be exacerbated by conditions that increase intra-abdominal pressure such as ascites, chronic cough, constipation, urinary outflow obstruction and heavy lifting.

I & S : Dependent on hernia type.

Terms used to describe hernias

- *Reducible*: the hernia will easily return to the cavity where it is normally contained.
- *Irreducible/incarcerated*: it is not possible to reduce the hernia, although its contents are viable and not obstructed.
- *Sliding*: the viscus forms part of the wall of the sac.
- *Obstructed*: the bowel in the hernia becomes obstructed (the second commonest cause of SBO).
- *Strangulated*: the contents of the sac become stuck and irreducible. The blood supply to the contents is compromised causing ischaemia. Patients have symptoms of SBO and the hernia is a tender inflamed swelling.

Hernia types: inguinal versus femoral

	Direct	Indirect	Femoral
Sex	M > F	M > F	F > M
Relation to pubic tubercle	Above and lateral	Above and medial	Below and lateral
Descent into scrotum	Possible	Not possible	Not possible
Reduction	Reduce spontaneously	May not reduce spontaneously	Does not reduce spontaneously
Control (pressure over deep ring)	No	Yes	No
Risk of strangulation	Low	Higher	High

EMQs and MCQs for Surgical Finals, 1st edition.   © Hye-Chung Kwak, Imran Bhatti, Jaskarn Rai, Farhan Rashid, Bachittar Singh Jassar, Murthy Nyasavajjala, Viren Asher, Jon Lund and Mike Larvin. Published 2011 by Blackwell Publishing Ltd.

Inguinal hernia

D: Protrusion of a swelling in the groin above the pubic tubercle.

I & S: This type of hernia is very common; it is estimated that 7% of patients will develop an inguinal hernia during their lifetime. Inguinal hernias comprise 75% of all hernias and are 25 times more common in men than women. They may become apparent in two different forms: direct or indirect.

A & P:

- Indirect inguinal hernia may be congenital due to failure of obliteration of the processus vaginalis. It can also be acquired when the sac passes into the deep ring though the inguinal canal and it may occasionally emerge through the superficial ring into the scrotum.
- Direct inguinal hernia is only acquired and occurs as a result of weakness in transversalis fascia found in Hasselbach's triangle. Hasselbach's triangle is bordered medially by the lateral aspect of rectus muscle, laterally by the inferior epigastric artery and inferiorly by the inguinal ligament.

C F & D: Hernias present as a bulge in the groin which may become more prominent by coughing, straining or standing up. They are often painful and usually disappear on lying down. Diagnosis is often clinical; USS and CT may be required.

T & M: Patients may be treated conservatively or offered surgical repair, either laparoscopically or by an open method (usually a mesh technique).

P: See under femoral hernia.

Femoral hernia

D: Protrusion of a swelling in the groin below and lateral to the pubic tubercle.

I & S: The incidence is highest in middle age and in the elderly. Femoral hernias account for 3% of all hernias. M/F ratio 1 : 4.

A & P: Femoral hernias occur in the femoral canal, medial to the femoral vein, a space occupied by lymphoid tissue and fat. In older women, loss of body fat leaves a space into which bowel can protrude. Femoral hernias often present as an emergency.

C F & D: Femoral hernias are more common in frail elderly women, although they can present in children. The incidence of strangulation of the femoral hernia is high. Femoral herniation is often found to be the cause of SBO.

The obvious finding may be a lump in the groin found below and lateral to the pubic tubercle. The cough impulse is often absent and should not be relied on to make the diagnosis. The differential diagnosis includes inguinal hernia, lymph node, aneurysm of the femoral artery, saphena varix, psoas abscess.

T & M: All femoral hernias should be repaired because of the high risk of strangulation.

Repair is performed by obliterating the femoral canal with a non-absorbable suture (stitching the inguinal and pectineal ligaments together) or by placing a mesh plug in the femoral ring. With any method, care should be taken to avoid pressure on the femoral vein which would restrict increased venous return in situations of leg activity causing oedema.

P: Inguinal and femoral hernia:

The overall operative mortality for strangulated hernia is 10%. Adequate preoperative resuscitation is crucial.

Umbilical hernia

D: Umbilical hernias may occur as a congenital malformation, which is commonly seen in male infants of African descent. They may also be seen as an acquired defect in obese patients as a result of increased intra-abdominal pressure.

I & S: M/F ratio (children) 1.7 : 1, (adults) M < F. Umbilical hernias account for about 15% of hernias in women.

CF & D: When seen in children as a congenital malformation, although sometimes large these hernias tend to resolve with conservative treatment by the age of 5 years. Obstruction and strangulation are rare because the underlying abdominal defect is large. Diagnosis is usually made on clinical examination.

T & M: Acquired defects may be repaired surgically. Congenital hernias tend to resolve with time.

P: Recurrence is likely when the hernia is larger than 2.5 cm and repaired without a mesh.

Incisional hernia

D: A protrusion of a viscus when the weakness in the wall containing it is due to an incompletely healed surgical wound.

I & S: Occurs after 2–10% of abdominal surgeries and is more common in adults. M/F ratio 1 : 2.

CF & D: Patients present with swelling at the incisional site with or without pain. It is more likely to occur in a patient with jaundice or cachexia, in those taking corticosteroids or those with a chronic cough. Poor surgical technique also plays an important role. Diagnosis is made on clinical examination.

T & M: The defect with an incisional hernia is often large and the risk of strangulation is low, although their unsightly appearance encourages patients to opt for surgical repair.

P: Recurrence risk after incisional hernia repair is as high as 20–45%.

MCQs (Answers, see p. 289)

1 Which of the following is the most common type of hernia in females?
   a Femoral hernia.
   b Obturator hernia.
   c Richter hernia.
   d Umbilical hernia.
   e Indirect inguinal hernia.

2 Which of the following statements about the abdominal wall layers is correct?
   a The internal oblique muscle fibres continue into the scrotum as cremasteric muscle.
   b The lymphatics of the abdominal wall drain into the ipsilateral axillary lymph nodes.

c Scarpa's fascia holds little strength in wound closure.

d The transversalis fascia is an important layer of the abdominal wall in preventing hernias.

e The inguinal canal is an oblique passage through the abdominal wall which conveys the spermatic cord in men and the round ligament in women.

3 Regarding hernia, which of the following are true and which are false?

a Femoral hernias arise below and medial to the pubic tubercle.

b Indirect hernias initially protude laterally to the inferior epigastric vessels.

c An indirect hernia occurs when the bowel protudes directly through a defect in the anterior abdominal wall.

d Indirect hernia is the commonest type of hernia in males compared with females.

e The deep inguinal ring is located at the mid inguinal point.

4 The following statements are true regarding the indications for treatment of inguinal hernias?

a A truss maintains a hernia in a reduced state reducing the risk of incarceration and strangulation.

b Most adult hernias remain stable in size, therefore delay rarely affects the technical aspects of surgical repair.

c Urgent operations as a result of hernia complications are associated with significant morbidity and mortality compared with elective repair.

d There is a direct relationship between the length of time that a hernia is present and the risk of major complications.

e Recurrent severe pain around the hernia site is an indication to expedite surgery.

5 In advising a patient preoperatively of the potential complications of surgical repair of inguinal hernia, which of the following statements are true?

a Wound infection increases the risk of recurrent hernia.

b Recurrence following primary hernia repair should occur in less than 10% of cases.

c Severe symptoms due to nerve entrapment can occur.

d The most common vascular injury from surgery is the femoral artery.

e Surgery can result in testicular infarction from damage to the testicular artery.

6 Regarding umbilical hernias in adults, which of the following are true and which are false?

a Incarceration is common with umbilical hernias.

b A paraumbilical hernia typically occurs in multiparous females.

c The presence of ascites is a contraindication to repair umbilical hernias electively.

d Most umbilical hernias in adults are the result of a congenital defect carried into adulthood.

e Recurrence is more likely if the hernia defect is greater than 2.5 cm.

Part 5   Pelvis

15   Gynaecology

Ectopic pregnancy

D : The presence of pregnancy outside the uterine cavity. Most ectopic pregnancies are located in the fallopian tube (98.3%), followed by abdomen (1.4%), ovary (0.15%) and cervix (0.15%).

I & S :   1 in 100 pregnancies.

A & P :   **Distortion of anatomy of the fallopian tube because of adhesions due to either pelvic infection or pelvic surgery. Sexually transmitted infections caused by** *Chlamydia* **or gonorrhoea are the commonest causative factor for ectopic pregnancy.** Other risk factors include:

- previous ectopic pregnancy
- presence of intrauterine contraceptive device (IUCD)
- previous abdominal or pelvic surgery or infection.

Most patients with ectopic pregnancy will have no risk factors as these are only present in 25–50%. Therefore, any woman of childbearing age presenting with lower abdominal pain and/or vaginal bleeding and/or amenorrhoea should have a urine pregnancy test and, if positive, should have appropriate investigations to rule out ectopic pregnancy.

C F & D :   **Investigations should include TVU examination and HCG estimation.** The presence of intrauterine pregnancy on TVU practically rules out ectopic pregnancy, as the presence of pregnancy inside and outside the uterus (heterotypic pregnancy) is rare in spontaneous conception but is relatively common in pregnancies conceived by IVF techniques.

T & M :   Conservative, medical or surgical.

Conservative management

Suitable for asymptomatic and stable patients with no obvious adnexal mass or fluid on USS and HCG < 1000 IU/L. The patient requires regular measurement of HCG levels to confirm its decline and should be warned of the symptoms of abdominal pain or bleeding, which may then need intervention.

Medical management

Includes IM administration of methotrexate in hemodynamically stable patients with adnexal mass < 4 cm in size with minimal free fluid on USS and no fetal

---

EMQs and MCQs for Surgical Finals, 1st edition.   © Hye-Chung Kwak, Imran Bhatti, Jaskarn Rai, Farhan Rashid, Bachittar Singh Jassar, Murthy Nyasavajjala, Viren Asher, Jon Lund and Mike Larvin. Published 2011 by Blackwell Publishing Ltd.

cardiac activity. HCG should be < 3000 IU/L with no contraindications to methotrexate therapy and the patient should be able to regularly return for follow-up for several weeks.

Surgery

Involves removal of the ectopic pregnancy with the fallopian tube (salpingectomy) or without the fallopian tube (salpingostomy) either by laparotomy or laparoscopy. Most ectopic pregnancies are managed laparoscopically, with laparotomy generally indicated in haemodynamically unstable patients with large amounts of blood in the peritoneal cavity (haemoperitoneum) and showing signs of hypovolaemic shock. Salpingectomy is generally performed if the contralateral tube is healthy, while salpingostomy is generally reserved for patients with a damaged tube on the other side as salpingostomy is associated with a higher chance of subsequent ectopic pregnancy than salpingectomy.

P :   Fatal to the fetus. Early treatment has a better prognosis for the mother.

Pelvic inflammatory disease

D :   Infection of the genital tract due to ascending infection from endocervix leading to endometritis, salpingitis, parametritis, oopheritis, tubo-ovarian abscess and pelvic peritonitis and abscess. PID can often lead to long-term sequelae like chronic pelvic pain, tubal infertility and ectopic pregnancy.

I & S :   PID is a common cause of morbidity, diagnosed in about 1 in 60 women under the age of 45 years. The exact incidence is unknown as most cases go unnoticed as they are asymptomatic.

A & P :   STIs caused by *Chlamydia trachomatis* and *Neisseria gonorrhoeae* are the most common organisms involved, although *Mycoplasma genitalium, Gardnerella vaginalis* and other anaerobes may be implicated as well.

Risk factors

- Age less than 25 years
- Multiple sexual partners
- Past history of sexually transmitted diseases
- Termination of pregnancy
- New sexual partner (within previous 3 months)
- Insertion of IUCD in past 6 weeks

C F & D :   Often presents with non-specific symptoms. A high index of suspicion is essential for early treatment as the sequelae of untreated PID has a huge impact on the woman's life. The following symptoms and signs are suggestive of PID:

- bilateral lower abdominal tenderness
- abnormal cervical or vaginal discharge
- fever (<38°C)
- abnormal vaginal bleeding (post-coital, intermenstrual)
- deep dyspareunia

- cervical motion tenderness and adnexal tenderness on bimanual vaginal examination.

Diagnosis

- Pregnancy test should always be performed to rule out ectopic pregnancy.
- Vaginal and cervical swab taken for gonorrhoea and *Chlamydia* testing.
- Urine samples: rapid testing of organisms can also be done using PCR.
- Raised ESR or CRP can support the diagnosis.
- Laparoscopy is the gold standard for detection of PID, although 15–30% of cases of PID may not have any findings. Laparoscopy also enables biopsy of the tissues, drainage of pus and can also indicate the severity of disease.
- TVU has been shown to be helpful in detecting tubo-ovarian masses and can help to differentiate appendicitis from PID in some cases, but there is insufficient evidence to justify its routine use at present.

The following conditions should be considered while assessing women with lower abdominal pain:

- ectopic pregnancy
- acute appendicitis
- endometriosis
- ovarian cyst torsion
- irritable bowel syndrome (and other GI disorders)
- functional pain of unknown origin
- UTI.

T & M : Empirical treatment of PID with antibiotics has been recommended as delay in treatment leads to long-term sequelae that can have detrimental effects on the health of the woman.

Outpatient treatment

Patients with mild and moderate PID can be treated with antibiotics (I dose IV ceftriaxone followed by oral doxycycline and metronidazole for 14 days) on an outpatient basis.

Inpatient treatment

Admission of patients is justified in the following circumstances:

- clinically severe disease
- other surgical conditions cannot be excluded
- tubo-ovarian abscess
- PID in pregnancy
- lack of response to therapy
- intolerance to oral therapy.

Intravenous antibiotic therapy should be commenced on admission and should be continued for at least 24 hours after resolution of symptoms.

Surgical management is indicated in patients with severe disease not responding to antibiotics and presence of pelvic abscess which should be drained.

Staff should provide detailed explanation of the condition, including the importance of completing the treatment and the long-term implications of the disease for patients and their partners. This information should also be provided as leaflets.

All women and their partners should be offered referral to the genitourinary medicine (GUM) clinic for STI screening and contact tracing. They should be advised to avoid intercourse until both have been fully treated. Use of condoms to reduce future episodes of PID should be advocated.

Initial follow-up of patients should be done at 72 hours to assess response to therapy and to exclude the need for parenteral or surgical treatment. Subsequently the patient should be seen at 4–6 weeks to ensure:

- compliance with antibiotics
- adequate response to treatment
- screening and treatment of sexual contacts
- to advise about safe sexual practices and explain significance of PID and its sequelae.

P : Antibiotics will treat the infection but the effects of the infection are permanent.

Ovarian cyst

D : Ovarian cyst is a fluid-filled sac of more than 2 cm that develops in the ovary. They can vary from pea size to huge cysts.

I & S : Ovarian cysts are present in most premenopausal women; around 15% present in the postmenopausal age group. Most cysts are innocent and resolve spontaneously. Ovarian cysts are classified as follows.

- *Functional cysts*: follicular cyst, corpus luteum cyst, haemorrhagic cyst
- *Benign cysts*: dermoid cyst, endometriotic cyst, cystadenomas
- *Malignant cysts*

Emergencies associated with ovarian cysts

- Torsion: dermoid cyst is usually associated with torsion due to the presence of a long pedicle, which makes it mobile.
- Haemorrhage: can occur in any type of cyst and is associated with rupture of a blood vessel in the cyst causing distension and pain.
- Rupture (rare) can present as an emergency in patients with ovarian cysts. Corpus luteal cyst can rarely undergo rupture causing haemoperitoneum (blood in abdominal cavity) necessitating laparotomy.

C F & D : Patients present with mild ache to sudden onset of severe lower abdominal pain associated with vomiting. The pain can radiate to the back and thighs and can be associated with fainting spells. Haemorrhage into the cyst can be associated with onset of menstruation, while rupture of corpus luteal cysts typically occurs premenstrually.

On examination the patient may be tachycardic with abdominal guarding and occasionally rebound tenderness. If large enough the cyst can be felt per vaginum and is very tender to touch.

Diagnosis

- USS examination of the pelvis is the mainstay in diagnosis of this condition. Haemorrhagic cyst can be seen as a thin-walled cyst with multiple echogenic areas suggesting the presence of blood. Torsion in an ovarian cyst is very difficult to diagnose on USS and is essentially a clinical diagnosis.
- Doppler examination has been shown to be helpful in some cases.

T & M:

- Conservative: haemorrhagic cysts are generally managed conservatively as they are self-resolving. Most patients require simple analgesics.
- Surgery: ovarian cysts that have either undergone torsion or rupture need laparoscopy or laparotomy to relieve the pain and avoid further bleeding. If the cyst has undergone necrosis as a result of interruption of blood supply due to torsion, then salpingo-oopherectomy is performed to remove the necrotic cyst. If the ovary is viable then rarely a cystectomy can be possible. Haemorrhagic corpus luteum can be removed to avoid further bleeding or occasionally may require oopherectomy.

MCQs

Ectopic pregnancy (Answers, see p. 291)

1 Which of the following are risk factors for ectopic pregnancy?
   a Previous ectopic pregnancy.
   b Use of combined OCP for contraception.
   c Fibroid uterus.
   d Multiple sexual partners.
   e Previous tubal surgery.

2 Regarding ectopic pregnancy, which of the following are true and which are false?
   a It is the presence of pregnancy outside the uterine cavity.
   b Can lead to hypovolaemic shock.
   c Is always associated with first pregnancy.
   d Can be present without any risk factors.
   e Always occurs in the fallopian tube.

3 Which of the following describe the signs and symptoms of ectopic pregnancy?
   a Lower abdominal pain with the last period 6 weeks ago associated with cervical excitation may suggest ectopic pregnancy.

b Can be diagnosed with certainty with history and clinical examination.
c Can be associated with left shoulder tip pain.
d Can be completely asymptomatic.
e Can present with bleeding.

4 Regarding the diagnosis of ectopic pregnancy, which of the following are true and which are false?
a Can always be made with certainty using TVU.
b Estimation of levels of HCG is helpful.
c Always leads to surgery.
d Should always be kept in mind when any childbearing woman presents with abdominal pain and/or bleeding.
e Can be ruled out if HCG < 5 IU/L.

5 Regarding the management of ectopic pregnancy, which of the following are true and which are false?
a Conservative management is possible in selected patients.
b Laparotomy is indicated in patients showing signs of hypovolaemic shock.
c Salpingostomy is preferred if the contralateral tube is normal.
d Salpingectomy increases the risk of subsequent ectopic pregnancy compared with salpingostomy.
e Administration of methotrexate helps to resolve ectopic pregnancy.

6 Regarding the management of ectopic pregnancy, which of the following are true and which are false?
a Methotrexate can be given to a patient with an adnexal mass > 3.5 cm and moderate amount of free fluid in abdomen.
b Conservative management is only indicated in patients with minimal symptoms and no adnexal mass.
c No follow-up is required after methotrexate treatment.
d Patients can get pregnant immediately after treatment with methotrexate.
e Emergency surgery is required for ruptured ectopic pregnancy.

PID (Answers, see p. 291)

1 Regarding PID, which of the following are true and which are false?
a Can be asymptomatic.
b Does not lead to long-term health problems.
c Is commonly seen in women in steady relationships.
d Can be associated with insertion of IUCD.
e Is caused by STI.

2 Regarding the diagnosis of PID, which of the following are true and which are false?
a PID can be associated with abnormal vaginal bleeding.
b Should only be treated after confirmation of diagnosis.
c Laparoscopy is considered the gold standard for diagnosis.
d Irritable bowel syndrome should be considered as differential diagnosis in patients suspected of PID.
e Can be made by testing for *Chlamydia* on a urine specimen.

3 Regarding the management of PID, which of the following are true and which are false?
a Empirical treatment is recommended based on clinical criteria alone.
b Can be treated on an outpatient basis.
c Partners of patients diagnosed with PID do not need treatment.
d Referral to GUM is essential for contact tracing.
e Intravenous antibiotics are essential.

4 Regarding the prevention of PID, which of the following are true and which are false?
a Use of a condom is recommended to prevent recurrence of infection.
b Avoidance of intercourse is essential until both partners have been fully treated to prevent reinfection.
c Treatment of contacts does not reduce risk of reinfection.
d IUCD helps prevent PID.
e Regular screening for PID.

5 Regarding follow-up of patients with PID, which of the following are true and which are false?
a Follow-up of patients is not essential after treatment.
b Advice on treatment of contacts and safe sexual practices should be given.
c Should be ideally done in GUM clinics.
d Long-term sequelae of PID should be explained and leaflets given on follow-up.
e It is important to assess response to treatment.

6 Which of the following are risk factors for PID?
a Multiple sexual partners.
b Past history of IVF.
c Termination of pregnancy.
d New sexual partner (within previous 3 months).
e Using barrier contraception.

Ovarian cyst (Answers, see p. 292)

1 Regarding ovarian cysts, which of the following are true and which are false?
a Are present in most premenopausal women.
b Can be asymptomatic.
c Are unlikely to regress spontaneously.
d Can be of varying sizes.
e Functional cysts are the most common type of ovarian cyst.

2 In ovarian cyst emergencies, which of the following are true and which are false?
a Torsion is associated with dermoid cysts.
b Torted ovarian cyst can undergo necrosis.
c Ectopic pregnancy should always be considered in differential diagnosis.
d Pain associated with haemorrhagic ovarian cyst can resolve spontaneously.
e Ovarian cysts can cause abdominal bloating.

3 In the diagnosis of ovarian cyst emergency, which of the following are true and which are false?

  a Torsion of ovarian cyst always presents with severe abdominal pain.
  b Haemorrhage in ovarian cyst can coincide with onset of menstruation.
  c USS of pelvis is the mainstay in diagnosis.
  d Haemorrhagic ovarian cysts can be palpated on vaginal examination.
  e Serum CA125 levels are routinely measured.

4 Regarding the management of ovarian cysts, which of the following are true and which are false?

  a Haemorrhagic ovarian cysts always need to be removed.
  b Most patients with haemorrhagic cysts need simple analgesics.
  c Ruptured corpus luteal cysts need removal to prevent further blood loss.
  d Laparotomy for cancerous ovarian cysts.
  e Conservative management for torsion of ovarian cyst.

5 Regarding torsion of ovarian cyst, which of the following are true and which are false?

  a Always necessitates removal of the ovary.
  b Can be diagnosed conclusively on USS.
  c Necrosis in the ovary is due to interruption of blood supply in the torted pedicle.
  d Is mostly a clinical diagnosis.
  e Typically presents with gradual lower abdominal pain lasting a few minutes.

EMQs (Answers, see p. 293)

1 Options:

  a Ectopic pregnancy.
  b Torted ovarian cyst.
  c PID.
  d Pelvic abscess.
  e Degeneration of fibroid.
  f Ovarian hyperstimulation syndrome.
  g Haemorrhagic ovarian cyst.

For each case below suggest the most appropriate diagnosis from the above list of options. Each option may be used once, more than once or not at all.

  (i) A 25-year-old woman presents to A&E with sudden-onset abdominal pain and distension that is getting worse. She has been previously diagnosed with polycystic ovarian syndrome and has been using clomifene citrate (fertility medication) as the couple have been trying for a pregnancy. Her last menstrual period was 4 weeks ago.

  (ii) A 30-year-old woman who has been seen by the gynaecologist previously for a dermoid cyst presents with sudden onset of lower abdominal pain and vomiting following lifting a heavy box. On examination she is tachycardic with severe abdominal tenderness and guarding.

  (iii) A 20-year-old woman who is in a new relationship is referred to the gynaecology clinic with lower abdominal pain and greenish-yellow foul-smelling discharge. She also complains of deep dyspareunia and post-coital bleeding. On examination, she is apyrexial and there is lower abdominal tenderness. She is very tender on vaginal examination especially on touching the cervix.

2 Options:
   a Ectopic pregnancy.
   b Torted ovarian cyst.
   c PID.
   d Pelvic abscess.
   e Degeneration of fibroid.
   f Ovarian hyperstimulation syndrome.
   g Haemorrhagic ovarian cyst.
   For each case below suggest the most appropriate diagnosis from the above list of options. Each option may be used once, more than once or not at all.
   (i) A 40-year-woman female who has had a copper IUCD inserted 1 week ago presents with lower abdominal pain and foul-smelling yellow discharge. She is pyrexial (38°C), tachycardic and hypotensive with guarding of the abdomen. Vaginal examination reveals a boggy mass in the pouch of Douglas which is fluctuant.
   (ii) A 27-year-old woman who had her last menstrual period 6 weeks ago comes in with sudden-onset lower abdominal pain radiating to the left shoulder. She has also been experiencing fainting spells off and on. On examination she is tachycardic and hypotensive, and there is marked cervical excitation. Her pregnancy test is positive.
   (iii) A 35-year-old woman with known history of ovarian cysts presents with gradually increasing lower abdominal pain which has got worse for the last 2 days. On examination there is tenderness and guarding in left iliac fossa. Vaginal examination reveals tender left adnexa and no masses. Urine pregnancy test was negative.
   (iv) A 30-year-old woman with a known history of fibroids presents with sudden onset of lower abdominal pain with vomiting. She is 10 weeks' pregnant and is worried about the baby. On examination she is tachycardic with a pulse of 100 bpm and BP 126/75 mmHg. A firm tender mass is felt just above the pubic symphysis.

3 Options:
   a Corpus luteal cyst.
   b Ovarian cyst rupture.
   c Placental abruption.
   d Uterine rupture.
   e Chorioamnionitis.
   For each case below suggest the most appropriate diagnosis from the above list of options. Each option may be used once, more than once or not at all.
   (i) A 28-year-old woman presents to the emergency department with sudden lower abdominal pain during the week 37 of gestation. An emergency ultrasound scan revealed blood clots behind the placenta.
   (ii) A 22-year-old woman who is 35 weeks' pregnant presents with severe abdominal and chest pain and vaginal bleeding. The obstetricians are called immediately because the fetus is noted to have severe bradycardia.

16 Urology

Urinary tract infection

D: Bacterial infection of the urine with $>10^5$ colony-forming units (CFU) in asymptomatic patients and $>10^2$ CFU in symptomatic patients.

I & S: Approximately 4% of females, prevalence in males being rare. Pregnancy increases the risk of recurrent UTI or progression of simple UTI to pyelonephritis.

A & P: The commonest causative agent is the gut coliform *Escherichia coli*.

T & M: Treatment is with antibiotics in symptomatic patients. Before treatment, culture of MSU should be checked to ensure correct sensitivity. Acute pyelonephritis requires inpatient IV antibiotics.

Chronic pyelonephritis as a result of recurrent infections of the kidney causes inflammation and glomerular fibrosis and can lead to hypertension and renal impairment. An extreme form of chronic pyelonephritis is xanthogranulomatous pyelonephritis, which is due to an excessive immune response and results in multiple parenchymal abscesses and reduced renal function often requiring nephrectomy.

P: Simple UTIs respond well to oral antibiotic use, with complete resolution of symptoms within a few days. Acute pyelonephritis can take longer, with several days of IV antibiotics and oral antibiotics for up to 14 days. Recurrent or severe UTI should be investigated for underlying pathology.

Renal colic

Renal colic is an acute and painful urological emergency, with patients presenting quickly to admissions departments and is a common surgical presentation to an F1 in the emergency, urological or surgical department.

D: Flank pain usually radiating to the groin caused by obstruction to the flow of urine due to kidney or ureteral stones.

I & S: M > F, $\approx$ 20–40 years of age.

A & P: Low urinary volume is a common cause of renal stones. Other causes include:

- hypercalciuria (calcium + oxalate/phosphate)
- hyperuricosuria (disorder of uric acid metabolism)
- cystinuria
- hyperoxaluria.

C F & D: Typically constant loin to groin pain associated with nausea and vomiting. Pyrexia and tachycardia may indicate severe UTI.

Distal ureteral stones cause pain that tends to radiate into the groin or testicle in the male or labia majora in female. The pain is referred from the ilioinguinal or genitofemoral nerves and so an obstructed stone in the intramural ureter can be confused with cystitis or urethritis causing pain at the tip of the penis (in men),

EMQs and MCQs for Surgical Finals, 1st edition.   © Hye-Chung Kwak, Imran Bhatti, Jaskarn Rai, Farhan Rashid, Bachittar Singh Jassar, Murthy Nyasavajjala, Viren Asher, Jon Lund and Mike Larvin. Published 2011 by Blackwell Publishing Ltd.

and sometimes various bowel symptoms such as diarrhoea and tenesmus. These symptoms can be confused with PID, ovarian cyst rupture, or torsion and menstrual pain in women.

Investigations

- Urine dipstick: microscopic haematuria +/− leucocytes +/− nitrites (associated with UTI); pH (consider uric acid stones if pH < 6, UTI if pH > 8).
- Blood tests: U&E (renal function); FBC (neutrophilia suggests infection) +/− blood cultures.

Imaging

- Plain X-ray of KUB: identifies calcifications and foreign bodies
- IVU: outlines entire urinary system and identifies stones and hydronephrosis
- Non-contrast CT of KUB: identifies stones and assesses stone density
- Renal USS +/− drainage: (i) detects hydronephrosis and large stones, (ii) percutaneous nephrostomy for obstructed kidney, (iii) excludes AAA and gallstones

---

T & M : Analgesia and hydration +/− treat UTI. Smaller stones are more likely to pass spontaneously; calculi larger than 7 mm are likely to require surgical assistance. In patients with recurrent stones, 24-hour urine collection for urinalysis (cause of stone formation) and stone chemical composition. Surgical options include double J-stent insertion or ESWL.

P : Depends on the cause of renal colic.

Prostate cancer

D : Cancer of the prostate gland.

I & S : Prostate cancer usually affects older males (>70 years) and is the most common cancer in males in the UK (excluding skin cancers).

A & P : Most prostate cancers are adenocarcinomas arising in the peripheral zone. Growth of the prostatic epithelium is under the influence of testosterone and its more potent form dihydrotestosterone (DHT). This conversion is controlled by the enzyme 5α-reductase.

C F & D : Most patients have mild urinary symptoms over many years. Some other symptoms include:

- urgency
- nocturia
- haematuria
- urinary retention
- bone pain in metastatic disease.

Diagnosis of prostate cancer is based on PSA, DRE and histology, although a clinical diagnosis can be made in advanced disease without histology. Tissue is obtained via transrectal ultrasound-guided biopsy.

T & M : Depends on the stage or grade of prostate cancer. In general:

- active surveillance for slow-growing cancers
- prostatectomy +/− radiotherapy (localized cancer)

- prostatectomy +/– radiotherapy and hormone therapy (advanced cancer)
- hormone therapy +/– radiotherapy (recurrent/metastatic disease).

Inhibition of androgens will stop growth effects on the prostate and therefore any hypertrophy or carcinoma of these tissues. The normal apoptotic measures will ensue and all hormonally sensitive prostate tissue growth subsequently arrests and the prostate involutes.

For prostate-confined disease in a patient with a life expectancy greater than 10 years, treatment is aimed at curative intent. In a surgically fit patient, this involves radical prostatectomy by open, laparoscopic or robotic methods. In a less fit patient, radical radiotherapy is treatment of choice. Other options include brachytherapy (implanted radioactive seeds), cryotherapy (implanting ice) or high-intensity focused ultrasound or active surveillance.

For metastatic prostate cancer, curative intent is not possible. The mainstay of treatment is hormonal ablation (removal of testosterone and DHT) following hormone relapse (12–18 months); if sufficiently fit, chemotherapy (docetaxel) is the next stage of treatment, offering increase in survival as well as improvement in symptoms.

P: Generally 81% 5-year survival.

Benign prostatic hypertrophy

D: Benign enlargement of the prostate gland. This condition is also known as prostatism or prostatic enlargement.

I&S: Common in males over 60 years of age.

A&P: The exact cause is unknown. The prostate gland grows with hormone exposure.

CF&D: Symptoms of BPH are very common in older males:

- urinary retention
- frequency
- urgency
- incomplete bladder emptying
- hesitancy
- nocturia
- terminal dribbling
- weak or interrupted urinary stream.

Investigations

- Urine dipstick
- Blood tests for U&E and PSA (high in BPH)
- Imaging (USS, IVU)
- Non-invasive urodynamic test (detects lower urinary tract obstruction); urine flow rate recording
- Post-void residual volume

T&M:

- Regular monitoring
- Medication: α-adrenergic blockers, 5α-reductase blockers
- Surgery: balloon dilatation, TURP, prostatectomy.

Brief overview of transurethral resection of the prostate (TURP)

This is the surgical procedure for relieving bladder outflow obstruction secondary to BPH. The indications for surgical intervention include the following.

- Acute urinary retention, failed voiding trials, recurrent gross haematuria (from BPH), UTI, and renal insufficiency secondary to obstruction.
- Failed medical therapy due to side effects are indications for surgical intervention.

In current clinical practice, most patients do not present with obvious surgical indications. Instead, they often have milder lower urinary tract symptoms and are therefore initially treated with medical therapy.

TURP has long been the most common method by which obstructing prostate tissue is removed through the urethra. This procedure is performed with regional or general anaesthesia and involves the placement of a working metal sheath in the urethra through which a hand-held device with an attached wire cutting loop is placed. Electric current is passed through this loop to either cut or coagulate tissue. This device is either visualized directly through an eyepiece or more commonly on a video monitor.

TURP is often successful (80–90%) but has significant side effects. TURP carries a significant risk of morbidity (18%) and mortality (0.23–6%).

P : Depends on length of symptoms and treatment.

Renal cell carcinoma

D : Renal cell carcinoma (RCC) is an adenocarcinoma of the renal cortex and the most common renal tumour.

I & S : RCC accounts for 85% of renal tumours and indeed 2% of all deaths from cancers. Generally affects older males (aged > 65years).

A & P : The known risk factors include renal failure and dialysis, smoking, hypertension, von Hippel–Lindau (VHL) syndrome, and polycystic and horseshoe kidneys.

Grading is by the Furhman system (I, well differentiated to IV, poorly differentiated) and staged with the TNM classification.

C F & D : Painless haematuria, mass, and vague symptoms such as weight loss and lethargy. Some patients have no symptoms. Investigations include USS abdomen, IVU, CT urogram and cystoscopy (rule out bladder cancer).

T & M : The gold standard of treatment for localized disease remains surgical (open or laparoscopic).

- Radical nephrectomy: for ipsilateral RCC aiming for excision of the RCC within Gerota's fascia and good surgical margins +/− ipsilateral adrenal glands +/− localized lymph nodes. The artery is ligated and removed prior to the vein to prevent organ swelling.
- Partial nephrectomy: for multifocal bilateral disease or with disease in a single kidney or for those with VHL syndrome.

For locally advanced disease, a multidisciplinary surgical approach is still the mainstay. Adjuvant options exist with radiotherapy or immunotherapy to reduce the presurgical tumour burden but have not yet proved to be of benefit.

For metastatic disease the prognosis is very poor and this is still a large group of patients at presentation (25%). The role for chemotherapy and hormone therapy is poor in this very resistant disease. Radiotherapy is helpful for palliation of painful metastasis. Cytoreductive surgery is helpful for reducing tumour burden but can relieve symptoms of pain and haematuria. In poor surgical candidates embolization is the alternative. New therapies have developed for metastatic RCC, with immunotherapy at the forefront; other treatment modalities include gene therapy, anti-angiogenic therapy and tyrosine kinase inhibitor treatment. Steroids also have a role in palliative care of RCC.

P : Poor prognosis, 5–30% at 5 years.

Bladder cancer

D : Cancer of the urinary bladder. The majority are epithelial, with transitional cell carcinoma representing the majority (90%) and squamous cell carcinoma (<10%) and adenocarcinoma (≈2%) the rest. Very rare tumours of the bladder include sarcoma, lymphoma, melanoma and phaeochromocytoma. Secondaries, which are usually adenocarcinoma in origin, arise from prostate, gut, ovary and colon.

I & S : More common in males. Malignant disease of the bladder is vastly more common than benign disease.

A & P : Smoking and exposure to chemicals (arylamines and polycyclic hydrocarbons) are the two main risk factors for developing bladder cancer.

Like all cancers the histological grading ranges from well differentiated to poorly differentiated and is assigned G1–G3 grading. For disease staging the TNM classification is used.

C F & D : Patients commonly present with painless haematuria. Other symptoms include frequency, urgency and dysuria. The following investigations are used to investigate microscopic or macroscopic haematuria:

- X-ray of KUB: shows up to 80% of renal calculi.
- USS of renal tract: good for imaging renal pathology including hydronephrosis and hydroureters of upper tracts. Bladder masses can be seen if full bladder. Prostate and lower urinary tracts not well visualized.
- Flexible cystoscopy: under local anaesthesia visualizes urethra, prostatic urethra and bladder surface. Good for viewing superficial tumour, chronic cystitis and abnormal prostatic urothelium.
- Urine can be sent for cytology.
- The above investigations are fairly exhaustive for excluding pathology in haematuria. However, they may also lead to further investigations such as IVU or CT to exclude a possible stone and other renal lesions.
- Cystoscopy under local anaesthesia: used to take biopsies of bladder lesions and laser ablation of small lesions can be done. For larger lesions, transurethral resection of bladder tumour (TURBT) is required.

T & M :

- Bacille Calmette–Guérin (BCG) vaccine (a modified strain of *Mycobacterium bovis*) is given intravesically for carcinoma *in situ*.
- TURBT +/– intravesical mitomycin C for superficial bladder cancers (used to reduce the risk of recurrence).

For muscle-invasive disease pT2a/3, the untreated 5-year survival is a miserable 3%. The options for bladder-confined disease are as follows:

- Radical cystectomy with urinary diversion: offers the best outcome for most aggressive bladder cancers but is a major undertaking for the surgeon and the patient.
- Less aggressive surgery in the form of a partial cystectomy or TURBT will require adjuvant systemic chemotherapy +/− radiotherapy. This is often an option for the elderly medically unfit.
- Radical radiotherapy: offers poorer results than radical cystectomy but is a choice for those unwilling to undergo radical cystectomy and retains the bladder with fewer problems.
- For metastatic disease surgery has no role and systemic chemotherapy is the only option. Radiotherapy has a role for palliative control of painful metastasis.

P: On average, 50–60% 5-year survival.

MCQs

UTI (Answers, see p. 295)

1 Which of the following organisms are responsible for UTIs?
a *Enterobacter* and *Klebsiella* spp.
b *Eschericha coli.*
c *Proteus* spp.
d *Pseudomonas* and *Candida* spp.
e *Staphylococcus saprophyticus.*
f All of the above.

2 Which of the following is the most common cause of unresolved bacteriuria (bacteria within the urine, which is normally bacteria free)?
a Initial bacterial resistance.
b Persistence of bacteria.
c Rapid reinfections.
d Recurrent urethral trauma.
e Staghorn calculi.

3 Which of the following are complications of urethral catheterization?
a False passage.
b Infection.
c Trauma.
d Paraphimosis.
e Urethral stricture.
f Raised PSA.
g Bleeding.
h Diuresis.
i Rectal perforation.

Renal colic (Answers, see p. 295)

1 Which of the following are characteristic symptoms of renal colic?
a Haematuria, cloudy or foul-smelling urine.
b Nausea and vomiting.

c Urgency of micturition.
d Associated fever or rigors.
e Patient lies immobile.
f Renal failure.

2 Which of the following statements regarding causes of renal calculi are true?
  a Calcium stones are the least common cause of renal calculi.
  b Increased oxalate may result from chronic UTI.
  c Cystinuria is a common cause of stones.
  d Increase in citrate or magnesium can predispose to stone formation.
  e Clot from bladder bleeding is a common cause of renal colic.
  f IV fluids should be started in all patients.
  g Analgesia is not always needed.
  h NSAIDs are contraindicated in renal colic.
  i AXR of KUB is of no use and USS is first line in renal colic.

3 Because stones in different parts of the renal tract can cause differing symptoms, it is important to rule out other pathologies. In upper ureteric and renal pelvis stones, the pain tends to radiate to the flank and lumbar areas. Which of the following would be the differential diagnosis on the right?
  a Renal colic.
  b Cholecystitis or cholelithiasis.
  c Hepatitis.
  d Acute pancreatitis.
  e Peptic ulcer disease and gastritis.

4 Mid-ureteral calculi cause pain that radiates anteriorly and caudally. Which of the following would be the differential diagnosis on the right?
  a Appendicitis.
  b Ovarian pathology.
  c Ectopic pregnancy, spontaneous miscarriage.
  d Acute diverticulitis.
  e Abdominal aortic aneurysm.

5 Which of the following are the common locations for a stone to obstruct?
  a Pelvi-ureteric junction.
  b As the ureters pass along the transverse processes of L2/L3.
  c Crossing the pelvic brim.
  d As the ureters cross the bifurcation of the iliacs.
  e Vesico-ureteric junction.

Prostate cancer (Answers, see p. 296)

1 Regarding prostate cancer, which of the following statements are true and which are false?
  a The incidence of the disease in the under-sixties is very rare.
  b The incidence does not increase with age.
  c Risk factors include Afro-Caribbean descent and positive family history.

d The disease can present as bladder outflow obstruction with lower urinary tract symptoms.

e Prostate metastasis is often found in the lungs.

2 Regarding prostate cancer, which of the following statements are true and which are false?

a Histology is graded using the Duke staging and the TNM classification.

b There is no formal screening.

c Active surveillance is only an option in advanced disease.

d Surgery is far superior to radiotherapy as treatment for localized disease.

BPH (Answers, see p. 297)

1 Which of the following statements about BPH is true?

a The cells increase in a hyperplastic process.

b Castrated males cannot get BPH.

c PSA is an accurate determinant for BPH.

d The prostate reaches its maximum size during puberty.

e BPH initially leads to a distended floppy bladder and increasing residual volume.

f DRE allows you to feel the whole prostate.

2 Which of the following are complications/risks of TURP?

a Bleeding.

b Hyponatraemic, hypochloraemic metabolic acidosis.

c Urethral stricture.

d Retrograde ejaculation.

e Erectile dysfunction.

f All of the above.

RCC (Answers, see p. 298)

1 Regarding renal cell cancer, which of the following statements are true and which are false?

a The most common presentation of RCC is the classic triad of haematuria, pain and mass.

b Night sweats are a rare sign.

c Right-sided varicocele is a sign of tumour extension into the right renal vein.

d Paraneoplastic syndromes are a rare manifestation of late disease.

Bladder cancer (Answers, see p. 298)

1 Which of the following statements about the symptoms of bladder cancer are true?

a Microscopic haematuria is a common feature of bladder cancer in the under-fifties.

b Macroscopic haematuria is a sign of significant disease and often associated with abdominal pain.

c Recurrent UTI and pneumaturia are often caused by colovesical fistula secondary to bladder cancer.

d Signs of locally invasive disease include palpable mass, pallor, fatigue, anuria, lower limb oedema.

Miscellaneous (Answers, see p. 299)

1 Priapism is an acute emergency that occurs due to inability to drain the cavernosal blood supply. In one-third of cases the cause is sickle cell disease, while other causes include leukaemias, trauma, neurological conditions and the side effects of drugs. Treatment is often conservative, usually asking the patient to climb stairs repeatedly (arterial steal phenomenon) until detumescence occurs. Which of the following are treatment options for priapism?

a Ice.

b Antihypertensives.

c Sympathomimetics.

d Sildenafil.

2 Painful lumps in the scrotum include torsion of testes, strangulated inguinal hernia and epididymo-orchitis. These can also present painlessly especially if left over time and there is tissue damage. Which of the following result in painless lumps in the scrotum?

a Inguinal hernia.

b Hydrocele.

c Epididymal cyst.

d Spermatocele.

e Varicocele.

f Testicular tumour.

g Haematoma.

EMQs (Answers, see p. 299)

UTI

1 UTI is a common condition seen in many different medical specialities and all age groups but there are various peaks in incidence.

a Young adults.

b Children.

c Elderly.

d All age groups.

Match the age groups listed above to the most likely cause of UTI listed below.

(i) Anatomical differences in the sexes.

(ii) Bladder outflow obstruction.

(iii) Congenital (vesicoureteric reflux).

(iv) Strictures, tumours and stones.

2 Options:

a Acute cystitis.

b Acute pyelonephritis.

c Acute bacterial prostatitis.

d Chronic bacterial prostatitis.

For each case below suggest the most appropriate diagnosis from the above list of options.

(i) Dysuria, low back pain, perineal discomfort.

(ii) Dysuria, perineal pain, deep suprapubic pain recent.

(iii) Pyrexia, malaise, loin pain, dysuria, rigors, haematuria.

(iv) Urinary frequency, urgency, dysuria, suprapubic pain, malaise and haematuria.

3 Urethral catheterization of the bladder is performed for the treatment and diagnosis of certain urological and non-urological conditions. As a junior doctor you will be called to the ward to catheterize both male and female patients. The options are:

a Short-term catheter.

b Long-term catheter.

c Intermittent self-catheter.

d Seek urological guidance.

e None of the above.

For each situation below suggest the most appropriate intervention from the above list of options. Each option may be used once, more than once or not at all.

(i) Acute retention of urine.

(ii) Chronic retention of urine.

(iii) UTI.

(iv) Monitoring of urinary output.

(v) Collection of uncontaminated urine in males.

(vi) Instillation of intravesical treatment.

(vii) Decompression of neurogenic bladder.

(viii) Intraoperative monitoring for general anaesthesia patient.

(ix) Post radical prostatectomy.

Prostate cancer

1 Options:

a Diethylstilbestrol.

b Gonadotrophin-releasing hormone analogues.

c Castration.

d Docetaxel.

e Steroids.

Match each of the mechanisms of action listed below with the most appropriate treatment from the above list of options. Each option may be used once, more than once or not at all.

(i) Activates then competitively blocks pituitary receptors.

(ii) Initial surge of FSH and LH and subsequently androgens, and resulting increase in prostate cancer growth ('tumour flare').

(iii) Competitively targets androgen receptors.

(iv) Reduces inflammation associated with metastasis.

(v) Removes production of testosterone.

(vi) Member of the taxane group of chemotherapeutic agents used in hormone-refractory prostate cancer.

BPH

1 Options:

a Alpha blockers (α_{1a}).

b Side effects of alpha blockers.

c Mode of action of 5α-reductase inhibitors.

d Side effects of 5α-reductase inhibitors.

Match each of the desc riptions listed below with the most appropriate drug from the above list of options.

  (i) Induce relaxation of the smooth muscle within the prostate.

 (ii) Prostatic enlargement results from the potent androgen 5α-DHT. In the prostate gland, type II 5α-reductase metabolizes circulating testosterone into DHT. DHT binds to androgen receptors in the cell nuclei stimulating cell growth and proliferation.

(iii) Orthostatic hypotension, dizziness, fatigue, ejaculation disorder, nasal congestion.

(iv) Reduced libido, ejaculatory disorder and erectile dysfunction.

RCC

1 Options:

  a Grawitz's tumour.

  b Oncocytoma.

  c Hypernephroma.

  d Angiomyolipoma.

  e Clear cell carcinoma.

  f Hamartoma.

Match each of the descriptions listed below with the most appropriate tumour from the above list of options.

  (i) A rare renal tumour that is radiologically difficult to distinguish from renal cell carcinoma.

 (ii) Another name for renal cell carcinoma.

(iii) This tumour is composed of blood vessels, smooth muscle and fat.

Miscellaneous

1 Torsion of testes is the twisting of the testes on its pedicle (blood supply and cord structures). Thus the arterial supply is occluded and the testis undergoes ischaemia. If prolonged this will result in tissue death with loss of the affected testicle. Testicular torsion can occur at any age, although the incidence is greatest in adolescence. The options are:

  a Epididymo-orchitis.

  b Strangulated hernia.

  c Testicular tumour.

  d Torsion of testes.

Match the symptoms listed below to the diagnoses above. What is the treatment for each presentation?

  (i) Increased temperature, increased WCC, urethral discharge, dysuria, testicular and groin pain and onset of days.

 (ii) Hard tender lump unilaterally, onset over a week.

(iii) Sudden onset of severe testicular pain, nausea and vomiting, recent trauma.

(iv) Groin scrotal swelling, tender, inflamed, change in bowel habit.

Part 6   Vascular
17   Vascular

Abdominal aortic aneurysm

D : The normal diameter of the abdominal aorta is 16–22 mm. AAA has a diameter of more than 3 cm or twice the size of the lumen above the aneurysm. It is most commonly located infrarenally.

I & S : Incidence in males is four times greater than in females, with the highest prevalence in males over 65 years old. In England and Wales, there are upto 10000 ruptured AAA (RAAA) per year.

A & P : It is thought to be due to a degenerative process of the aortic wall due to higher intraluminal pressure, or to genetic predisposition, infection, trauma, arteritis or connective tissue disorders. The diameter of the aneurysm expands approximately 10% per year and the risk of rupture increases as the diameter of the aneurysm increases.

Risk factors

- Hypertension
- Hyperlipidaemia
- Family history
- Smoking: 90% of patients have smoked during their lifetime

CF & D : AAA is asymptomatic in 75% of cases, but the possible symptoms include epigastric and back pain, and malaise associated with weight loss. An expanding pulsatile mass in the abdomen is an AAA. A triad of abdominal pain, shock and pulsatile abdominal mass makes the diagnosis of RAAA; 15% of aneurysms will rupture, with only 1–2 in 10 surviving. Half the patients with aortic rupture will die before they reach hospital and 90% die before reaching the operating theatre.

Presenting features in RAAA

- Acute abdominal/back pain
- Pulsatile abdominal mass
- Hypovolaemic shock

EMQs and MCQs for Surgical Finals, 1st edition.   © Hye-Chung Kwak, Imran Bhatti, Jaskarn Rai, Farhan Rashid, Bachittar Singh Jassar, Murthy Nyasavajjala, Viren Asher, Jon Lund and Mike Larvin. Published 2011 by Blackwell Publishing Ltd.

Rare presentations

- Distal embolic episodes
- Aortocaval fistula
- Aorto-intestinal fistula

T & M : Consider open surgery if symptomatic, rapidly expanding aneurysm (>1 cm/year), AAA diameter > 6 cm, or ruptured. The surgeon will replace the diseased aorta using a synthetic graft made of Dacron or Teflon. It is important to select patients with a higher risk of rupture compared with the risk of operation. In order to plan the operation, a CT abdomen is needed to assess AAA size, its relation to the renal arteries, and identify the involvement of iliac vessels. Note that RAAA requires open surgery.

Endovascular repair (EVAR) of AAA involves placement of prosthetic graft by a transfemoral/transiliac approach. This is suitable in approximately 60% of AAA (this figure is improving with advancing technology and techniques).

P : Mortality for emergency surgery is over 50%, mortality for elective surgery is under 5%.

Screening

In February 2009, the National Screening Committee launched AAA screening (AUS) for men aged 65. It is being introduced gradually and is expected to be fully up and running by 2013.

Useful hints and tips

In all suspected cases of leaking AAA, assess the patient using the ABCDE approach. After clearing the airway and breathing, insert two large-bore cannulas (16G or above) in both antecubital fossa and insert a urinary catheter to monitor UO, which is a measure of end-organ perfusion. Do not infuse too much fluid too quickly, as a sudden increase in blood pressure will disrupt any clots formed around the bleeding site.

Popliteal artery aneurysm

D : Popliteal artery aneurysm (PAA) has a diameter of more than 2 cm and accounts for four-fifths of all peripheral aneurysms.

I & S : The most common peripheral aneurysm. M > F. The general rule for PAA: greater than half the PAAs are found to be bilateral, up to half are associated with a coexistent AAA, and more than half the PAAs are asymptomatic.

A & P : Same aetiology, pathology and risk factors as for AAA (i.e. atherosclerosis in 90%). PAAs tend to thrombose rather than rupture (only 5% rupture).

CF&D:

> **Symptoms and signs**
> • Rest pain: progressive thrombosis of PAA.
> • Acute ischaemia: emboli or acute thrombosis.
> • DVT/venous insufficency: compression of popliteal vein and other surrounding veins.
> • Foot drop: compression of peroneal nerve, other neurological symptoms depending on the compressed nerve.
> • Rupture: 5% will rupture due to weak vessel wall with atherosclerosis.

Diagnosis is incidental (pulsatile mass found behind the knee). Half of patients will be symptomatic and undergo USS and then an angiogram to accurately define the vasculature and anatomy.

T&M: Surgical: bypass the PAA before it becomes completely thrombosed, use vein as bypass graft (higher long-term patency and therefore preferred) or synthetic PTFE grafts. There is still approximately 1% risk of limb amputation due to complications such as graft thrombosis.

P: Usually depends on the condition of the rest of the arteries but if left alone, there is a high chance of complications (outlined above). The 5-year patency for vein grafts is upto 94% and for prosthetic grafts upto 42%.

Carotid artery disease

D: Stenosis (abnormal narrowing) caused by atherosclerosis and plaque formation in the carotid arteries. If it affects the internal carotid artery (ICA), there is an increased risk of CVA, transient ischaemic attack (TIA) and retinal infarction.

I&S: Higher in males aged < 75 years and in females aged > 75 years.

A&P: Atherosclerosis can cause carotid artery stenosis, plaque rupture and thrombosis. Plaque and thrombus can embolize (break up into emboli) and occlude smaller branches causing TIAs and CVAs.

CF&D: Asymptomatic, amaurosis fugax, TIA and CVA. Patients with symptomatic 70% carotid artery stenosis have a greater than 30% risk of CVA and death, in a 2–3 year period, even with optimum medical treatment.

Diagnosis is with duplex USS. Other useful imaging may include angiogram, CTA, MRA, depending on the information required.

T&M: Carotid angioplasty and stenting, carotid endarterectomy.

> **Studies for evidence-based practice**
>
> *Surgery for asymptomatic stenosis*
> • Asymptomatic Carotid Atherosclerosis Study
> • Asymptomatic Carotid Surgery Trial

> *Surgery for symptomatic stenosis*
> - North American Symptomatic Carotid Endarterectomy Trial (NASCET)
> - European Carotid Surgery Trial
>
> Both studies included subjects with greater than 60% reduction in luminal diameter.

P: Patients are at high risk of developing ischaemic TIA and CVA from embolization, thrombosis and low flow.

> **Definitions**
>
> - *Amaurosis fugax*: temporary unilateral loss of vision due to temporary occlusion of the ICA and hence insufficient flow to the ophthalmic artery.
> - *Duplex USS*: combines ultrasound (sound waves reflecting off blood vessels) with Doppler ultrasonography (sound waves reflecting off moving objects) to create a dynamic picture.
> - *Emboli*: undissolved material carried in the bloodstream from one place to another.

Amputations

D: Irreversible removal of a limb or part of a limb that is no longer functional or is life-threatening.

I & S: Approximately 5500 annually in the UK. Mostly in males age > 65 years.

A & P: Atherosclerosis (plaque formation and progression) eventually blocks the vessel, and poorly controlled diabetes accelerates small-vessel disease and neuropathy. The combination leads to ischaemia.

C F & D: The patient's symptoms and clinical and radiological findings dictate the need for amputations, e.g. the poorly controlled diabetic patient with chronic ischaemia who has failed angioplasty to improve the circulation to the lower limb.

> **Indications for amputation**
>
> *Upper limb*
> - 5% of all amputations
> - More than half due to trauma
>
> *Lower limb (Western world)*
> - Peripheral vascular disease (85%, half have diabetes)
> - Failed arterial reconstruction
> - Unsalvageable limb associated with intractable rest pain
> - Trauma
> - Tumour for cure or palliation
> - Infection, with gangrene and non-healing ulcers

T & M : There are essentially many types of amputation, but we focus here on the two main types of lower limb amputation for end-stage peripheral vascular disease (EPVD).

	Transtibial/below-knee amputation	Transfemoral/above-knee amputation
Gold standard	Yes, procedure of choice	No, but most common for EPVD
Limb length	Preserved	Shorter limb length preserved
Mobility and rehabilitation	Most (80%) will walk	Less than half will walk, others will be wheelchair bound
Quality of life	Better. Preserving the knee joint provides better balance and ability to transfer	Poorer
Life expectancy	Live longer	5-year survival is less than in patients with Dukes B colon cancer
Complications	'Phantom limb' Progress to above-knee amputation Flexion contracture of knee predisposes to pressure ulcers Can impair sitting and transfer	'Phantom limb' Pressure ulcers Can progress to amputation at a higher level if the stump becomes ischaemic

P : As above. The healed mature amputation stump requires a well-fitting prosthesis.

> **Definitions**
>
> - *Below-knee amputation*: the posterior reconstructive transtibial flap method is commonly used.
> - *Phantom limb*: after amputation of a limb, the patient continues to experience pain from where the amputated limb used to be. This condition is very difficult to treat.

Varicose veins of the lower limbs

D : Swollen superficial veins due to incompetent valves. The deep venous system lies within muscles, and on contraction of the leg muscles venous blood is pumped towards the heart. The superficial veins (long and short saphenous veins) lie superficially and drain the skin and subcutaneous tissue of the lower limbs. The deep and superficial veins are connected by perforating veins which have one-way valves to prevent backflow of blood from the deep veins when muscle contracts.

I & S : 20-30% chance of developing varicose veins in lifetime in adult females, 10–15% in adult males. M/F ratio 1 : 4.

A & P : Incompetent valves, obstructed venous outflow tracts and inefficient muscle pump are the anatomical abnormalities found; there may be a weakness of the vein wall or congenital absence of valves (rare). Venous hypertension develops. Risk factors include age, female, heredity, obesity, familial, occupation (standing), trauma (bone fracture) to underlying vessels, DVT, pregnancy and idiopathic.

C F & D : Leg pain and heaviness, ankle swelling, night cramps or itching. Diagnosis is with duplex USS, for direction of blood flow and abnormal vein structure.

T & M : Conservative. Surgery for pain, phlebitis or skin changes.

Conservative

- Graduated compression stockings to relieve swelling and aching.

Conservative/surgical

- Injection sclerotherapy: chemical used to damage vessel wall. Needs 4–6 weeks of conservative treatment.
- Foam sclerotherapy: foam for larger vessels.

Surgical

- Ligation and stripping: tie off and remove the long saphenous or short saphenous vein.
- Endovenous laser ligation: heat used to close up the vein.

P : Left untreated, severe chronic venous disease develops (venous hypertension), which is associated with lipodermatosclerosis (chronic inflammation and fibrosis of the skin and subcutaneous tissues), pigmentation, ulcers, eczema and phlebitis. After surgery, varicose veins can recur due to incomplete procedure or vein regrowth.

Definitions

- *Doppler ultrasound test*: sound waves reflected off moving objects (e.g. blood cells) allows evaluation of blood flow through a vessel.
- *Duplex ultrasonography*: combines Doppler flow information and conventional imaging information (sometimes called B-mode) to allow physicians to see the structure of blood vessels. Duplex ultrasound shows blood flowing through vessels and measures the speed of blood flow. It can also be useful for estimating the diameter of a blood vessel as well as the degree of obstruction, if any, in the vessel.

Diabetic foot

D : Diabetic patients develop foot problems due to direct damage to their nerves and blood vessels caused by high blood glucose levels.

I & S : Foot ulcers affect 1 in 10 diabetics during the entirety of their condition. M > F.

A & P : High blood glucose dampens WBC function and, more importantly, damages the vascular endothelium, accelerating atherosclerosis, resulting in poor macro- and micro-circulation. Diabetics are at increased risk of developing infections, peripheral neuropathy, retinopathy and renal impairment/failure.

Risk factors of diabetic foot

- Infections of soft tissues: bacterial/fungal infections due to ingrown toenails for example are inadequately treated with antibiotics due to the poor circulation, becoming gangrenous limb-threatening infections.
- Poorly fitting footwear: blisters and cuts can become infected.
- Peripheral neuropathy: patient cannot sense minor trauma; left unnoticed may become severe lesions.
- Smoking: increased atherosclerosis and vasoconstriction of peripheral circulation leads to poor circulation and poor wound healing.

CF&D : There may be an obvious large wound/ulcer associated with erythema and pyrexia.

Symptoms and signs

- Pain or persistent pain: claudication on exercise (arterial diagnosis), underlying infection. Feel for a pulse to exclude ischaemic foot.
- Limp or difficulty in walking: infection, ill-fitting shoes, Charcot's joints (neuropathic).
- Warm erythema and migrating erythema: spreading cellulitis due to infection. Do not confuse with dependent hyperaemia in ischaemic limbs.
- Discharging pus: foul-smelling pus due to infection. Often associated with persistent pain and erythema.
- Swelling: infection, poor venous return. Feel for crepitus (gas in soft tissue).
- Pyrexia, rigors, confusion: bacteraemia, sepsis from infection.

Investigations

- Blood: FBC (look for ↑WCC), U&E (renal function), random glucose (may need to treat hyperglycaemia in sepsis), CRP (inflammatory reaction).
- Foot X-ray: soft tissue gas (gas gangrene), osteomyelitis, Charcot's joints.
- Duplex USS: to assess blood flow to the foot.

T&M : The main emphasis is on prevention and early recognition and treatment. This includes daily foot checks, daily moisturizing, regular toenail cutting, well-fitting footwear and good glycaemic control.

Treatment

- Angiogram and angioplasty to improve blood flow to aid healing.
- Débridement: clean the wound, remove pus, dead necrotic tissue and infected bone. May require skin grafting.

P: Depends on the problem. Smokers, older patients with longer history of uncontrolled diabetes, and those with gangrenous infections and large ulcers have poorer outcome.

> • Note: Approximately 90% with diabetes have type 2 diabetes.
> • Most complications of diabetes are related to vascular impairment.

Peripheral vascular disease

D: Arterial disease affecting the peripheral circulation; if severe enough causes ischaemic limb.

I&S: In the UK, approximately 5% of patients over age 50 are affected. M > F.

A&P: Smoking, diabetes, hypertension and hypercholesterolaemia are risk factors for atherosclerosis. Progressive atherosclerosis and plaque formation narrows and weakens the arteries, leading to PVD.

CF&D:

> **Symptoms and signs**
>
> • Intermittent claudication brought on by exercise, relieved by rest, usually in legs
> • Weakness, tiredness in legs, tingling or numbness
> • Leg pain at night relieved by hanging the leg down
> • Impotence
> • Non-healing ulcer
> • Gangrene

Ankle–brachial pressure index (ABPI) is one of the bedside tests used to assess PVD. Using hand-held Doppler (HHD) to hear the blood flow at the same time is useful.

> **ABPI**
>
> • > 1: rigid +/– calcified vessels (e.g. diabetics)
> • 1: normal
> • < 0.9: ischaemia
> • < 0.6: severe ischaemia
>
> Take care when interpreting ABPI in diabetics because they have higher ABPIs due to calcified vessels.
>
> **HHD**
>
> • Normal vessel: triphasic arterial signal
> • Ischaemic vessel: monophasic sound

Investigations

- Duplex USS: sound waves interpreted into images of blood flow.
- MRA: non-invasive imaging.
- CTA: contrast required, visualize vessels and treat.
- DSA: inject contrast to outline arteries, look for stenosis and blockages, can perform angioplasty and insertion of stent at the same time.

Fontaine classification of PVD

Stage I   Asymptomatic
Stage II   Intermittent claudication
Stage III   Rest pain/nocturnal pain
Stage IV   Necrosis/gangrene

T & M :

- Lifestyle modifications: diet and exercise, weight reduction, smoking cessation.
- Anti-atherosclerotic medication: antihypertensives, cholesterol-lowering drugs, antiplatelet drugs, tight glycaemic control.
- Interventional radiology: angioplasty and stent insertion is the gold standard procedure for stenosis or blocked peripheral arteries.
- Surgical: elective bypass procedure.

P :   Lifestyle modifications and management of risk factors can reduce symptoms and improve the circulation/prevent deterioration. Left untreated, PVD leads to amputation in approximately 1% per year, and critical ischaemia requiring intervention in 10% per year.

- Note: In a patient with healthy blood vessels, BP in the legs should be higher than in the arms.
- Stop metformin 48 hours before any iodinated contrast is given as metformin can alter renal function and precipitate lactic acidosis.

Acutely ischaemic limb

D :   A very short history (hours) of rest pain and pulselessness +/− other features.
I & S :   Depends on the cause of limb ischaemia.
A & P :   There is underlying atherosclerosis. The acute event is caused by thrombus, embolus or acute trauma.

Thrombus

- Origin: atheromatous debris
- Risk factors: hypotension/sepsis

> **Embolus**
>
> • Origin: cardiac, atheroma, FB/tumour
> • Risk factors: after myocardial infarction/AF

CF&D: A full cardiovascular examination is needed, including looking for chronic skin changes, listening for heart murmurs and bruits in the vessels, feeling for all pulses.

> **The 6 Ps**
>
> • Pain: indicates acute ischaemia
> • Pallor: advanced ischaemia may be associated with peripheral cyanosis
> • Pulseless: pulses not palpable due to decreased or obstructed flow
> • Perishing with cold: compared with 'normal' limb
> • Paraesthesia: nervous damage indicates limb-threatening ischaemia, treat urgently
> • Paralysis: muscle damage indicates limb-threatening ischaemia, treat urgently

Diagnosis of acute ischaemia is clinical.

T&M: Admit the patient with acute limb ischaemia. Take a good history, insert IV line and take bloods at the same time for FBC, U&E, inflammatory markers; ABG for metabolic state; ECG for arrhythmia or acute ischaemia; ABPI. Imaging of vascular tree may be required for thrombotic causes; Doppler USS to assess blood flow; CTA with contrast to look for arterial insufficiency.

> **Treatment**
>
> • The general rule in surgical and medical treatment: start heparin (prevents fibrin formation and clot propagation)
> • Embolic cause: embolectomy +/− fasciotomy and warfarin
> • Thrombosis: angiography or bypass surgery +/− fasciotomy

P: This condition is associated with high morbidity and mortality.

MCQs

AAA (Answers, see p. 302)

1 Regarding AAA, which of the following are true and which are false?
   a AAA has a diameter of 22 mm.
   b It is commoner in females.
   c Approximately 90% are located infrarenally.
   d There is an increased risk of AAA with Marfan's disease.
   e Arterial disease is a risk factor.

2 Which of the following are risk factors for AAA?
   a Smoking.
   b Hyperlipidaemia.
   c Positive family history.
   d Hypertension.
   e Respiratory disease.

3 Regarding AAA, which of the following are true and which are false?
   a Retroperitoneal RAAA has a better prognosis.
   b 50% of patients with AAA also have PAA.
   c RAAA will commonly present with abdominal pains radiating to the back.
   d EVAR is associated with higher morbidities postoperatively.
   e After an open AAA repair, the patient may require an embolectomy.

4 Regarding ruptured AAA, which of the following are true and which are false?
   a Approximately 15% of AAAs rupture.
   b 90% of patients die before reaching hospital.
   c Renal colic must be excluded first.
   d Loss of consciousness is a good prognostic indicator.
   e The initial management is erect CXR.

5 Which of the following are presentations of AAA?
   a Bleeding per rectum.
   b Loss of consciousness.
   c Bilateral lower limb ischaemia.
   d Tearing chest pain and pain between the scapulae.
   e Grey Turner's sign.

6 Regarding EVAR, which of the following are true and which are false?
   a All AAAs are amenable to EVAR.
   b Is associated with increased complication rates.
   c There is a 1% risk of AAA rupture after EVAR.
   d Complications include graft migration.
   e There is only one type of graft used for EVAR.

PAA (Answers, see p. 303)

1 Regarding PAA, which of the following are true and which are false?
   a PAA has a diameter greater than 2 cm.
   b It accounts for 80% of all aneurysms.
   c They are not associated with AAA.
   d The risk of rupture is greater than 20%.
   e Bypass surgery is indicated when the PAA becomes thrombosed.

2 Regarding PAA, which of the following are true and which are false?
   a PAA is usually bilateral in half the cases.
   b Foot drop is one of the presentations for PAA.

c A venous graft is preferred when performing a PAA bypass procedure.
d There is a 10% risk of amputation due to PAA thrombosis.
e Rest pain suggests progressive thrombosis of PAA.

3 Regarding bypass grafts, which of the following are true and which are false?
a Vein grafts can only be used when PTFE graft has failed.
b Only lower limb veins may be used as grafts.
c PTFE grafts have a lower risk of failure than vein grafts.
d Antibiotics are given after the graft has been successfully anastamosed.
e Heavy vicryl sutures are used to anastomose the graft.

Carotid artery stenosis (Answers, see p. 304)

1 Which of the following are risk factors for carotid artery disease?
a Anorexia.
b Diabetes.
c Hypotension.
d Cigarette smoking.
e Atrial fibrillation.

2 Which of the following are symptoms of carotid artery disease?
a Amaurosis fugax.
b Slurred speech.
c Difficulty swallowing.
d CVA.
e Asymptomatic.

3 Which of the following are used in the diagnosis of carotid artery disease?
a Hand-held Doppler probe.
b Doppler ultrasound.
c DSA.
d MRA.
e Plain neck X-ray.

4 A 61-year-old smoker is admitted under the medics with slurred speech and visual disturbances. On questioning the patient, he tells you that he has hypercholesterolaemia and hypertension, and that he has had one similar episode 6 months ago. What is the investigation of choice?
a Doppler ultrasound.
b Tilt table test.
c HbA_{1c} blood test.
d CT brain.
e Echocardiography.

5 A 55-year-old man who had a TIA 1 week ago has been referred to the vascular team with 75% right carotid artery stenosis. What is the best method for reducing his risk of CVA?

a Encourage dieting.
b Carotid endarterectomy.
c Start antihypertensives.
d Cardiac angioplasty.
e Carotid angioplasty.

6 A 60-year-old woman is 1 day post carotid endarterectomy and is complaining of a hoarse voice. What is the most likely cause?
a Trauma caused by endotracheal tube.
b Dry mouth and throat.
c Viral laryngitis.
d Greater auricular nerve damage.
e Recurrent laryngeal nerve damage.

Amputations (Answers, see p. 305)

1 Regarding amputations, which of the following are true and which are false?
a It is a reversible procedure.
b There are only two types of amputations in the lower limb.
c This is the first-line treatment for an infected diabetic foot.
d Trauma is the commonest reason for an amputation in the UK.
e There are no associated complications associated with amputations.

2 Regarding below-knee amputations, which of the following are true and which are false?
a The mortality associated with BKA is higher than those with AKA.
b There is a greater chance of rehabilitation compared to AKA.
c Flexion contracture is one of the complications associated with BKA.
d Is the procedure of choice for EPVD.
e Is the only option for EPVD.

3 Regarding above-knee amputations, which of the following are true and which are false?
a Is the procedure of choice for EPVD.
b The 5-year survival is better than those with Dukes B colon cancer.
c The majority of patients will become wheelchair bound.
d 'Phantom limb' is one of the complications associated with AKA.
e Involves less metabolic stress and is therefore better than BKA.

Varicose veins (Answers, see p. 305)

1 Which of the following are symptoms of varicose veins?
a Cold legs.
b Joint pains.
c Leg weakness.
d Dry, itchy skin over the varicose vein.
e Swollen legs.

2 Regarding varicose vein surgery, which of the following are true and which are false?

a The recurrence rate after varicose vein surgery is up to 60%.
b The surgical procedure is called ligation and stripping.
c Is safer than sclerotherapy.
d Is usually a day-case procedure.

3 Which of the following are used in the diagnosis of varicose veins?
  a Lower limb X-rays.
  b MRA.
  c Doppler scan for blood flow.
  d Duplex scan for images of vein structure.
  e CTA.

4 Which of the following are involved in the management of varicose veins?
  a Compression stocking.
  b Sclerotherapy.
  c Hormone replacement therapy.
  d Vein transplantation.
  e Endovenous laser treatment.

5 Which of the following are the complications of varicose veins?
  a Chronic venous insufficiency.
  b Haemosiderin deposition.
  c DVT.
  d Leg ulcers.
  e Bleeding.

6 When consenting a patient for varicose vein surgery, which of the following complications must be explained?
  a Bleeding.
  b Wound infection.
  c Damage to sensory nerves.
  d Thromboembolism.
  e Anaesthetic complications.

Diabetic foot (Answers, see p. 306)

1 Which of the following can cause foot infections in diabetics?
  a Trauma.
  b Foot deformities.
  c New shoes.
  d Heel blisters.
  e Daily feet examination.

2 Regarding Charcot's foot, which of the following are true and which are false?
  a Occurs in type 1 diabetics.
  b Occurs in type 2 diabetics.
  c Describes the beginning of diabetic neuropathy.
  d Results in internal fractures.
  e Is easy to diagnose.

3 A 70-year-old diabetic with known PVD and chronic bilateral foot ulcers presents to the outpatient clinic with increasing right foot pain. On examination, both his femoral pulses are present. What is the best management option?
a Patient education.
b Regular clinical examination.
c Surgical débridement of ulcers.
d Amputation.
e Angiogram +/– angioplasty.

4 A 66-year-old diabetic woman who has had previous femoral artery to femoral artery cross-over surgery presents with increasing left foot pain. On examination, pulses are present in both groins and in the graft. What investigation should you request?
a Duplex scan.
b Angiogram.
c MRA.
d CTA.
e Radionuclide scan.

5 A 55-year-old man with diabetic peripheral neuropathy presents with a neuropathic ulcer on his heel. What is the management?
a Amputation.
b Analgesia and antibiotics.
c Special footwear and regular clinical examination.
d Bypass surgery.
e Débridement of non-viable tissue and wound care.

6 A 48-year-old diabetic patient has been admitted with DKA. On examination, there is an erythematous, boggy area on his left foot over a small ulcer which is the likely cause of his DKA. What is the best management after resuscitating the patient?
a USS to look for a collection.
b CT scan to assess the bones and look for infection.
c Ask for surgical consult with a view to surgery.
d MRA to assess the soft tissues.
e Plain foot X-ray to look for osteomyelitis.

Peripheral vascular disease (Answers, see p. 307)

1 Regarding investigations for PVD, which of the following are true and which are false?
a DSA is the first-line investigation for patients with PVD.
b DSA is only used if intervention is planned at the same procedure.
c The only disadvantage of DSA is allergic reaction to iodinated contrast and exposure to ionizing radiation.
d Duplex ultrasound requires contrast to visualize the vessels.
e MRA cannot be used in patients with metallic implants.

2 Regarding chronic lower limb ischaemia, which of the following are true and which are false?

a ABPI is less than 0.9.
b Rest pain is worst when standing.
c Ulcers classically present on the shin.
d Toe pressures are helpful in diabetic patients.
e Pentoxifylline has proven to be very useful.

3 Other causes of PVD include which of the following?
   a Emboli.
   b Inflammatory.
   c Infective.
   d Acquired.
   e Trauma.

4 A 29-year-old white male who is a heavy smoker presents with a 2-week history of rest pain in his left foot associated with redness and swelling. Which of the following management options are appropriate?
   a The history of claudication is important.
   b Take blood tests to exclude infection in his foot.
   c Ask the patient to stop smoking.
   d Examine for all peripheral pulses and for an AAA.
   e Arrange an urgent duplex scan.

5 A thin 55-year-old farmer presents to the vascular outpatient department with a 2-year history of worsening buttock claudication and impotence associated with back pain. He has been smoking 30 cigarettes per day for over 30 years. All his peripheral pulses are present but the femoral pulses are weak. Which of the following management options are appropriate?
   a Ask the patient to stop smoking.
   b Abdominal USS.
   c MRA.
   d Book immediately for theatre.
   e Advise lifestyle modifications.

6 Which of the following medications may be appropriate for a patient with PVD?
   a Aspirin.
   b Atenolol.
   c Folic acid and vitamin B_6.
   d Insulin.
   e Simvastatin.

7 A 56-year-old smoker presents with a 2-year history of right leg pain worsened by exercise and relieved with rest. The symptoms are getting worse and he would like surgery for the pain. What is your next management option?
   a Take a thorough history and examine the patient.
   b Request an MRI scan to rule out sciatica.
   c Request USS to measure the abdominal aorta.
   d Advise exercise, analgesia and reassure patient.
   e Duplex ultrasound to locate site of lesion.

Ischaemic limb (Answers, see p. 309)

1 A 60-year-old diabetic arteriopath presents with a pulseless pale right foot associated with shortness of breath. Which of the following features indicate acute limb ischaemia?
   a Onset of sudden foot pain during rest, in the last 3 hours.
   b Pain on/off in the last 1 year.
   c Leg pain on exertion relieved with rest.
   d Worsening leg pain over the last 3 months.
   e Leg pain after a fall onto the leg.

2 Which of the following are symptoms and signs of acute limb ischaemia?
   a Pallor.
   b Pulseless.
   c Persistent hypotension.
   d Paralysis.
   e Pigmentation.

3 Which of the following factors predispose to acute thrombosis?
   a Hypertension.
   b Thrombocytopenia.
   c Malignancy.
   d Polycythaemia.
   e Sinus tachycardia.

4 Which of the following are causes of acute limb ischaemia?
   a Obesity.
   b Trauma.
   c Popliteal aneurysm.
   d Iatrogenic injury.
   e Embolism.

5 A 65-year-old woman who is usually chair-bound is admitted with a 2-week history of continuous left foot pain which is getting worse, and which is only mildly relieved by hanging her left leg from the side of her bed. Her history includes meningioma with associated seizures, CVA affecting the left side of her body, and diet-controlled diabetes. On examination, she has fixed contractures at the left knee and hip; her left foot smells infected, with erythema and oedema, no pulses on left side except the popliteal artery. There are monophasic signals on HHD. On elevating her leg, there is blanching. What are your immediate management options?
   a Analgesia and keep NBM.
   b Duplex followed by MRA +/− angioplasty.
   c BKA.
   d AKA.
   e Book this patient for femoral embolectomy.

6 A 72-year-old man with type 2 diabetes and a history of previous CVA affecting the right side of his body was admitted with a 1-month history of increasing left

leg pain and 1 week of black discoloration of the first web space. He has an exercise tolerance of 50 m and suffers from nocturnal rest pain. He had been mobile until pain. On HHD there are dampened biphasic signals in the foot vessels, indicating limited blood flow. What is your management?

a Admit for duplex to exclude superior femoral artery occlusion.

b MRA+/– angioplasty.

c Amputation of big toe.

d BKA.

e Femoral embolectomy.

EMQs (Answers, see p. 310)

1 Diagnosis of aneurysms. Options:

a Leaking AAA.

b PAA.

c Ultrasound.

d CT abdomen.

e MRA.

g Thoracic aneurysm.

h DVT.

For each case below choose the single most likely diagnosis or investigation from the above list of options. Each option may be used once, more than once or not at all.

(i) A 60-year-old smoker, with no other medical problems, presented with a 24-hour history of generalized back pain radiating to the groin. On examination, there is a tender pulsatile mass palpable in his epigastric region, and he has 3+ bloods on his urine dipstick.

(ii) A 70-year-old woman has recently been diagnosed with a 4.5-cm diameter abdominal aorta and requires 6-monthly follow-up to check the size of the aorta.

(iii) A 45-year-old man with haemophilia B presents with continuous left leg pain, worse on exercising. On examination, there is an adequate left femoral pulse but there are no pulses palpable distally.

(iv) An 80-year-old man with a 7-cm diameter abdominal aorta is complaining of vague abdominal and back pains for 3 weeks, associated with episodes of dizziness.

(v) A 55-year-old man has a severe chronic foot ulcer, associated with a thrombosis in the right popliteal artery. He requires an operation to alleviate his symptoms.

2 Peripheral vascular disease. Options:

a ABPI.

b Pseudoaneurysm.

c Berger's test.

d Gangrene.

e Amputation.

f DVT.

For each case below choose the single most likely diagnosis or investigation from the above list of options. Each option may be used once, more than once or not at all.

(i) Mr C. is a 50-year-old man who was discharged yesterday after a right total knee replacement 3 days ago. He now presents with a very tender, enlarged, engorged right lower limb associated with sensory loss over the L5 distribution. On examination, both distal pulses are weak and there is a prominent popliteal pulse.

(ii) Mr P. is a 68-year-old man who had a partial gastrectomy for adenocarcinoma 5 months ago. He has developed a tender swollen left leg with patches of dark blue discoloration over his toes in the last 24 hours.

(iii) Mrs J. is a 64-year-old retired hairdresser who has presented with a 2-week history of worsening left leg pain. Her husband is increasingly worried as her left leg has become very swollen, blue and blistered.

(iv) Mr T. is a 29-year-old smoker who presents to vascular clinic with worsening painful leg pain. You examine him on the couch. His legs are pale, hairless and cold to touch but on moving the legs into a dependent position, there is reactive hyperaemia. Pulses are difficult to feel on both sides but audible with HHD. What is the next bedside test?

(v) A 90-year-old man with extensive PVD and uncontrolled diabetes is admitted with right toe infection. On examination, the toe is black and smelly and the foot is cellulitic, with erythema extending proximally towards the knee.

3 Vascular operations. Options:
a Femoro-femoral cross-over.
b Angioplasty +/− stent.
c Femoral endarterectomy.
d Femoro-distal bypass.
e Axillo-bifemoral bypass.
f Amputation.

For each case below choose the single most likely operation from the above list of options. Each option may be used once, more than once or not at all.

(i) A 56-year-old man with a history of IDDM presents with gradually worsening left leg pain associated with a non-healing ulcer on his big toe. The pain is worse on exercise and better on resting. He has failed medical therapy and on MRA there is a femoral artery stenosis.

(ii) A 62-year-old man had an angioplasty and stenting of his right femoral artery 8 months ago but is now complaining of intolerable resting right leg pain associated with mottling discoloration in his foot. There is a high suspicion of occluded femoral artery.

(iii) A 70-year-old man who is fit and well has presented with right leg claudication. The MRA has revealed a calcified aorta with total occlusion of the right iliac artery.

(iv) A 59-year-old woman has had bilateral BKAs after a car accident 10 years ago. She now presents with non-healing bilateral stump pressure ulcers associated with rest pain. MRA shows extensive aortic atherosclerosis and bilateral iliac artery stenosis.

(v) A 49-year-old man presents with right leg rest pain which is gradually getting worse, disturbing his sleep and making him house-bound. On investigation, he has a short stenosis in the distal right femoral artery and a right popliteal aneurysm.

4 Varicose vein clinic. Options:
a Problem in the deep venous system.
b Problem in the superficial venous system.
c Saphenofemoral ligation and stripping of the long saphenous vein and multiple avulsions.
d Sclerotherapy.
e Compression hosiery/compression bandaging.
For each case below choose the single most appropriate answer from the above list of options. Each option may be used once, more than once or not at all.

(i) A 30-year-old woman presents with extensive right-sided varicose veins associated with heaviness and aching. She previously had a fracture of the right tibia 5 years ago in a car accident. On bilateral Perthes' testing, both limbs become engorged and painful.

(ii) A 50-year-old woman presents with a 30-year history of extensive bilateral varicose veins associated with itching. The mid-thigh tourniquet test causes most of the varicose veins to disappear and duplex ultrasound excludes deep venous cause for her varicose veins.

(iii) A 61-year-old obese woman who had a DVT 4 years ago presents for the first time with ulceration in the gaiter area associated with eczema and pigmentation.

(iv) A 39-year-old woman who had a varicose vein operation 2 years ago (stripping and ligation of long saphenous vein) presents with varicose veins below her left knee.

(v) A 63-year-old woman who is usually fit and well has presented in vascular clinic with recurrent superficial thrombophlebitis.

Part 7 Orthopaedic
18 Orthopaedics

Brachial plexus injury (see Appendix 3)
Usually classified as birth injury or later life injury.

Birth
D : Injury to brachial plexus roots (C5 to T1) during birth (resulting in Erb's or Klumpke's palsy).
A & P : Obstetric (delivery-related) trauma. Most are postganglionic (trunk injury).

Lesion	Example	Clinical features
Upper root	Paralysis of abductors and external rotators. Occurs during delivery	Erb's palsy (C5, C6 +/− C7): extended elbow and wrist and finger flexion, palm faces up ('waiter's tip' position of hand and arm) Sensation loss C5, C6
Lower root	Weakness in pronators of forearm, wrist and finger flexors. Horner's syndrome if cervical sympathetic chain involved. Accounts for <1% of brachial plexus palsies	Klumpke's paralysis (C8, T1): weak intrinsic muscles of the hand, leading to claw hand. Sensation loss C8, T1

C F & D : Diagnosis is clinical, plus MRI and electromyography.
T & M : Physiotherapy, nerve grafting (from 3 months onwards), contracture surgery (later still).

Adult
D : Brachial plexus lesions due to adult trauma to upper limbs and neck.
I & S : Young adults, M > F.
A & P : Usually traction injury from motorcycle accidents, direct trauma after fall, penetrating gunshot or knife injury. Suspect brachial plexus injury if pain around neck and shoulder with neurovascular symptoms/findings in upper limbs.

EMQs and MCQs for Surgical Finals, 1st edition.   © Hye-Chung Kwak, Imran Bhatti, Jaskarn Rai, Farhan Rashid, Bachittar Singh Jassar, Murthy Nyasavajjala, Viren Asher, Jon Lund and Mike Larvin. Published 2011 by Blackwell Publishing Ltd.

CF&D: Diagnosis is clinical, plus MRI (anatomical patter of injury) and electromyography (extent of functional damage).
T&M: Depends on the cause.

Conservative treatment

- Some stretch injuries, low-velocity gunshots

Surgery

- Immediate exploration of penetrating injuries with a view to end-to-end repair
- Immediate débridement and delayed repair for blunt injuries
- Nerve grafting for preganglionic (root avulsion) injuries

P: Most recovery spontaneously as postganglionic. Overall prognosis depends on the initial injury, age of patient and type of management. Preganglionic injuries have poorer outcome.

Radial nerve injury or entrapment (see Appendix 3)
D: The radial nerve (C5–C8, sensory from T1) is predominantly a motor nerve responsible for extending the fingers, wrists and elbow. Injury to the radial nerve results in wrist drop. Testing the extension of these gives clue as to the level of injury.
I&S: Radial nerve injury can occur at any age. No gender predilection. Radial nerve entrapment is the least common of the three major nerves of the upper limbs.
A&P: Varies (see table below).

Lesion	Cause	Outcome and treatment
Very high	Pressure in axilla affecting lower half of brachial plexus ('Saturday night' palsy) Fracture/dislocation of humerus	Unable to extend wrist or fingers, sensory loss over dorsum of first web space and thumb base. Usually complete recovery over weeks/ months. Splint wrist and finger drop
High	Fracture mid-humerus (radial nerve in radial groove) Prolonged tourniquet usage	Motor: wrist drop (loss of wrist/digit extensors), forearm supinators. Spares triceps Sensory: variable, dorsoradial region hand, dorsal aspect of radial 3½ digits
Low	Fracture at elbow, forearm or radius	Motor: loss of extension of the carpophalangeal joints Sensory territory: as above

(cont'd)

Lesion	Cause	Outcome and treatment
Chronic compression	Posterior interossous nerve compression	Weak wrist and digit extensors Sensation posterior aspect wrist

CF&D: History/examination. Nerve conduction/velocity studies confirm location. MRI may be required.

T&M: Depends on the level and cause of injury. Conservative (immobilization and analgesia) or surgery for entrapment; trauma may require exploration.

P: Nerves grow 1 mm/day. Prognosis best with neuropraxia; worst for neurotmesis.

Ulnar nerve palsy (see Appendix 3)

D: Ulnar nerve supplies half of flexor digitorum profundus (FDP), the lumbricals to ring and little fingers and all interossei. Ulnar nerve injury anywhere along its course can result in claw hand.

I&S: Can occur at any age, more likely in older patients. M = F.

A&P: Trauma, rheumatoid arthritis, diabetes, ganglion, tumour may all cause ulnar nerve palsy.

CF&D: History and examination. Tinel's sign at elbow (tap the ulnar nerve in the ulnar groove and over the cubital tunnel): the test is positive if the patient experiences paraesthesia over the areas supplied by the ulnar nerve.

Diagnosis is with USS (measure nerve diameter before and after compression), conduction studies and MRI can localize injury.

Lesion	Cause	Result
Elbow	Ulnar half of FDP is paralysed and the fingers are therefore straighter	Motor: wasting interossei on hand dorsum, weakness of finger and thumb abduction and adduction resulting in mild claw hand. Positive Froment's test (see below). Sensory loss little finger and ulnar half ring
	The ulnar nerve may be irritated in cubital tunnel by repeated activities	Cubital tunnel syndrome: numbness and tingling, weakness +/− clawing in ring and little fingers
Wrist	Fracture: there is unopposed action of the extensors and FDP, causing clawing	As above but more marked Claw hand: MCP hyperextension ring/little finger, flexion same interphalangeal joints. Less in Guyon's entrapment
	Irritation of ulnar nerve as it passes Guyon's canal	Numbness/tingling little finger, ulnar half ring

T & M : Analgesia, splint, elbow pads, corticosteroid injections, physiotherapy. Operative decompression can provide good relief. Elbow decompression may require anterior transposition if nerve subluxing.

P : 95% of patients have good outcome from surgery.

> **Froment's test for ulnar nerve palsy (any level)**
>
> Ask the patient to grip a piece of paper between thumb and the proximal phalanx of the index finger. If paper pulls out easily test is positive.

Carpal tunnel syndrome

D : Compression of median nerve as it passes under flexor retinaculum (carpal tunnel) at wrist.

I & S : Affects 1 in 20 females and 3 in 10 males, usually aged 45–65 years.

A & P : Oedematous inflamed tissues in carpal tunnel compress nerve. Hereditary, an increased risk in rheumatoid arthritis, diabetes, acromegaly, lupus and hypothyroidism, plus other rare causes.

C F & D : Symptoms worse at night as wrist is flexed in sleep, or when wrist flexed (e.g. reading). Paraesthesia in thumb, index finger, middle finger and half ring finger. Palm unaffected as palmar branch arises proximal to wrist, passes anterior to retinaculum. Thenar eminence wasting if severe.

Diagnosis with Tinel's test (light tap over wrist reproduces sensory symptoms), Phalen test (hyperflexing wrist for 60 s), nerve conduction studies, MRI.

T & M : Treat primary medical problem such as rheumatoid arthritis; wrist splint, corticosteroids, carpal tunnel decompression surgery (divide flexor retinaculum).

P : The majority of patients recover completely after surgery.

> **LOAF: motor branch of the median nerve supply**
>
> First two Lumbricals and thenar eminence muscles (Opponens pollicis, Abductor and Flexor pollicis brevis).

Shoulder dislocation

D : Usually anterior glenohumeral joint dislocation occurs after the humeral head moves anteriorly away from the glenoid cavity of the scapula, often with tearing of the capsule and glenoidal labrum (fibrocartilagienous 'lip'). Posterior dislocations are very rare.

> Posterior shoulder dislocations are uncommon and caused by trauma (epileptic seizures or electrocution). There may be a posterior bulge but they are easily missed due to the subtle signs. AP X-ray may give a misleading impression of the humeral head sitting in the glenoid, and may show the 'light bulb' sign (due to internal rotation, the greater tuberosity is not seen).

I & S : Approximately 95% are anterior, generally healthy young male adults or older females.

A & P :   Caused by direct trauma or falling onto hand.

C F & D :   Always assess for neurovascular compromise.

Look
- Loss of curved contour of deltoid muscle +/– anterior bulge
- Patient supports affected upper limb using other hand

Feel
- The humeral head is displaced anteriorly

Move
- Severe pain so reluctant to move, difficult abduction and internal rotation
- Assess deltoid power post reduction

Radiography
- AP and axillary lateral view or trans-scapular 'Y' view to assess relation of humeral head to glenoid and any associated fracture
- Humeral head under the coracoid process on AP view indicates anterior dislocation. Humeral head in front of the 'Y' on axillary lateral view

Neurovascular
- Check arterial circulation: radial, brachial and axillary pulses
- Check axillary nerve (sensation of 'regimental badge' area over deltoid); radial nerve (test extension of thumb, wrist, elbow, and sensation over hand dorsum)

Diagnosis is usually clear on history and examination of both shoulders, confirmed by radiographs.

T & M :   Non-operative reduction under sedation/LA using Hippocratic method, or reduction under GA. Surgical repair/reconstruction may be required for recurrence. Repeat radiographs after reduction to confirm position, then immobilize to allow healing of muscles and ligaments.

P :   Return to normal in 6–8 weeks with physiotherapy. Higher chance of recurrence in younger patients; up to 50% under 40 years will recur. MRI to diagnose predisposing bony/soft tissue defect.

Hippocratic method of reduction

1 Hold the affected arm by the wrist and apply traction at 45° angle.
2 Ask assistant to provide countertraction by wrapping a sheet around the patient's torso.

Colles' fracture

D :   The most common form of distal radial fracture, usually about 2.5 cm from the articular surface. There is posterior angulation and translation, impaction, radial angulation, supination +/– an associated ulnar styloid fracture. In combination this produces the classic dorsally displaced 'dinner-fork' deformity.

I & S : The most common upper limb fracture; bimodal age distribution (teenagers and elderly).

A & P : Caused by falls onto outstretched hand, other trauma.

C F & D : History (acute pain, 'pins and needles', numbness). Look, Feel and Move ('dinner fork' deformity, bruising, swelling, tenderness). Check ulnar styloid and radial head at elbow to rule out associated fractures. Neurovascular examination mandatory.

Diagnosis with plain AP and lateral X-rays. Fractures divided into intra-articular (involving joint), more difficult to treat, and extra-articular; distal radial angulation and displacement; comminuted (more than two bone fragments), also more difficult to treat. If bone breaches skin (compound fracture) patient must be taken to theatre as soon as possible.

T & M : Minimally displaced/deformed, backslab applied; deformed/displaced, closed reduction to restore anatomy before backslab applied. Full cast once swelling subsided. Post-reduction X-ray to assess reduction. Follow-up in orthopaedic fracture clinic.

P : Usually heals in 6–8 weeks.

- *Smith's fracture*: reverse deformity to Colles' fracture, with volar (towards palm) displacement of the distal segment resulting in 'garden spade' deformity.
- *Barton's fracture*: intra-articular fracture of the wrist, oblique fracture line runs into the joint causing the hand and anterior part of distal radius to move forward.

Smith's and Barton's fractures reduced in opposite direction to Colles'. Above elbow cast applied with wrist dorsiflexed, forearm supinated. May require open reduction (and anterior plate).

Fractured neck of femur

D : This is a common serious fracture, and may disrupt the blood supply to the femoral head. It is associated with a high morbidity and mortality (10%). The blood supply to femoral head depends on cervical vessels in the joint capsular retinaculum which is damaged in displaced fractures; on intramedullary vessels which are always torn; and on the ligamentum teres, which contributes minimally in old age or may be absent.

I & S : In the UK, about 75 000 hip fractures annually, 80% in females, average age 80 years.

A & P : Usually elderly ladies with osteoporosis and prone to falls, or minor trauma in patients with osteoporosis or osteomalacia; in young patients, high-velocity trauma.

C F & D : History, typically an elderly female unable to weight-bear/mobilize due to pain after a fall on the affected side. Examination: lower limb shortening, adduction and external rotation, tender anterior and lateral hip joint, all movement painful. AP X-ray pelvis (to show both hips), follow Shenton's lines from the top of obturator foramen to the inner femoral neck; lateral X-ray assesses displacement. If no fracture is seen but high clinical suspicion, consider MRI (marrow oedema), bone scan (fracture uptake) or CT (good for comminuted fracture).

Two groups of fractures according to level

Group	Subdivisions	Description and treatment
Intracapsular (femoral neck)	Subcapital	The proximal segment often loses its blood supply, risk of avascular necrosis (AVN)
	Transcervical	
	Basicervical	*Garden's classification*:
		I /II: undisplaced neck of femur (I incomplete, II complete). Conservative or dynamic hip screw
		III/IV: displaced neck of femur (III in contact, IV no contact). Require hemiarthroplasty or total arthroplasty (hip replacement)
Extracapsular (trochanters)	Intertrochanteric	The joint capsule and blood supply is intact, heals better
	Subtrochanteric	Dynamic hip screw (DHS): reduces pain and helps early mobilization

T & M : Assess initially with ABCDE algorithm, insert two large-bore IV cannulas, take FBC, clotting and G&S, resuscitate patient with warm IV crystalloids, oxygen, and ensure adequate analgesia. Aim of surgery is to avoid AVN and allow rapid mobilization.

P : Surgical prognosis is good.

Treatment of femoral head fractures by Garden classification

Mnemonic: 1 and 2, screw; 3 and 4, head to the floor
Garden I/II fractures can be treated with internal fixation using screws and Garden III (partially displaced) or IV (total displacement) fractures can be reduced (closed or open) and internally fixated, or treated with total or partial primary prosthetic replacement of the hip joint.

Osteoarthritis of knee

D : Degenerative joint disease with progressive loss of hyaline articular cartilage with new bone formation and capsular fibrosis.

I & S : OA affects 8.5 million in UK. M/F ratio 1 : 2, usually >50 years old.

A & P : Primary OA occurs with loss of water content in cartilage; secondary OA occurs with trauma, obesity, gout and diabetes.

C F & D : History and examination. Pain, usually worse at night (hyperaemia, venous stasis), stiffness, decreased range of movement, localized swelling. Look for knee movement, deformity, e.g. fixed flexion, varus or valgus, synovitis or effusion. Blood tests to exclude other forms of arthritis such as rheumatoid arthritis.

Four cardinal radiological features: subchondral cysts, osteophytes, loss of joint space, subchondral sclerosis (new bone formation). MRI has little to add to plain radiographs in OA.

T & M : Lifestyle (gentle exercise, lose weight), medical (capsaicin cream, analgesia, intra-articular steroid injection), surgical options for severe OA.

> **Surgical procedures**
>
> - *Arthroscopy*: can be used for diagnosis; irrigation for loose bodies, débride cartilage. Provides temporary relief.
> - *Osteotomy*: for localized OA, realigns joint. Good pain relief but may require arthroplasty in the future.
> - *Arthroplasty*: total or partial knee replacement. Improves pain and restores function.
> - *Arthrodesis*: fusion of the joint. Improves pain.

P : Pain is relieved and mobility improved by surgery.

MCQs
Brachial plexus injuries (Answers, see p. 313)

1 Which of the following are causes of brachial plexus injuries?
   a Stab injury to the neck.
   b Low-energy trauma.
   c Fall onto the shoulder.
   d Obstetric trauma.
   e Gunshot wounds.

2 Which of the following are good prognostic indicators in brachial plexus injury?
   a Older age.
   b Preganglionic injury.
   c Postganglionic injury.
   d Lack of patient understanding.
   e Female.

3 A 30-year-old man came off his motorcycle at high speed 2 weeks ago, landing on his right shoulder. He sustained multiple injuries including bilateral upper limb fractures and head and neck injuries. He has had both upper limbs internally fixed. He has recovered from a period of coma managed conservatively and is now fully awake, but complaining of intractable burning pain down his right arm. What is the most likely cause of his pain?
   a Incorrect positioning during upper limb surgery.
   b Oedema after upper limb surgery.
   c Simple musculoskeletal pain.
   d Inadequate analgesia.
   e Brachial plexus injury.

Radial nerve injury or entrapment (Answers, see p. 313)

1 Typically in a 'Saturday night' palsy, which of the following are present?
   a There is wrist extension.
   b There is elbow extension.
   c There is finger extension.
   d The hand is pronated (palm down).
   e Decreased sensation in the hand.

2 Fracture dislocation of the humerus after trauma is a cause of radial nerve injury. What are the complications of open reduction and internal fixation of the humerus?
a Infection.
b Damage to the nerve during surgery.
c Wound dehiscence.
d Venous thrombosis.
e Non-union of humerus.

3 A 22-year-old man who smells of alcohol has presented to the emergency department with numbness and diminished sensation to his left arm and hand. He tells you that he woke up to find weak and numb wrist and fingers. What would you like to do next?
a A thorough neurological examination.
b Nerve conduction studies.
c MRI scans of his brachial plexus.
d FBC and electrolytes.
e Call the trauma team.

Ulnar nerve palsy (Answers, see p. 314)

1 Which of the following are causes of ulnar nerve palsy?
a Idiopathic.
b Drugs used in general anaesthesia.
c Trauma.
d Compression during surgical procedures.
e Rheumatoid arthritis.

2 Which of the following should be used in the diagnosis of ulnar nerve palsy?
a Nerve conduction studies.
b Ultrasound.
c History and examination.
d MRI.
e Histological analysis.

3 Which of the following are complications of ulnar nerve palsy?
a Deformity of the forearm.
b Partial loss of sensation in the hand.
c Pain on moving the digits.
d Weak wrist muscles.
e Intractable pain.

4 Which of the following indicate a poor surgical prognosis in ulnar nerve surgery?
a Young age.
b Multiple trauma patients.
c The presence of ulnar nerve responses.
d Atrophy of muscles innervated by the ulnar nerve.
e Diabetes.

Carpal tunnel syndrome (Answers, see p. 314)

1 Which of the following are risk factors for carpal tunnel syndrome?
   a Wrist fracture.
   b Pregnancy.
   c Occupation.
   d Male sex.
   e Anorexia.

2 Which of the following are symptoms of carpal tunnel syndrome?
   a Weakness.
   b Numbness.
   c Pins and needles.
   d Burning sensation.
   e Ischaemia.

3 Which of the following should be used in the diagnosis of carpal tunnel syndrome?
   a Tinel's test is usually positive.
   b X-ray.
   c Nerve conduction studies.
   d Radionuclide scans.
   e Ultrasound scans of the wrist.

4 Which of the following are used in the non-surgical treatment of carpal tunnel syndrome?
   a NSAIDs.
   b Corticosteroid injection.
   c Elbow back slab.
   d Shoulder exercises.
   e Wrist splints.

5 A 45-year-old diabetic woman presents to outpatient clinic with a 6-month history of 'pins and needles' in her dominant hand, together with clumsiness of her thumb and index finger. Diabetes is present and has been well controlled for some time. What is the next option?
   a Further investigations.
   b Change her antidiabetic medications.
   c List her for a median nerve decompression.
   d Advise conservative measures.
   e Refer to physiotherapist.

6 A 29-year-old woman who is 8 months pregnant presents to the neurology outpatient department with a 3-month history of burning pains in both her hands. Her symptoms are worse at night when the pain wakes her from sleep. What is your management of this patient?
   a Refer to hand clinic for median nerve decompression.
   b Advise analgesia and light exercises.

c Wrist splint to be worn at night time.
d Refer for further investigations.
e Corticosteroid injection.

Shoulder dislocation (Answers, see p. 315)

1 Which of the following are causes of shoulder dislocation?
 a Contact sports.
 b Falls.
 c Throwing an object.
 d Epileptic fits.
 e Reaching to catch an object.

2 A 22-year-old inebriated man presents to A&E with a painful right shoulder after a fall. There is an anterior bulge in the shoulder and trans-scapular 'Y' X-ray reveals a humeral head in front of the 'Y'. What is the diagnosis?
 a Posterior dislocation.
 b Undisplaced fracture of the scapula.
 c Fractured clavicle.
 d Anterior shoulder dislocation.
 e Acromioclavicular subluxation.

3 In dislocated shoulder, the arm is typically held in which of the following positions?
 a Abduction and external rotation.
 b Adduction and forward flexion.
 c Adduction and internal rotation.
 d Abduction and internal rotation.
 e Adduction and external rotation.

4 Which of the following are complications of anterior dislocations?
 a Damage to the rotator cuff.
 b Associated fracture of humeral head.
 c Damage to the axillary nerve.
 d Associated fractured sternum.
 e Biceps tendon ruptures.

5 A 70-year-old woman tripped and fell onto her right hand while shopping in town. On first glance, there is an obvious deformity of her right upper arm and shoulder. What is the next step in the management?
 a X-ray the right shoulder.
 b X-ray her right shoulder and right humerus.
 c Examine her distal pulses and neurology.
 d Phone her relatives and ask them to come to hospital.
 e Give analgesia and record the patient's observations.

6 A 19-year-old man has presented to A&E with a painful and deformed left shoulder. The X-ray confirms anterior dislocation of his shoulder which is

reduced by the on-call orthopaedic doctor. This is the sixth time he has had this problem this year. What is the next best management?

a Refer to the orthopaedic shoulder specialist with a view to further management.

b Educate the patient and ask him to be careful.

c Request an MRI of his shoulder to look for a cause of the recurrent dislocations.

d Advise the patient to wear a collar and cuff at all times.

e Refer him to the physiotherapist.

Colles' fracture (Answers, see p. 316)

1 Which of the following are risk factors for Colles' fractures?

a Osteoporosis.

b High-velocity trauma.

c Diabetes.

d Osteoarthritis.

e Osteomalacia.

2 Which of the following are signs of Colles' fracture?

a Oedema.

b Deformity.

c Crepitus.

d Non-tender.

e Erythema.

3 Which of the following are general complications of fractures?

a Fat embolism.

b Compartment syndrome.

c Avascular necrosis.

d Lymphatic damage.

e Neurovascular damage.

4 Which of the following are complications of a Colles' fracture ?

a Volkmann ischaemic contracture.

b Compressive neuropathy.

c Cubital canal syndrome.

d Carpal tunnel syndrome.

e Rheumatoid arthritis.

5 A 60-year-old woman fell onto her dominant hand and presents with pain in her right wrist associated with 'pins and needles'. On examination there is a very obvious deformity of the right wrist and you see bone protruding through skin. What is your immediate line of management?

a Analgesia and observations.

b Book theatre immediately.

c Splint the wrist.

d Carry out regular neurovascular observations.

e Antibiotics.

6 A 22-year-old student has had an accident while skateboarding. He presents with pain and deformity of his left wrist. There is no neurovascular compromise, no tenderness of his ulnar styloid or radial head, and X-rays reveal intra-articular fracture of his radius with displacement of his distal radius. What is the best line of management?

a Apply a back slab and discharge.

b Attempt haematoma block and reduction of fracture.

c Book the patient for fixation with K-wire.

d Request a CT for further evaluation of the fracture.

e Group and save.

7 A 45-year-old woman has fallen on her dominant hand while out celebrating her birthday. She has broken both bones in her right wrist in several places and has associated pins and needles. The X-rays confirm the complex fracture sustained by this patient. What is the management?

a Conservative management.

b K-wire fixation.

c Bone grafting.

d Open reduction and internal fixation (ORIF).

e External fixation.

Fractured neck of femur (Answers, see p. 316)

1 Which of the following are risk factors for hip fracture?

a Smoking.

b Active lifestyle.

c Corticosteroid use.

d High body weight.

e Alcohol abuse.

2 Which of the following should be used in the investigation of hip fracture?

a CT pelvis is the preferred initial investigation.

b MRI hips may help to diagnose hip fracture.

c X-ray is the preferred initial investigation.

d A bone scan may help to diagnose a suspected hip fracture.

e PET is the gold standard investigation in non-pathological hip fractures.

3 A 45-year-old woman fell whilst walking in town. She has severe pain in her left hip and knee and she cannot weight-bear on the left side. On examination, there is a discrepancy in lower limb length and X-rays reveal a minimally displaced transcervical fracture of her left hip. Which option is best for this patient?

a Left hip hemiarthroplasty.

b Conservative management including traction.

c Left total hip replacement.

d Left dynamic hip screw.

e Left intramedullary nail.

4 An 88-year-old woman with dementia is found on the floor in the morning by the nursing home staff. She was mobile using a walking (Zimmer) frame but now cannot bear weight at all. X-rays show a Garden grade IV fracture of the right femur. The family would like to discuss her management. Which procedure will need to be explained to her?

a Right hemiarthroplasty.
b Right total hip replacement.
c Conservative treatment.
d Right dynamic hip screw.
e Right Thomas splint.

5 Hemiarthroplasty is indicated in which of the following situations?
a Low risk of non-union.
b High risk of AVN.
c A femoral neck fracture in a previously fully mobile patient.
d A femoral neck fracture in a medically fit patient.
e Failure after dynamic hip screw insertion.

6 Internal fixation of femoral neck fractures is indicated in which of the following?
a All young patients.
b Limited expected lifespan.
c Medically fit patients.
d Subcapital fractures.
e Intertrochanteric fractures.

7 Which of the following are complications of hip fracture surgery?
a Disturbed balance.
b Sural nerve injury.
c Chronic pain.
d Pulmonary embolism.
e Infection.

8 A 71-year-old man has tripped at home overnight and was found this morning on the floor by his cleaner. He looks dehydrated, and his left lower limb is deformed with mottled discoloration and feels very cold. What is your initial management (after ABCDE approach)?
a Take bloods for FBC, electrolytes and G&S.
b Insert two large-bore IV cannulas and give warmed fluids to resuscitate patient.
c Request senior orthopaedic help for further management.
d Examine the neurovascular status of his leg and complete a systemic examination.
e Request an immediate AP and lateral X-ray of his left hip.

OA of knee (Answers, see p. 318)

1 Which of the following are risk factors for OA?
a Old age.
b Obesity.
c Pregnancy.
d Hyperthyroidism.
e Hereditary.

2 Which of the following are complications of OA of the knee?
a Popliteal cyst.
b Majority experience long-term disability.
c Loss of stability.
d Sudden flare-ups.
e Increased mobility.

3 A 60-year-old woman who underwent a previous right patellectomy presents with feeling unwell, with fever and rigors associated with an inflamed hot and tender right knee. All movement is restricted and there is a high suspicion of septic arthritis. She denies trauma or any other medical problems. Once you have taken a thorough history and examination, what is your management?
a Analgesia and splint leg.
b X-ray.
c Aspirate the knee effusion.
d Take her to theatre for immediate exploration.
e Blood cultures.

4 A 60-year-old on warfarin for AF has presented to A&E with a 3-day history of swollen right knee which is increasingly painful and restricting his movement. It is neither erythematous nor hot to touch. There is no neurovascular deficit. The patient is tachycardic and rolling around in pain, and analgesia seems to be ineffective. What is the next step in management?
a Aspirate the knee.
b Check the INR.
c Cross-match.
d X-ray the right knee.
e Call a senior colleague for help.

5 A 31-year-old martial arts expert presents to the emergency department with a painful swollen left knee after intensive training. On examination the knee is locked in 30° flexion and he cannot fully extend. How should this be managed?
a Analgesia and rest.
b X-ray knee.
c Take to theatre for exploration of knee.
d Arthroscopy.
e Book an orthopaedic outpatient appointment.

6 A 69-year-old man with known OA has presented to the orthopaedic outpatient department with a large lump on the back of both knees. The knees are still painful but now the lump is getting larger and causing tightness behind the knee. How is this best managed?
a Aspiration and corticosteroid injection.
b Arthroscopic surgery.
c Total hip replacement.
d Analgesia.
e Ultrasound.

EMQs (Answers, see p. 319)

1 Hand and wrist. Options:
  a Barton's fracture.
  b Bennett's fracture.
  c Colles' fracture.
  d Fracture of the fifth metacarpal.
  e Fracture of the terminal phalanx.
  f Lunate dislocation.
  g Scaphoid fracture.
  h Smith's fracture.

For each description below choose the single most appropriate answer from the above list of options. Each option may be used once, more than once or not at all.

  (i) A fracture common after a clenched fist hits a brick wall.
  (ii) The commonest carpal dislocation.
  (iii) There is posterior angulation of the distal radial segment.
  (iv) Describes a fracture to the base of the thumb.
  (v) A common fracture seen mainly in middle-aged and elderly females after a fall on the outstretched hand.

2 Elbow. Options:
  a Capitulum fracture.
  b Intracondylar fracture.
  c Lateral epicondylar fracture.
  d Medial epicondylar fracture.
  e Olecranon fracture.
  f Pulled elbow.
  g Radial dislocation.
  h Radial head fracture.

For each case below suggest the diagnosis from the above list of options. Each option may be used once, more than once or not at all.

  (i) A 38-year-old woman with diabetes fell on her right outstretched hand. She presents with pain in the elbow associated with bruising and swelling. The elbow is tender on forearm pronation and supination, and elbow extension is limited.
  (ii) An elderly male with Parkinson's disease accidently fell and landed on his left elbow. The back of his left elbow is swollen and tender.
  (iii) A distressed 3-year-old girl is brought into A&E with pain in her right elbow and limited range of movements.
  (iv) There is a risk of ulnar nerve injury.

3 Humerus. Options:
  a Distal humeral fracture.
  b Greater tuberosity fracture.
  c Lesser tuberosity fracture.
  d Middle third humeral shaft fracture.
  e Surgical neck fracture.
  f Proximal humeral fracture.

For each case below suggest the diagnosis from the above list of options. Each option may be used once, more than once or not at all.

(i) An 89-year-old woman fell onto her right arm at home. The whole arm is swollen with bruising tracking down from her upper arm to her elbow.

(ii) A motorcyclist is brought into A&E with an open fracture of his right arm. There is wrist drop and sensory impairment on the dorsum of his right hand.

(iii) A 70-year-old woman presents with problems with her U-slab. Which fracture is she likely to have?

(iv) An obese male has presented with non-union of his humeral shaft.

4 Shoulder. Options:
a Acromioclavicular subluxation.
b Anterior shoulder dislocation.
c Clavicular fracture.
d Posterior shoulder dislocation.
e Scapular fracture.
f Sternoclavicular dislocation.

For each case below suggest the diagnosis from the above list of options. Each option may be used once, more than once or not at all.

(i) A basketball player injured his right shoulder during practice. On X-ray, there is widening of the gap between the acromion and clavicle.

(ii) A middle-aged woman tripped and landed on her right shoulder. There is external rotation of the shoulder with diminished sensation over the 'regimental badge' area.

(iii) A 45-year-old man was violently hit over his right shoulder with a heavy blunt object during a robbery. There is full range of movement of his right arm, forearm and hand but there is pain over his right upper back.

(iv) An epileptic female is complaining of shoulder pain after a grand mal fit.

Part 8   Burns and plastics

19   Burns and plastics

Burns

D : Damage to the skin or other body parts caused by extreme heat, harsh friction, contact with electricity or chemicals/radiation. This damage to the skin interferes with its role as a protective barrier to regulate body temperature, keep out infectious organisms and maintain fluid balance. It causes major changes in the body's fluid and electrolyte balance.

I & S : In the UK, approximately 250000 persons per year are affected, commonest in children aged under 3.

A & P : Several factors determine the severity of the burn, including the cause, degree (depth) and extent of the burn as well as the part of the body involved.

Cause of burns

Thermal
- Exposure to dry heat (flames) or moist heat (steam, hot liquids). Includes frostbite.

Mechanical
- Friction/abrasion, for example skin rubbed against a coarse surface.

Electrical
- Contact with faulty electrical wiring. Electricity causes destruction along the conduction pathway.
- Check the patient for entrance and exit wounds (e.g. entrance through the right hand and exit through the left foot).
- There may be a coexisting thermal burn if the patient's clothes become ignited.
- Example: immersion in water that has been electrified.

Chemical
- Contact with acids/alkalis/vesicants destroys protein in tissues and leads to necrosis.
- Tend to be superficial burns, involving the outer layer of skin.

Radiation
- Sunburn or radiation treatment for cancer.
- Tend to be superficial burns, involving the outer layer of skin.

EMQs and MCQs for Surgical Finals, 1st edition.   © Hye-Chung Kwak, Imran Bhatti, Jaskarn Rai, Farhan Rashid, Bachittar Singh Jassar, Murthy Nyasavajjala, Viren Asher, Jon Lund and Mike Larvin. Published 2011 by Blackwell Publishing Ltd.

CF&D: Burn thickness affects cell function. Therefore, classifying the degree of burn helps to determine the type and extent of intervention needed.

> *First-degree burn*
> - Also known as partial-thickness burn. Involves the superficial layer of the epidermis.
> - Pink, dry and painful, without blistering. There may be some oedema.
>
> *Second-degree burn*
> - Also known as deep partial-thickness burn. Involves both the epidermis and dermis.
> - Tender swollen red area with blisters. On applying pressure, there is blanching.
>
> *Third-degree burn*
> - Also known as full-thickness burn. Involves the epidermis, dermis and tissue below the dermis.
> - Painless dry leathery skin. There is no blanching on applying pressure.

There should be a high suspicion of inhalation injury and potential airways obstruction in any patient admitted with a burn injury.

Calculating the body surface area will aid estimation of fluid requirements and resuscitation.

Calculating the body surface area (BSA): rule of 9s for adults

	Front	Back
Head	4.5%	4.5%
Right arm	4.5%	4.5%
Left arm	4.5%	4.5%
Right leg	9%	9%
Left leg	9%	9%
Genitals (any involvement)	1%	–
Torso and abdomen	18%	–
Thorax and buttocks	–	18%

T&M: The ABCDE approach is followed in the management of burns patients. Once airways and breathing is cleared, insert large-bore cannulas in the antecubital fossa for IV fluids; give warm isotonic fluids 2–4 mL/kg per %BSA for second- and third-degree burns in the first 24 hours.

> **Investigations**
>
> - Blood tests: FBC, U&E, clotting profile, G&S. ABG to estimate carboxyhaemoglobin levels.
> - X-ray: for associated injuries (fractures, pneumothorax).

Interventions

- Analgesia: offered to patient for pain and distress.
- Urinary catheter: measures UO, estimates end-organ perfusion.
- Wound care: clean, débride loose tissues, blisters and dead tissue, apply silver sulfadiazine and an occlusive cotton gauze dressing. Early burn wound excision and skin grafting may be required. Tetanus prophylaxis.
- Transfer to burns centre if chemical burns, inhalation injury, significant full/partial-thickness burns and burns involving the face, hands, feet or genitalia.

Note: patients being transferred to a regional burns unit should have the wound covered with Clingfilm. Topical agents are not advised as it may interfere with assessment of the burn at the burns unit.

P: Most superficial burns heal within 14 days leaving minimal scarring. However, older patients and those with inhalation injuries with greater BSA involvement have a poorer outcome.

Plastics

Skin grafts

Definition of grafts

- *Autograft* is from the person who requires the skin graft
- *Allograft* is from another human source or skin substitute
- *Xenograft* is from an animal source

D: A piece of healthy skin/part of skin taken from one area (donor site) and placed over the affected area (recipient site) without transfer of blood supply.

A & P: Used to replace damaged skin in chronic wounds, burns, trauma, and plastic/reconstructive surgery.

CF & D: There are essentially two forms: split-skin grafts and full-thickness skin grafts.

Split-skin graft (Thiersch grafts)
Epidermis and a small part of the dermis.

Meshed split-thickness graft
The skin is put through a machine that makes small diamond-shaped cuts so that the grafted skin is larger. The skin may also be perforated with a surgical knife to increase the size. In both forms of split-skin graft, blood and fluids are drained away from under the skin graft.

Full-thickness graft (Wolfe graft)
Includes all the layers of the skin. All grafts require very good blood supply to survive.

T & M : The wound needs to be free of bacteria, debris, blood clot and dead skin before the skin graft is placed over the wound and the graft secured in place with sutures around the edges. The wound is covered with ointment and mesh gauze for gentle pressure, and bandaged to keep the graft in place. The donor site and skin graft should not be disturbed, and movement and stretching is avoided. The skin graft is dressed and left for 2–7 days, and redressed until full healing established.

Advantages

- It covers the wound and tissue underneath
- Helps healing
- Reduced pain during change of dressings
- Reduced infections
- Reduced scarring
- Minimizes contractures over joints

Disadvantages

- Infection
- Graft failure and rejection
- Contracture

P : In split-skin grafts, the hair follicles remain over the donor site and are responsible for regrowth of the epithelial lining. In full-thickness grafts, hair follicles, sweat glands and sebaceous glands regenerate respectively. Recovery of sensation depends on the cause of immediate damage.

Composite graft

This includes skin with fat or skin with cartilage usually used for reconstruction of the eyelid, nose and fingertips.

Flaps

D : Tissue transfer along with its blood supply.

Types of flaps

- Rotational: triangular or rectangular flaps are raised bearing no relation to the blood supply.
- Axial: much longer flaps based on blood supply to the skin.
- Pedicle: these are swung around the axial blood supply.
- Free: these have their blood supply restored by microsurgery to the recipient site.
- Composite: osseocutaneous flap (with bone) or myocutaneous (with muscle).

Advantages
- Greater tissue choice available
- Minimizes donor site morbidity

Disadvantages
- Specialist technique
- Failure involves large tissue loss

MCQs (Answers, see p. 320)

1 Regarding split-skin grafts, which of the following are true and which are false?
  a Common donor sites include buttock, thigh and arm.
  b The donor wound site heals by granulation and epithelialization.
  c Once the graft is harvested, it is secured over the donor site with sutures around the edges.
  d Skin grafts may be applied even in presence of infection.
  e The graft obtains its nutrition from the serum of the recipient site.

2 Regarding full-thickness grafts, which of the following are true and which are false?
  a Common donor locations include pre- and post-auricular, supraclavicular and inguinal fold of skin.
  b Light pink colouring of the graft after a few weeks is a sign of partial loss of graft.
  c The full-thickness tissue is removed with an elliptical incision.
  d Donor site is closed by primary suturing.
  e Can be used to cover the defect after excision of facial skin lesions.
  f It is better to have some underlying fat with the full-thickness skin graft.

3 A patient has been brought in by ambulance with severe burns to his legs. Which of the following management options is required?
  a Clear the airway first.
  b The patient will require a blood transfusion after the airways are cleared.
  c Insertion of intravenous lines should be avoided to prevent further skin damage.
  d A catheter is inserted only if the patient is haemodynamically stable.
  e Send blood tests for U&E.

4 Which of the following suggest burn wound infection?
  a The patient has a fever and there is pain associated with progressive erythema and swelling in the skin surrounding the burn wound.
  b A ventilated burns patient is septic and there is a sweet smell from the burns wound.
  c A patient has increasing pain and blue/green discharge from the wound.
  d The full-thickness skin graft over the wound has dark patches.
  e Pale insensate skin.

5 Which of the following are causes of graft failure?
  a Haematoma.
  b Seroma.
  c Bacterial infection.
  d Poor surgical technique.
  e Shear forces.

6 Regarding burns, which of the following are true and which are false?

a Burns result in reduced capillary permeability.

b There is microthrombosis formation.

c Circumferential burns predispose the patient to renal failure.

d Fourth-degree burns can occur in electrical burns.

e Nil by mouth is recommended.

EMQs (Answers, see p. 321)

1 Options:

a Composite skin graft with fat.

b Axial flap.

c Fasciocutaneous flap.

d Primary closure.

e Healing by second intention.

f Trapezius myocutaneous graft.

g Rectus abdominis myocutaneoous graft.

h Thiersch graft from right thigh.

i Thiersch graft from right arm.

j Transpositional flap.

k Wolfe graft.

For each case below suggest the best mode of closure from the above list of options. Each option may be used once, more than once or not at all.

(i) A 16-year-old girl presents with a linear lacerated incised wound on her left cheek. There is no active bleeding. This was inflicted by broken glass after an altercation with friends at a local pub.

(ii) A 36-year-old woman develops post-burn contracture over the flexor aspect of the right elbow. This will need surgical correction as it is gradually increasing functional restriction.

(iii) A 54-year-old factory worker narrowly escaped a machine injury at work. However he lost the upper half of his proximal phalanx.

(iv) A 63-year-old needs excision of his large inner canthal basal cell carcinoma.

(v) A 65-year-old needs wide local excision for recurrent squamous cell carcinoma of the neck.

2 Parkland formula for burns. Options:

a 1 L.

b 2.2 L.

c 2.8 L.

d 4.5 L.

e 5.6 L.

f 6.3 L.

g 6.5 L.

h 7.4 L.

For each case below suggest the required volume of fluid from the above list of options. Each option may be used once, more than once or not at all.

(i) A 70-kg man is admitted with 20% second-degree burns. What is the fluid requirement in the first 24 hours?

(ii) A 56-kg woman with significant cardiovascular comorbidities is found in her home with third- degree burns to both forearms. You calculate the surface area as 9%. How much fluid is required in the first 8 hours?

(iii) A 90-kg construction worker has been involved in an industrial accident and is brought into A&E with 25% burns. He has had half the 24-hour fluid requirement. How much fluid does he require in the next 16 hours?

(iv) A 6-year-old boy weighing 20 kg has sustained second-degree burns to both legs (front and back). How much fluid does he require in the first 24 hours?

(v) An unconscious 88-kg woman with second-degree burns to her front torso and abdomen (18% BSA) has been brought into A&E by her boyfriend. What is her fluid requirement in the first 24 hours?

Part 9   Useful procedures
20   Useful procedures

Abscess

D :   An abscess is a localized tissue infection marked by a collection of pus. Most abscesses present in breast, buttocks or the perianal area. They begin by breaching the normal skin barrier, which is followed by invasion of microorganisms into the underlying tissues.

A & P :   Some of the most common causative organisms include *Streptococcus*, *Staphylococcus*, enteric bacteria (perianal abscess) or a combination of anaerobic and Gram-negative organisms.

C F & D :   Localized pain, swelling, fluctuancy and erythema. Clinical diagnosis, although sometimes difficult especially where blood vessels are normally expected. In such circumstances, needle aspiration of the swelling may be considered.

T & M :   Abscesses resolve by drainage. Smaller abscesses (<5 mm) may resolve by conservative measures (warm soaks) to encourage drainage. Larger abscesses require incision and drainage

P :   Good with incision and drainage.

Indications
- Large abscess on the skin which is palpable.

Equipment and materials
- Local anaesthetic (1 or 2% lidocaine) with 10-mL syringe and needle for infiltration
- Skin preparation solution
- Scalpel
- Draping
- Culture swab
- Sterile saline wash
- Kaltostat packing
- Gauze

Procedure
1 Obtain informed consent and explain the steps of the procedure.
2 Apply skin preparation solution over abscess site.
3 Drape around the abscess to create a sterile field.
4 Infiltrate the skin with local anaesthetic.

EMQs and MCQs for Surgical Finals, 1st edition.   © Hye-Chung Kwak, Imran Bhatti, Jaskarn Rai, Farhan Rashid, Bachittar Singh Jassar, Murthy Nyasavajjala, Viren Asher, Jon Lund and Mike Larvin. Published 2011 by Blackwell Publishing Ltd.

5 Make a cruciate incision with a scalpel.

6 Allow the pus to drain and take a culture swab.

7 Break up the loculations within the abscess cavity with your finger.

8 Pack the abscess cavity with Kaltostat.

9 Place the gauze dressing over the wound.

Urinary catheter insertion (see Appendix 2)

This is a useful if not essential skill for all doctors. Catheters are sized in French (Fr/F/Ch) where the French size equals the circumference of the catheter in millimetres. The diameter of the catheter is one-third the French size. Catheters are available with or without balloons and in different materials (latex/silicon) and different lengths (short for females/long for males).

Inserting a urethral catheter gains access to the urinary bladder. This allows drainage/decompression of the bladder (retention or bladder outflow obstruction) as well as measurement of urine production. Catheters are also used to obtain clean samples of urine and during operative procedures which may be lengthy or involve a spinal anaesthetic.

Indications

- Urinary obstruction
- Weak bladder (neurological condition)
- Bladder irrigation
- Monitor urine output

Equipment and materials

Equipment required and ready on a sterile trolley.

- Sterile gloves
- Sterile drape/catheter drape
- Cleansing solution, e.g. Savlon/normal saline
- Cotton swabs/balls
- Sterile water (10 mL two-way/30 mL three-way) in syringe
- Foley catheter (usually 12–18Fr)
- Lubricant (Instillagel/lidocaine)
- Collection bag (leg bag 500 mL/irrigation bag 2 L/manometer 1 L)

Procedure

1 Explain procedure to patient and gain verbal consent.

2 Assist patient into supine position with legs flexed at knees with hips externally rotated and ankles together. Males can be sat up to 45° with legs slightly apart.

3 Prepare the sterile field and apply sterile gloves, empty catheter pack on to field and check balloon patency.

4 Thoroughly clean the external male or female genitalia using cotton balls/gauze in appropriate cleansing solution using sterile forceps in right sterile hand. The genitalia should only be handled by the left non-sterile hand when needed. Remember the aseptic non-touch technique and only use each cotton piece once and place away from the sterile working field. Do not touch anything with the left hand once it becomes desterilized.

5 Drape the patient keeping only the genitalia exposed. Apply lubricant to the tip of the catheter and insert into the urethral meatus. For best effect lubricants containing anaesthetic are left for at least 10 min.

6 In the female, hold the labia apart with the left hand and insert the catheter with the right hand. In the male hold the penis with the left hand perpendicular to the body and apply minimal traction.

7 Identify the urethral meatus and insert catheter with right hand. Once urine is draining from catheter tip, advance the catheter further by 5–7.5 cm.

8 Inflate the catheter balloon using water (not saline) and connect to catheter drainage bag. Pull foreskin back.

9 Dispose of equipment appropriately.

Document procedure in the medical notes, listing the following points:
- Indication for catheter, i.e. retention of urine/haematuria.
- Size and type of catheter, i.e. male 14Fr two-way latex.
- Amount and type fluid in balloon, i.e. 10 mL water.
- Residual volume and assessment of urine, colour/concentration/presence of blood.

Issues
Contraindications to catheter insertion include pelvic trauma and post radical prostatectomy. Catheters can cause tissue trauma and infection and false passage formation in male prostatic urethras.

For questions refer to Urology (Chapter 16).

Examining stomas
The term 'stoma' is derived from the Greek for mouth and for the surgeon it means an artificial opening to the abdominal wall in order to divert the flow of faeces or urine. There are 100 000 patients with stomas in the UK and approximately 65% of them are permanent. The most common stomas are colostomy (end or loop), ileostomy (end or loop) and urostomy (ileal conduit).

Stomas are created in the following circumstances:
- if there is no distal bowel present (i.e. in abdominoperineal resection)
- if there is poorly functioning distal bowel present (i.e. incontinence)
- if distal bowel needs to be rested for defunctioning (e.g. distal surgical anastomosis, distal fistula in CD or inoperable rectal cancer)
- if primary anastomosis would be unsafe to perform (e.g. acute diverticulitis or peritonitis).

End colostomy
Formed to manage rectal carcinoma, diverticular disease or faecal incontinence.

- Abdominoperineal resection: in the case of a very low rectal tumour both rectum and anus are resected and the cut end of the remaining sigmoid colon is brought to the left iliac fossa of the abdominal surface.
- Hartmann's procedure: the upper rectum and sigmoid are resected and the non-functioning part of the rectum is sewn or stapled and left inside the abdomen as a stump. The distal part of the bowel (i.e. descending colon) is

brought out to the left iliac fossa. As the rectum has not been removed, mucus and some old stool will be passed. If the colostomy is temporary, then a second operation is needed to reconnect the two ends of the bowel.

Less frequently, two stomas may be created. The distal stoma opens into the non-functioning portion of the colon, called a mucus fistula which produces only mucus. This is usually small, flat, pink-red in colour and moist.

Loop colostomy

Formed to defunction inflamed diverticular disease, to defunction a distal anastomosis or to relieve distal obstruction. A loop of colon (usually transverse) is brought to the abdominal surface and supported by a rod, which is removed in 5 days. The bowel is partially divided to produce two openings consisting of an afferent and efferent limb. The stoma site is usually high on the abdomen because the transverse colon is usually used.

End ileostomy

Formed following the removal of the entire colon, rectum and anus (pan-proctocolectomy).

The ileum is resected just short of the caecum and a short segment of bowel (6–7 cm) is brought to the abdominal surface in the right iliac fossa. It is everted to form a spout to protect the skin from the irritant content of the ileal fluid.

Following panproctocolectomy the end ileostomy is permanent. An end ileostomy may also be temporary when an emergency subtotal colectomy is carried out and part of the sigmoid is left in place (e.g. for ulcerative colitis, acute ischaemic bowel and sigmoid bowel obstruction).

Loop ileostomy

Allows for defunctioning of a distal anastomosis or defunctioning of the anus (e.g. incontinence or perianal CD). Loop ileostomy has largely replaced loop colostomy as it is less bulky and easier to site and close.

Double-barrel stoma

Following the removal of the caecum, a double-barrel stoma may be created. This includes an end ileostomy and a mucous fistula (made up of the remaining colon) sited beside one another.

Urostomy

Urostomy is the surgical diversion of the urinary tract. The indications for a urostomy include bladder cancer, neuropathic bladder and resistant urinary incontinence.

Formation of an ileal conduit includes the isolation of a segment of ileum and anastomosis of the ureters. The open ileum is then brought to the skin as a spout.

Complications

Functional problems
- Increased output
- Constipation

Structural problems
- Stomal necrosis
- Skin excoriations
- Stomal prolapse
- Stomal retraction
- Parastomal hernia

The different types of stoma bags

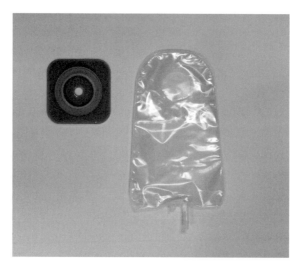

Urostomy bag is used to cover the urostomy. The colour of urine and the condition of the stoma can be evaluated through this clear bag.

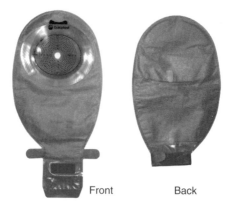

Front   Back

Front and back of a colostomy bag.

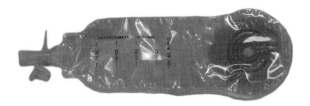

Fistula or drain bag.

MCQs (Answers, see p. 323)

1 Regarding abscesses, which of the following are true and which are false?
   a An abscess is a collection of pus caused by viruses.
   b Abscesses only develop in the skin.
   c A boil is an abscess.
   d Abscesses in the skin are not tender.
   e The skin surrounding the abscess is red and hot.

2 Which of the following are symptoms and signs of an abscess?
   a Tender.
   b The surrounding skin is cold to touch.
   c Pointing.
   d Fever and rigors.
   e Rupture of abscess.

3 Regarding pilonidal abscess, which of the following are true and which are false?
   a Means nest of hairs.
   b Is an infection of the pilonidal sinus.
   c Is typically situated near the natal cleft.
   d Is more common in those with physically demanding jobs.
   e An acute pilonidal abscess requires antibiotics.

21 Clinical scenarios

MCQs (Answers, see p. 324)
Choose the single best answer.

1 Mrs D. is a 78-year-old woman with a history of ischaemic heart disease, oste-oarthritis and type 2 diabetes. She had a fall at home injuring her left lower limb and buttocks. The patient was able to get herself back up but has been finding it increasingly difficult to mobilize due to the pain. On inspection, the patient has an externally rotated and shortened left leg with extensive bruising and oedema over the lateral left thigh.

1a What is the most likely diagnosis?
  a Soft tissue injury only.
  b Fracture of left neck of femur.
  c Pelvic fracture.
  d Hip dislocation.
  e Left knee dislocation.
  f Fracture of right neck of femur.

1b Which imaging is required to make a diagnosis?
  a CXR.
  b Lumbar spine X-ray.
  c AP X-ray of right hip.
  d Knee X-ray.
  e AP and lateral X-ray of left hip.

1c What is the initial management of this patient?
  a Thomas splint.
  b Analgesia.
  c Back slab.
  d Catheterization.
  e Blood tests.

2 Mrs P. is an 82-year-old woman with severe osteoarthritis and rheumatoid arthri-tis. She has been complaining of increasing lower back pain affecting her mobil-ity. She finds that a hot-water bottle applied directly onto her skin helps relieve the pain. In an attempt to do so, she accidently spilled the boiling water over her back. On examination, there are large blisters and erythema over her back. The area is approximately three times the size of her hand and is very painful.

2a What degree of burn has Mrs P. suffered?
  a First-degree burn.
  b Second-degree burn.

EMQs and MCQs for Surgical Finals, 1st edition. © Hye-Chung Kwak, Imran Bhatti, Jaskarn Rai, Farhan Rashid, Bachittar Singh Jassar, Murthy Nyasavajjala, Viren Asher, Jon Lund and Mike Larvin. Published 2011 by Blackwell Publishing Ltd.

    c Third-degree burn.

    d None of the above.

  2b What is the percentage burn suffered by Mrs P?

    a 3%.

    b 9%.

    c 4.5%.

    d 2%.

    e 1%.

3 Mr. T. is a 30-year-old physiotherapist who is usually fit and well. He drank 5 pints of beer and fell asleep at home in front of the television. The flat next door caught fire and Mr. T. was found with lots of soot on his face and in his airways.

  3a How do you initially manage this conscious patient with soot and oedema in his mouth/upper airways and nasal passages?

    a Insert IV access and administer fluids.

    b Follow the ABCDE approach.

    c Give oral fluids.

    d Keep patient cool.

    e Calculate carbon monoxide in the blood.

  3b The patient develops hoarseness and noisy breathing in the A&E resuscitation room. What is the next step?

    a Intubate.

    b Surgical tracheostomy.

    c Start inhalers.

    d Call the anaesthetist.

    e Wait for the medical registrar.

4 Mr O. is a 73-year-old alcoholic who presented with a 3-week history of painless jaundice, lethargy and weight loss. He has never been abroad and says that his stools have become pale and his urine is darker than usual. On examination, the patient has a large body habitus and his abdomen is distended, with the presence of a tender smooth liver and palpable distended gallbladder. Urine dipstick testing reveals bilirubin +++. The blood investigations are as follows (see Appendix 2 for reference ranges): Hb 14.3 g/dL, WBC 18 × 10^9/L, MCV 87 fL, Hct 0.4, sodium 135 mmol/L, potassium 3.5 mmol/L, bilirubin 312 μmol/L, ALP 1298 U/L, ALT 280 U/L, albumin 30 g/L, calcium 2.3 mmol/L, urea 16 mmol/L, creatinine 150 μmol/L, CRP 276 mg/L, CA19-9 10 013 U/mL.

  4a What is the likely cause of his jaundice?

    a Gallstones.

    b Cholangiocarcinoma.

    c Hepatitis.

    d Gastric cancer.

    e Cholecystitis.

    f Ascending cholangitis.

    g Colon cancer.

  4b USS shows dilated CBD and no gallstone. What is the next line of treatment for his condition?

    a Emergency laparotomy.

    b ERCP with brushings.

   c Percutaneous insertion of stent.

   d Repeat liver function tests every 6 hours.

   e Monitor urine output.

4c The patient requires an invasive procedure. What blood test is essential before the procedure?

   a APTT.

   b Factor VIII.

   c INR.

   d Platelets.

   e Vitamin K.

4d ERCP reveals a growth within the CBD. Which investigation would be required next?

   a CT abdomen and chest.

   b USS abdomen.

   c MRCP.

   d Endoscopy.

   e Mesenteric angiography.

5 Mr B. is a 49-year-old mechanic with a history of hypertension. He presented with a 12-hour history of upper abdominal pains associated with nausea and retching. On examination, he was restless, tachycardic and hypotensive. It was difficult to examine his abdomen due to his central obesity but there was definite localized tenderness over the epigastric region.

5a What differential diagnosis do you need to consider? There may be more than one answer.

   a Gastritis.

   b Leaking abdominal aortic aneurysm.

   c Biliary colic.

   d Myocardial infarction.

   e Peptic perforation.

   f Acute pancreatitis.

5b What tests do you need to order? There may be more than one answer.

   a Erect CXR.

   b AXR.

   c ABG.

   d Thyroid function tests.

   e OGD.

   f Blood glucose (to exclude DKA).

   g ECG.

   h FBC, U&E, amylase, CRP.

   i USS.

   j Echocardiography.

5c Mr B's blood tests are as follows (see Appendix 2 for reference ranges): WBC 19×10^9/L, Hb 15 g/dL, platelets 343×10^9/L, MVC 94 fL, sodium 140 mmol/L, potassium 4 mmol/L, urea 12 mmol/L, creatinine 90 μmol/L, ALT 60 U/L, ALP 80 U/L, amylase 2986 U/L, CRP 150 mg/L, troponin 0.01 ng/mL. What is the most likely diagnosis based on these blood results?

   a Gastritis.

   b Biliary colic.

c Cholecystitis.
d Peptic perforation.
e Acute pancreatitis.
5d Which of the following are important in the immediate management of Mr B's care:
    a Intravenous fluids.
    b Central line access.
    c Catheterization.
    d Epidural.
    e Nasogastric tube.
    f Intubation and ventilation.
    g Analgesia.
5e What is the appropriate investigation to exclude gallstones?
    a USS abdomen.
    b CT abdomen.
    c MRCP.
    d ERCP.
    e EUS.

6 Mrs K. is a 26-year-old nurse who has been complaining of increasing episodes of RUQ pain radiating to her side and back. Her observations reveal pyrexia and tachycardia. On examination, the patient is lying still in bed and holding her right side. The abdomen is soft with the presence of a palpable gallbladder and positive Murphy's sign.
6a What are the differential diagnoses?
    a Biliary colic.
    b Cholecystitis.
    c Empyema of gallbladder.
    d Mucocele.
    e Gastritis.
    f Acute pancreatitis.
    g Perforation.
    h All the above.
6b Mrs K. has become jaundiced in the last 48 hours associated with rigors and swinging pyrexia. On USS abdomen the gallbladder is compressing the CBD (Mirizzi's syndrome). What is the next management of choice?
    a ERCP.
    b Laparotomy.
    c Lithotripsy.
    d Laparoscopic cholecystectomy and CBD exploration.
    e Percutaneous drainage of gallbladder.
6c What is the most common cause of pancreatitis in the UK?
    a Alcohol.
    b Gallstones.
    c ERCP.
    d Drugs.
    e Viral.

7 Mrs G. is a 59-year-old farmer with a recent diagnosis of rosacea. Her past history includes appendicectomy and she is currently not on any medications. Mrs G. complains of acute generalized abdominal pains associated with incessant projectile vomiting that has now settled. On examination, there is an appendicectomy scar, the abdomen is minimally distended and generally tender with very active bowel sounds. DRE is unremarkable.

7a Which of the following factors are important in helping to reach the diagnosis?

  a Site of pain.
  b Onset of pain.
  c Character of pain.
  d Radiation of pain.
  e Exacerbating factors.
  f Relieving factors.
  g All the above.

7b The patient opened her bowels this morning and had lunch and dinner as usual. The severe abdominal started again as she making herself ready for bed. She describes the pains as intermittent, coming and going in waves every 2–3 min with no exacerbating factors and relieved by vomiting. The abdomen is slightly distended but soft and non-tender. What are the differential diagnoses?

  a Small bowel obstruction.
  b Gastroenteritis.
  c Appendicitis.
  d Inflamed Meckel's diverticulum.
  e Volvulus.

7c The patient has a plain AXR which shows very non-specific bowel gas patterns. Which of the following diagnoses can be excluded?

  a Perforated viscus.
  b Bowel obstruction.
  c Ectopic pregnancy.
  d Malignancy.
  e Pancreatitis.
  f Acute GI bleed.
  g None of the above.

7d You re-examine the patient as she is complaining of further vomiting and find that she has tinkling bowel sounds. You have a high suspicion that this patient has small bowel obstruction. What resuscitation is appropriate?

  a Two large-gauge cannulas in the antecubital fossa.
  b Transfuse 2 units of blood.
  c Start intravenous fluids.
  d Catheter for input and output measurements.
  e NGT.
  f Analgesia and antiemetic.
  g All the above.

7e The patient has persistent symptoms. There is moderate abdominal distension with tenderness. Which investigation would you order?

  a Repeat AXR.

b USS abdomen.
c CT abdomen and pelvis.
d Repeat LFTs and bone profile.
e Echocardiogram.

7f A CT with oral contrast demonstrates dilated loops of bowel more than 3 cm proximal to the obstruction with collapse of bowel distally and bowel wall thickening. The operative findings are as follows: small bowel obstruction caused by scar tissue from the appendicectomy site (adhesional) with patches of ischaemia seen on the adjacent small bowel. The lesion was resected and the patient was given an ileostomy due to the poor viability of the remaining small bowel. What is the commonest cause of small bowel obstruction in adults?
a Hernias.
b Tumours.
c Adhesions.
d Obesity.
e Aneurysms.

8 An 89-year-old man from a nursing home is admitted with general deterioration associated with pain in RUQ. His past history includes type 2 diabetes, myocardial infarction 4 years ago, COPD and asthma, BPH with long-term catheter *in situ*. On examination, he is holding the right side of his abdomen and palpation reveals localized guarding and rebound tenderness in RUQ. The abnormal vital signs include a temperature of 38.2°C and respiratory rate of 30–34/min with Sao_2 of 88% on air.
8a What are the differential diagnoses?
a Gallbladder: cholecystitis, cholangitis, empyema, mucocele.
b Liver: hepatitis, abscess.
c Large bowel: hepatic flexure tumour, perforated diverticular disease, diverticulitis.
d Appendicitis.
e Pancreatitis.
f Small bowel: tumour, perforation.
g Pneumonia.
h All the above.
8b To exclude mesenteric ischaemia, which investigation is most appropriate?
a CT abdomen.
b Mesenteric angiography.
c CXR.
d CT chest.
e USS abdomen.
8c The patient was admitted to the surgical ward for possible mesenteric ischaemia. What is the cause of mesenteric ischaemia?
a Portal vein thrombosis.
b Abdominal aortic aneurysm.
c Superior mesenteric artery occlusion.
d Renal artery stenosis.
e Cystic artery occlusion.

9 A 78-year-old man with a known AAA of 3.5 cm is admitted with acute right-sided leg pain associated with loss of sensation on the dorsum of his foot. His drug history includes warfarin for AF. On examination, the right foot is cold and pale. The sensation is diminished over the dorsum of the right foot and power is maintained at 5/5.

9a What vital part of the examination have you omitted?

   a Rectal examination.

   b ABPI.

   c Berger's test.

   d Peripheral pulses.

   e Abdominal examination.

9b All the pulses on the left side are present and normal, but you can only feel a very weak right femoral pulse and no other pulses are palpable on the symptomatic side. What do you suspect is going on in his right limb?

   a Acute right leg ischaemia.

   b DVT.

   c Ruptured Achilles tendon.

   d Osteoarthritis of his right knee.

   e Muscle cramp.

9c What investigations do you need to order before considering further treatment?

   a Clotting profile.

   b LFTs.

   c FBC.

   d Glucose.

   e U&E.

9d The INR (1.6) is below the therapeutic range. What could be the cause of this patient's problem?

   a Embolus.

   b DVT.

   c Varicose veins.

   d Myocardial infarction.

   e Lymphoedema.

Answers

1 Preoperative assessment: answers

MCQs

1 b

2 c

3 b

4 c The elimination half-life of warfarin is 40–70 hours. All non-vascular post-surgical patients need to be considered for thromboembolic prophylaxis such as low-molecular-weight heparin and thromboembolic deterrent stockings (TEDS).

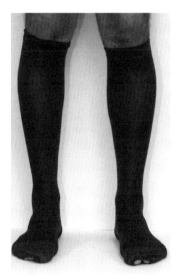

A surgical patient wearing thromboembolic deterrent stockings (TEDS)

5 c The aortic murmur needs to be assessed before surgery.

6 e No investigations are required for a fit and healthy patient having a procedure under LA.

EMQs and MCQs for Surgical Finals, 1st edition. © Hye-Chung Kwak, Imran Bhatti, Jaskarn Rai, Farhan Rashid, Bachittar Singh Jassar, Murthy Nyasavajjala, Viren Asher, Jon Lund and Mike Larvin. Published 2011 by Blackwell Publishing Ltd.

2 Neurosurgery: answers

MCQs
Head injury
1 a False.
  b True. His GCS is 12/15 (E3M5V4).
  c False. HI is classified as mild (GCS 14–15), moderate (GCS 9–13) and severe (GCS 3–8). He therefore has a moderate HI.
  d False. The cervical spine should be immobilized and not put on traction.
  e False. He should have head CT directly; there is no role for skull X-ray in patients with moderate head injuries.

2 a False. His GCS is (4/15) E1V1M2.
  b False. Hypotension in the acute setting in head-injured patients is not usually due to the HI but rather systemic injuries. All trauma patients should undergo assessment and management along ATLS guidelines, i.e. sequential assessment of airway (and cervical spine), breathing, circulation and disability.
  c False. Raised ICP is related to hypertension. Cushing's response is bradycardia and hypertension, which implies brainstem dysfunction.
  d True. The pupil dilates on the side of the expanding lesion and is an important localizing sign. It indicates herniation of the medial temporal lobe through the tentorium, which damages cranial nerve III resulting in pupillary dilatation with impaired reaction to light.
  e False. Steroids are contraindicated in HI. Patients treated with corticosteroids were 18% more likely to die from their brain injury than those who did not take steroids (CRASH trial).

3 a False. CSF leaks occur in 2% of all skull fractures and in 20% of temporal bone fractures. They can usually be treated conservatively, and tend to settle within 48 hours. Antibiotics are only commenced in the presence of infection; very occasionally intracranial repair of CSF leaks is required.
  b False. The clinical signs of base of skull fractures include bruising around the orbit (raccoon eyes), bruising over the mastoid (Battle's sign) and leakage of CSF from the nose (otorrhoea) or ear (rhinorrhoea). CSF can be identified by its glucose content, and ring appearance on a pillow sheet, or verification of β_2-transferrin presence.
  c True. The correct treatment for this injury is craniotomy to washout the 'compound' (open) depressed skull parietal fracture, as the chance of infection is increased. If the bony fragment is depressed greater than the skull thickness, it should be elevated to avoid pressure on the cortical surface as this could give rise to seizures.
  d False. Extradural haematoma. The extradural space is a potential space. In extradural haematomas, blood collects between the dura and skull and has

the ability to rip apart the firm attachment between them and push aside the relatively soft brain parenchyma.

4 a False.
  b True.
  c False.
  d False.
  e False
Mannitol acts by increasing intravascular pressure by drawing fluid from the interstitial spaces and from the brain cells. Therefore, ICP is reduced by a decrease in the total brain fluid content. To maintain optimal CPP, BP may have to be raised or lowered by inotropes and not by mannitol. Mannitol does not produce glucose.

5 a False.
  b True.
  c False.
  d False.
ICP monitors are introduced into the brain parenchyma through a small twist-drill burr hole in the skull. The most important factor associated with the development of ICP-related infection is the duration of monitoring. Patients who develop infections are commonly monitored for longer than 8 days. Suspicion of raised ICP is an indication for ICP monitoring, and not a complication. ICP is elevated in the presence of seizures, and not a complication.

6 a False. CPP = MAP − ICP
  b True. The adult skull can accommodate up to 100 mL of expanding volume without a significant rise in ICP.
  c False. Lowering P_{CO_2} is one of the ways to decrease ICP.
  d False. This can lead to cerebral hypoxia and brain death.
  e True. The neurosurgeons may need to carry out a decompressive craniectomy.

EDH

1 e Becoming uncooperative and abusive, and fitting, will lower the patient's GCS. Before taking this patient to the radiology department he must be triply immobilized as there is a high chance of associated cervical spine injury; one must liaise closely with radiologist and radiographers, nursing staff and porters to ensure safe transfer of the patient. Most importantly, one must be prepared for a sudden drop in GCS during transfer or during scanning. Ask the anaesthetist for escort and assistance. This young male had a very thin layer of extradural blood associated with a small full-thickness temporal bone fracture which was treated conservatively.

2 a True. CSF leak due to basilar skull fracture and tear in the dura.
  b False. The lowest GCS is 3.
  c True. Spinal EDH may cause complete cord compression.
  d False. According to the Munro–Kelly doctrine, a rise in the volume of blood will raise the ICP.

e True. The patient may be dead on arrival to hospital. Posterior fossa haematomas are contained in a very confined space and can result in rapid deterioration and death.

3 b The paediatric trauma team includes anaesthetists, general surgeons, orthopaedic surgeons, paediatric doctors, nurses and radiographers. The ATLS guidelines should be followed when managing this sick patient. This young girl was found to have a very large extradural frontal haematoma that required urgent evacuation.

4 a False. Brain oedema.
b True.
c True.
d True.
e False. This is the result of primary head injury.

SDH

1 a True.
b False. EDH is caused this way.
c True.
d True. The brain is generally more 'tight' in the cranium, thus allowing less room to accommodate the haematoma, whereas the aged brain is generally more atrophic.

2 a False. Subdural hygromas are subdural fluid collections associated with chronic SDH, post trauma and neurosurgical intervention. Hygromas often progress to haematomas. It is difficult to distinguish between hygromas and haematomas on head CT scan and therefore MRI is advised.
b False. Males have a higher incidence of acute SDH.
c False. Older patients are at greater risk of developing acute SDH after trauma.
d True. Up to one-third of patients with severe head trauma develop acute SDH.
e True.

3 a True. MRI demonstrates the extent, its location, whether it is multi-compartmentalized and its probable age. On the other hand, CT is more readily available and quick to perform.
b True. The blood of patients with diabetes has a higher osmotic pressure and has increased platelet aggregation.
c True. This collection of CSF develops a membrane with new vessels, which can haemorrhage.
d False. The chronic SDH has defective clot formation and haemorrhage.

4 a True.
b True. Brain atrophy increases the chance of shearing the bridging veins due to increased space between dura and brain surface.
c True. With its attendant risk of repetitive trauma, cerebral atrophy and coagulopathy.

d False. Intracranial hypotension associated with CSF shunts or CSF leaks increases the chance of developing chronic SDH.

e False. Thrombocytopenia is a risk factor for developing chronic SDH.

5 d A high INR must be corrected before surgery or there is a risk of the blood re-accumulating and the patient requiring further evacuations.

6 d Assess the patient following the ABCDE approach and then undo the dressing to examine the wound. The dressings may be wet with blood or CSF. In both cases an extra skin stitch may be required to stop the leak of CSF or blood.

SAH

1 a True. This reduces the incidence of cerebral ischaemia and infarction by about one-third. The mechanism whereby they act remains uncertain.

b False. In normal subjects a drop in BP results in cerebral vasodilatation to maintain cerebral blood flow. However, after SAH, autoregulation is often impaired with the risk of cerebral ischaemia.

c True. Treatment with inotropes increases cardiac output and BP. Since autoregulation can be affected in SAH, increasing BP can increase cerebral blood flow.

d False. Haemodilution can improve both cerebral blood flow and oxygen delivery by decreasing blood flow viscosity.

2 a False. Haemoglobin takes at least 6 hours to be broken down and to give a straw-coloured appearance to the CSF, or else the CSF should be uniformly blood-stained.

b True. If severe and fluctuating may reflect ischaemic hypothalamic damage.

c True. Due to catecholamine release following ischaemic damage to the hypothalamus. This adrenergic release causes prolonged myocardial contraction and decreased cardiac compliance.

d False. Usually enforced after SAH, although there is no evidence that this reduces the rebleed risk.

3 All true. About 20% of those who suffer an aneurysmal SAH develop a rebleed within 2 weeks. Other treatable complications include hydrocephalus, as blood within the subarachnoid space hinders the normal flow and absorption of CSF. If it persists, a ventricular shunt may be required. Vasospasm (an idiopathic narrowing of intracranial arteries) and epilepsy may account for a drop in conscious level.

4 a True. In the initial phase of SAH, dramatic increases in ICP are noted for several minutes, which cause venous congestion due to impairment of venous drainage to the cavernous sinus.

b True. Due to a blood clot within the ventricular system.

c True. Due to obstruction of the arachnoid villi hence minimizing absorption of CSF.

d True. The origin of cerebral aneurysms is still incompletely understood. Aneurysms are devoid of the muscularis media, which weakens the vessel wall. There are genetic links and higher incidence in patients with abnormalities of collagen morphology such as Marfan's syndrome and neurofibromatosis type 1.

   e False. Giant aneurysms are less likely to rupture due to multiple layers of thrombus reinforcing the inner wall.

5 a True.
   b True. Impaired or loss of consciousness occurs in up to 40% patients.
   c False. The patients have nuchal stiffness but not whiplash (soft tissue injury after a forceful jerk).
   d False. The patients are usually agitated and restless.
   e False. Rashes can indicate infection.

6 d Follow the ABCDE approach: ensure adequate oxygenation, hydration, BP control and analgesia. Check for electrolyte imbalances (low sodium), reassess the GCS and call the senior neurosurgeon before taking the patient to CT to look for rebleed, hydrocephalus and area of ischaemia (after vasospasm).

CSF

1 a False. It is 10–20 cmH$_2$O.
   b True. CSF contains lower concentrations of glucose than blood serum.
   c False. Nasal mucous secretions also contain glucose. To confirm CSF rhinorrhoea, analyse using immunoelectrophoresis.
   d True.
   e False. High protein content indicates infection.

2 a True. Radioisotope material is injected into the lumbar subarachnoid space and images are acquired up to 72 hours after injection.
   b False. This can demonstrate skull fracture but the better option is CT cisternogram after injection of contrast.
   c True. Collect the CSF and send for analysis.
   d False. Ultrasound is not useful in diagnosing CSF leaks.
   e True.

3 a True. Approximately 85% stop within 1 week.
   b True. Bed rest, stool softeners and lumbar drainage can help to assist spontaneous closure of traumatic CSF leak.
   c True.
   d False.
   e False. The preferred elevation is between 45 and 70°.

4 a True. The overall risk of meningitis associated with traumatic CSF leaks is 25%.
   b True.
   c True. In cases of non-traumatic CSF leaks, the problem usually persists for several tears.

d False. This is a contraindication. A thorough assessment is needed to make sure patients with cardiovascular comorbidities are stable enough for GA.

Hydrocephalus and lumbar puncture

1 a True. Coagulopathy may precipitate an epidural haematoma and compression of the thecal sac.

b True. Lumbar puncture cannot be performed in obstructive hydrocephalus.

c False. Obtaining a CSF sample is vital to aid diagnosis. A long-standing complication of meningitis is communicating hydrocephalus, which can be treated by CSF drainage (lumbar puncture, lumbar drain, or shunt).

d True. Performing a lumbar puncture in the presence of an intracranial mass could induce tentorial herniation as a result of creating a pressure gradient. If CSF is obtained by another route such as EVD or during shunt insertion, cytology may reveal tumour cells.

e False. MRI is the essential diagnostic tool to assess a prolapsed disc causing compression of the cauda equina. Cauda equina syndrome requires prompt neurosurgical intervention in the form of a laminectomy.

2 a False. CSF has a glucose concentration of 60 mg/dL compared with 90 g/dL in plasma.

b True. The osmolarity of CSF and plasma is identical (295 mosmol/L).

c True. The sodium concentration in CSF and plasma is identical (138 mmol/L).

d False. CSF has a pH of 7.33 compared with plasma which is 7.41.

e False. 0.3 mL/hour.

f True.

3 a True. Due to ventricular enlargement causing pressure on the frontal lobes.

b True. Typically gait disturbances are due to ventricular enlargement causing pressure on the pyramidal tracts passing round the ventricles towards the internal capsule.

c True. Due to ventricular enlargement causing pressure on the cortical centre for bladder control.

d True.

e False.

Normal-pressure hydrocephalus can be idiopathic or secondary to trauma, meningitis or radiation. There is evidence of ventricular enlargement (hydrocephalus) on imaging, in the presence of normal CSF pressure. Following treatment, symptoms resolve. Treatment involves CSF diversion in the form of a ventricular shunt.

4 a False. This is commonly associated with infection and inflammation.

b True. This can be one of the symptoms of hydrocephalus.

c True.

d False.

e True. Other symptoms include blurred/double vision, cognitive deterioration, drowsiness and incontinence.

5 a False. Acute hydrocephalus occurs over days, chronic hydrocephalus occurs over months or years.
b True.
c False. Obstruction to CSF flow describes non-communicating obstructive hydrocephalus.
d True. The space-occupying lesion distorts the anatomy of the ventricles.
e True. Communicating hydrocephalus occurs when there is defective absorption of CSF and there is full communication between the ventricles and subarachnoid space. This can happen after SAH blocking the arachnoid villi.

6 a False.
b False.
c True. Tumours can obstruct CSF anywhere along its path.
d True.
e True. This may cause hydrocephalus in adults

EMQS

1 a 2
b 3
c 4
d 1
e 1
f 2

Management of acute trauma patients should be in accordance with the ATLS guidelines. The ATLS guidelines dictate that Airway assessment along with cervical spine immobilization is the first priority (these two go hand in hand). Assessment of Breathing, followed by Circulation, Disability and finally Exposure and secondary survey. In this case, following airway management and cervical spine immobilization, he should be aggressively resuscitated with warmed crystalloids intravenously via two large-bore cannulas. Inotropes are never given in the acute setting as persistent hypotension is always thought to be caused by bleeding until proven otherwise. Hypoglycaemia is a cause of agitation, and should always be considered as part of Disability. GCS assessment forms part of the Disability assessment. This patient is likely to have spinal shock in view of the mechanism of injury, clinical findings of paraplegia, hypotension and bradycardia (disruption of sympathetic outflow).

2 (i) a, e This lady has multiple metastatic lesions.
(ii) d This man has a primary glioma affecting the left motor strip of the parietal lobe.
(iii) c This man has an intracerebral haematoma affecting the left occipital lobe
(iv) e A small abscess in the cerebellum was found. Cerebellar signs are dysarthria and ataxia.
(v) b Frontal lesion affects personality and expressive speech (broca's area)

3 **(i) c** This case describes a myelopathy. These patients typically have neck pain that may radiate down both upper limbs and associated sensory and motor deficits. Half the patients can experience sphincter disturbance.

   (ii) b This is cauda equina. He has a central disc prolapse at L5/S1 compressing the cauda equina. He has classic red flag symptoms, and requires an urgent MRI scan and neurosurgical intervention.

   (iii) e L5 nerve root impingement gives rise to paraesthesia and weakness in plantar flexion.

   (iv) d L3/4. L4 nerve root impingement gives rise to weakness of knee extension and paraesthesia over knee.

   (v) a This typically affects sensation over the radial side of arm and weakness in extensor muscles.

4 **(i) b** Blood is hyperdense and looks white on CT scan, as it is denser than surrounding tissue. Hyperdense material is typically bone, contrast material or calcification.

   (ii) c Air is hypodense and looks black on CT scan.

   (iii) a Contrast head CT is required to diagnose an abscess, and it typically enhances and is hyperdense.

   (iv) a

   (v) d T1-weighted MRI scans are better at looking at soft tissue

3   Ear, nose and throat: answers

MCQs
Epistaxis

1   **a**   Little's area is also known as Kisselbach's area or plexus. It receives blood from the ethmoid artery, a branch of the ophthalmic artery arising from the internal carotid artery.

2   **a**   False. Blowing the nose decreases the effects of local fibrinolysis and removes clots, which aids examination.
   b   True. Reducing the haemorrhage will aid examination and help locate the bleeding site.
   c   True. A posterior source of bleeding is more likely if there is bleeding from both nostrils, absence of bleeding seen in Little's area, and dripping blood seen in the posterior pharynx.
   d   True. The nose is supplied by both the internal carotid artery (ethmoid arteries) and external carotid artery (sphenopalatine and greater palatine arteries). Posterior haemorrhage originates from branches of the sphenopalatine artery (branch of maxillary artery, thus external carotid artery) in the posterior nasal cavity or nasopharynx.
   e   False. Cautery with silver nitrate or diathermy should only be used for one nostril at any one time, as there is an increased risk of perforation or necrosis of nasal septum.

3   All true. Local trauma (nose picking) is the commonest cause. Other causes of epistaxis include foreign bodies in children such as peanuts, small beads and nasogastric tubes.

4   **a**   Bilateral nasal packing will prevent drainage of the sinuses, therefore increasing the risk of sinusitis and possible toxic shock syndrome (inflammatory response to bacterial toxins). Amoxicillin is the antibiotic of choice for prophylaxis.

5   **d**   You need to resuscitate the patient following the ABCDE algorithm. The airways need to be protected if GCS is 8 or below, oxygenation needs to be optimized by administering high-flow oxygen. This woman has bled significantly and has hypovolaemic shock secondary to bleeding, so the next most important step is to administer IV fluids, institute cardiovascular monitoring, take FBC and G&S for cross-match. Once stabilized, continue with history and rest of the examination.

> For a quick preoperative assessment remember the mnemonic AMPLE: **A**llergies, **M**edications, **P**ast medical history, **L**ast meal, **E**vents.

6 a True. Tight packing may cause pressure necrosis.
  b True. Aspiration of blood can cause aspiration pneumonitis/pneumonia.
  c False. Nasal packing should aid haemostasis.
  d True.
  e True. Nasal packing can be very uncomfortable for the patient and may exacerbate hypoventilation, resulting in hypoxia. Patients with pre-existing respiratory comorbidities need to be admitted for regular monitoring.

7 a False.
  b True.
  c True.
  d False.
  e False.
  Aspirin and warfarin affect coagulation. The other drugs do not increase the risk of epistaxis.

Earache (otalgia)

1 All true. Chronic suppurative otitis media is diagnosed when there is discharge from the ear for >2 weeks following an ear infection. This can lead to further complications such as mastoiditis and meningitis. URTIs and allergies can cause swelling at the back of the nose where the eustachian tube normally drains; this can trap fluid which becomes infected by bacteria (in most cases) and viruses. Children have shorter and more horizontal eustachian tubes, increasing the risk of fluid accumulation and infection compared with adults. Glue ear is chronic otitis media with fluid accumulation; 90% of residual fluid in the middle ear will disappear in 3 months.

2 All true. These are all typical symptoms of otitis externa.

3 a False. Otitis externa rarely causes perforation of the eardrum. If perforation is discovered this indicates otitis media.
  b True. Middle ear infection can cause ischaemia of the eardrum associated with increased pressure in the middle ear. The combination can tear the eardrum.
  c False. Tympanic membrane perforations usually heal spontaneously but iatrogenic or patient instrumental perforations are less likely to heal.
  d True. A history, or the presence, of tympanic membrane perforation is a contraindication to ear irrigation due to the risk of introducing infection.
  e True. Purulent discharge can also be present in otitis externa, but in tympanic membrane perforation there is a greater volume of discharge.

Surgical intervention is required in patients with tympanic membrane infections if they suffer recurrent infections or hearing loss. Swimmers also need the tympanic membrane repaired as they are at risk of introducing water into the ear, which reduces earwax acidity and encourages infections, as well as possibly introducing water-borne bacteria.

4 a True. The fluid usually disappears in 1–3 months. Most (90%) will resolve in 1 year.

b True. This is the commonest symptom. There is hearing loss as fluid dampens the vibrations transmitted by the bones, stapes, incus and malleus. This can interfere with the child's development of speech, language and learning.

c False. Glue ear is common in children up to the age of 6. In England, 90% of all children will have at least one episode of glue ear by the time they are 10 years old.

d False. Half the cases of glue ear occur after otitis media infection in the winter months.

e True. Treatment is required for symptoms lasting more than 3 months. The patient will need audiometry to test hearing and tympanometry to assess fluid in the middle ear. There are a few surgical options including grommets and adenoidectomy. A small incision is made in the tympanic membrane to insert the grommet; this drains the fluid and helps maintain air pressure in the middle ear. The grommet is pushed out as the tympanic membrane heals (in 9–15 months). At the same time as grommet insertion, the adenoids are removed to prevent closure of the eustachian tubes due to enlarged adenoids.

5 a True. The aim of surgery is to remove all infection and restore hearing; the cholesteatoma can be removed in a single or multiple stages.

b True. Squamous keratinized epithelium, which is the normal lining of the ear canal and outer surface of the eardrum, invades the middle ear space in the presence of perforated eardrum (due to infection or trauma).

c False. Cholesteatoma can destroy the bones of hearing as they contain enzymes that become activated by moisture, and leads to conductive hearing loss.

d True. Cholesteatoma will eventually erode into the inner ear and cause dizziness and sensorineural hearing loss. Other complications of cholesteatoma associated with infection include hydrocephalus secondary to lateral sinus obstruction, meningitis and brain abscess.

e True. Firstly, audiometry is required to test the hearing, followed by temporal bone CT to examine the extent of cholesteatoma.

6 a True. Trauma causes separation of the anterior auricular perichondrium from the underlying cartilage, leading to bleeding of underlying vessels.

b False. Surgical management is recommended for pinna haematoma.

c True. The presence of subperichondrial haematoma stimulates formation of new cartilage.

d False. The wound should be checked for reaccumulation of haematoma and any signs of infection.

e False. There is much debate about treatment of pinna haematoma. Needle drainage may require further incision and drainage. Incision and drainage of haematoma with pressure dressing is associated with less reaccumulation of haematoma and is the preferred treatment in many centres.

Foreign bodies

1 a False. This toddler is far too young to cooperate. Ask the parent to seal his or her mouth over the child's mouth and close the unobstructed nostril, then to blow a quick puff of air. This is not easy. If unsuccessful and the FB can be seen in the nostril, a suction device may be tried.

  b False. Trying to remove the object at home can push it deeper into the nose, therefore it is better to ask an ENT specialist to assess.

  c True. Inducing sneezing is one of the methods for removing FBs from the nostril, because there is great force on sneezing. It may dislodge the FB and push it out.

  d True. Choking is a rare complication when a nasal FB passes backwards into the airway, often during sleep when the cough reflex is depressed. It is potentially life-threatening.

  e True. A nasal FB can cause trauma and bleeding. The blood is swallowed and can be brought back up as fresh or altered blood depending on how long the blood has been in the stomach.

2 a True. This is a common presenting symptom in adults.

  b True. Children are curious and may swallow or inhale an FB; wheezing, stridor, coughing or hoarseness may be the only symptoms.

  c False. X-rays may reveal radio-opaque objects such as coins and batteries but many bones are radio-opaque and seeds and nuts are radiolucent, thus difficult to see. Diagnosis is mostly based on history, clinical suspicion and findings. X-rays are used selectively to demonstrate radio-opaque FBs and exclude perforation (surgical emphysema).

  d False. The airway can be compromised in an attempt to retrieve the FB. Therefore the patient should ideally be taken to a fully equipped theatre and sedated with an anaesthetist present, before endoscopic removal is attempted by an experienced ENT surgeon.

  e False. Complications include complete airway obstruction, laryngeal oedema, oesophageal perforation, chronic erosion and abscess formation.

3 a True. An FB may block the ear canal.

  b False. Water causes the pea to swell and makes it harder to remove.

  c True. May be due to infection caused by the FB.

  d False. FB must first be removed before examination to confirm infection.

  e True. Mineral oil can be used to kill an insect prior to removal.

Tonsillitis and quinsy

1 a True. There is usually no need for treatment, and no complications.

  b True. The commonest cause is *Streptococcus* group A bacteria, but viral causes include influenza and parainfluenza viruses.

  c False. The incubation period is usually 2–4 days.

  d False. Coxsackievirus infection is associated with small blisters on the tonsil and roof of the mouth. These blisters become painful when they develop into scabs.

  e False. Viral infections are associated with milder symptoms and signs.

2 a True. Quinsy is thought to be a complication of untreated or inadequately treated acute exudative tonsillitis.
  b False. Tonsillitis is associated with otitis media.
  c False. Streptococcal throat infection can be associated with glomerulonephritis.
  d True. This is a rare condition usually caused by *Fusobacterium necrophorum*, which causes secondary infection and internal jugular vein thrombosis. The infected thrombus travels, causing metastatic abscess formation.
  e True. Large tonsillar swellings can cause obstructive airways compromise such as obstructive sleep apnoeas.

3 a False. Group A *Streptococcus* is usually predominant but infection may be mixed.
  b True. EBV also causes tonsillitis and this may lead to a peritonsillar abscess.
  c False. Two-thirds of patients have trismus (difficulty opening the mouth), which makes examination difficult.
  d True. The combination of pharyngeal oedema and trismus results in 'hot potato' voice.
  e False. The abscess pushes the uvula away from it; therefore the uvula deviates away from the lesion.

4 a True. Spread of mixed organisms into deeper neck tissues can lead to necrotizing fasciitis.
  b True. Spread of infection from the parapharyngeal space to the pericardial space can lead to pericarditis.
  c True. The abscess can become large enough to partially obstruct the airway.
  d True. Spread of infection from the parapharyngeal space to the mediastinum can lead to mediastinitis.
  e False. Spontaneous rupture of the abscess into the pharynx can lead to aspiration.

5 a False. A course of antibiotics is given and if there is no response or there is difficulty swallowing or airways compromise, a formal incision and drainage is recommended.
  b True. Gram staining is required to identify the type of organism (Gram negative or Gram positive); the pus is also cultured and assessed for antibiotic sensitivity.
  c False. In cases associated with recurrent tonsillitis, tonsillectomy is recommended.
  d False. Steroids are given to reduce symptoms.
  e True. There may be considerable discomfort.

6 a True. The 'cold steel' method describes tonsillectomy using sharp metal instruments, with haemostasis controlled by sutures or ligature (ties).
  b False. Antibiotics only treat tonsillitis caused by bacteria.
  c True. Diathermy (electrocautery) is used to dissect and coagulate tissues.
  d True. Coblation uses radiofrequency dissection to cut and seal the wound simultaneously.
  e True. Using laser energy is an option for tonsillectomy.

Parotid and parotid swellings

1 a False. Symptoms typically occur when eating, as the flow of saliva is obstructed leading to swelling and pain in the gland.

   b False. Stones near the opening of the duct can be massaged out without ductal dilatation. Excision of the duct is required for stones deep in the gland.

   c False. This condition is rare in children. It typically affects the middle aged (M = F).

   d True. Typically, ill-fitting dentures cause prolonged trauma to the duct opening, resulting in stenosis.

   e True. Stones are usually composed of calcium and magnesium phosphate, cellular debris and mucus. They are usually radio-opaque (80%) and thus seen on X-ray.

> Sialolithiasis is more commonly seen in submandibular gland (80%) which produces thicker mucous secretions and has a longer duct.

2 a True. This is an early complication of surgery. There may be a collection of saliva in the incision site which may discharge through the incision.

   b True. This is an early complication of surgery. There may be temporary or permanent damage to the facial nerve. In most cases of facial weakness or numbness the symptom resolves within 1 year.

   c False. There is facial asymmetry, with less fullness on the side of the operation depending on how much parotid gland was removed.

   d True. Most have injury to the greater auricular nerve resulting in numbness of the skin over the outer ear, which can be permanent.

   e True. This is a late complication of surgery. Due to aberrant regeneration of postganglionic secretomotor parasympathetic fibres onto postganglionic sympathetic fibres that supply the sweat glands on the face. Most report redness and gustatory sweating over the affected side of the face during eating.

3 a False. Most tumours affect the parotid gland and other large salivary glands.

   b False. Malignant salivary tumours are typically tender, fixed, hard lumps associated with neurovascular involvement.

   c True. From serous acinar cells of the parotid gland, it grows slowly and metastasizes late. Treatment involves superficial parotidectomy. Postoperatively, 90% survival at 5 years.

   d False. Salivary gland tumours in the smaller salivary glands are usually malignant (50%).

   e True. Account for one-third of malignant tumours of the salivary glands. Mostly occur in the parotid gland. Slow-growing and tend to spread to regional nodes. Low-grade forms have good prognosis after treatment (90% 5-year survival); high-grade forms have poor prognosis even after radiotherapy.

4 a False. It is an autoimmune condition affecting salivary and tear glands. This leads to dry mouth and dry itchy eyes, hoarse voice, dry cough, difficulty chewing and swallowing, and swollen salivary glands.

b False. Affects as many as 4% of the UK population; 90% are middle-aged and female.

c True. Ophthalmologists use Rose Bengal dye to assess the function of the tear glands. A similar test places blotting paper under the eyelid to detect wetness (Schirmer's test). Other diagnostic tests include blood autoantibodies, lip biopsy and microscopy.

d True. When medical management fails, tear ducts can be occluded with silicone plugs to prevent tears draining, thus increasing the quantity of tears remaining.

e False. There is an increased risk of non-Hodgkin's lymphoma.

5 a False. Sialadenitis is bacterial infection of the salivary gland, usually caused by *Staphylococcus aureus*.

b False. Usually affects the major salivary glands such as the parotid gland, due to obstruction of the duct by a stone or gland hyposecretion. Poor hygiene contributes to development.

c False. Usually presents with unilateral swelling, erythema and oedema of the overlying skin, pain and diffuse tenderness on examination. In severe cases, pus may be expressed from the duct, and the patient suffers from fever and rigors.

d True. Pus should be sent for MC&S and the patient should be started on antistaphylococcal antibiotics pending sensitivities. Any abscess should be incised and drained.

e False. This condition occurs more commonly in chronically ill patients with dry mouth (xerostomia), those with Sjögren's syndrome and those with history of radiation to the oral cavity and anorexia nervosa.

6 a False. The majority of parotid tumours are benign but the commonest parotid malignancy is mucoepidermoid carcinoma, which accounts for one-third of malignant salivary gland tumours.

b True. Involvement/invasion of the facial nerve suggests a poor prognosis.

c False. Parotid malignancy affects slightly more women than men.

d False. FNA is performed for cytology but CT/MRI is preferred to evaluate the parotid mass.

e True. Pain does not always indicate parotid malignancy, but pain in a confirmed case of parotid malignancy is a poor prognostic sign.

EMQS
ENT

1 **(i) f** Epiglottitis is usually caused by *Haemophilus influenzae* and is a surgical emergency because of the potential for complete respiratory obstruction. It most commonly affects children aged 3–7, presenting with drooling, problems in swallowing, stridor, use of accessory muscles associated with fever and tachycardia. Only an experienced ENT surgeon with a tracheostomy set at hand should attempt examination of the epiglottis. In the mean time sit the boy up as it may reduce oedema, reassure the boy and his parents, and administer oxygen if accepted by the child.

(ii) b This is infectious mononucleosis with associated splenomegaly. It is caused by EBV and usually affects young adults who have a range of symptoms and signs: fever, malaise and myalgia, sore throat (pharyngitis +/– tonsillitis), cervical lymphadenopathy, splenomegaly (often missed on examination) and hepatomegaly. The risk factors are kissing and blood transfusion. The patient requires symptom relief and is asked to avoid contact sports as there is an increased risk of splenic rupture with infectious mononucleosis.

(iii) e This man is an obese smoker; both are risk factors for GORD. He has a sore throat in the morning due to supine acid reflux whilst sleeping. He should be investigated to exclude laryngeal cancer.

(iv) a This is most likely to be a case of β-haemolytic *Streptococcus* causing exudative acute tonsillitis. Treatment is with antibiotics. Soothing lozenges and fluids may assist with symptoms.

(v) d This girl has a peritonsillar abscess on the left, pushing the uvula to the right. Examination and treatment will be difficult due to the limited mouth opening (trismus). Treatment will include intravenous antibiotics, rehydration and analgesia, needle aspiration +/– incision and drainage of peritonsillar space under GA.

2 (i) c Thrush is seen in the elderly, immunosuppressed, the very young and those on long-term antibiotics. This patient is undergoing radiation treatment, another risk factor. There may be much pain in the throat and on swallowing. Treat with an antifungal agent such as clotrimazole or fluconazole.

(ii) b Ulcerative tonsillitis is also known as Vincent's angina. It is an acute necrotizing infection of the pharynx caused by fusiform bacilli together with a spirochaete (*Borrelia vincentii*). The affected tonsil is ulcerated and covered by a pseudomembrane (necrotic superficial mucous membrane). Advise good oral hygiene and treat with antibiotics.

(iii) a Acute pharyngitis can be bacterial or viral in origin, and typically presents with sore throat and symptoms of upper respiratory infection. Viral pharyngitis is likely if there is a cough and runny nose. The throat usually looks red and swollen and there may be enlarged cervical lymph nodes. Treat with antibiotics for severe symptoms suggestive of bacterial infection, and advise rest and good hydration.

(iv) g Take a thorough history. This man probably has a fish or chicken bone stuck in the piriform sinuses or tonsils. He may need admission for endoscopic examination and removal of foreign body.

(v) e Ludwig's angina is an infection of the floor of the mouth, caused by severe dental caries. There is erythema and oedema under the chin, pain on moving the tongue, drooling if the patient is unable to swallow, and fever. In this case, the oropharynx is obstructed, and imminent airways obstruction is likely. An urgent tracheostomy with IV antibiotics and incision and drainage of the abscess is required.

Parotid

1 (i) d Parotitis is a rare *Staphylococcus aureus* infection of the parotid secretions/glands, most common in dehydrated elderly patients with poor oral hygiene, which is more likely when not eating properly such as with prolonged nasogastric intubation. Untreated cases can develop a large abscess with purulent discharge from the duct. Management includes fluid resuscitation, IV antibiotics, and good oral hygiene. Surgery is required for abscess drainage, in cases of neurovascular involvement, or failed medical therapy.

(ii) c This boy has mumps and acute pancreatitis, which is a rare complication. This can be confirmed by history and examination and antibody titres. A raised serum amylase may be salivary in origin, so lipase or diagnostic imaging may be required to confirm. Other complications of mumps include meningitis/encephalitis, orchitis and myocarditis.

(iii) h This condition is also known as adenolymphoma. This is a benign tumour associated with smoking. It affects males more than females (5 : 1). Treatment is superficial parotidectomy, which yields a very good prognosis.

(iv) e Pleomorphic adenomas can recur at the original site if the capsule is disrupted during surgery.

2   (i) c Gustatory sweating is a late complication of parotidectomy, caused by aberrant regeneration of postganglionic secretomotor parasympathetic fibres onto postganglionic sympathetic fibres that supply facial sweat glands. Anti-perspirant application may help, but further surgery can be an option.

(ii) d Damage to the greater auricular nerve is commonly unavoidable during parotidectomy; it usually leaves a variable degree of long-term numbness.

(iii) f The clear fluid can be serous fluid or saliva. After parotid surgery, a small suction drain is left in the wound under a pressure dressing; it is removed according to local practices. Most salivary fistulae heal spontaneously. In this patient, the drain was removed too early and a salivary fistula/ collection is present. The feeding collection will need to be drained with another drain. Persistent parotid salivary fistulae are difficult to manage, but some can be managed with anticholinergic medications.

(iv) g A salivary fistula is a risk factor for wound infection (and dehiscence). This clinical picture suggests a wound infection.

(v) a Temporary and permanent facial nerve damage can complicate parotid surgery. There is usually full recovery with time, and permanent facial nerve damage is very rare but disturbing to patients.

(vi) h As a junior doctor you should never be asked to consent for any surgical procedures (at least not without specific training), but you may be asked about operations by anxious patients and relatives who do not always remember what was explained in clinic. All surgical procedures have risks and complications, balanced by benefits and the risk and consequences of not operating. In parotid surgery, all the complications (a)–(g) should be explained. General risks such as thromboembolism and anaesthetic risks must also be covered.

4 Endocrine: answers

MCQs
Thyroid swellings

1 a True. Malignant nodules are usually rapidly growing painless nodules.
  b True. A lump fixed to surrounding structures usually indicates malignancy.
  c False. This is a sinister symptom; the recurrent laryngeal nerve is involved.
  d True. Multinodular goitre without a predominant nodule is associated with benign disease; however, a multinodular goitre with a dominant nodule is an indication of malignancy.
  e False. Cervical lymphadenopathy is associated with malignancy.

2 a True. Any suspicion of cancer after repeated investigations is an indication for resection.
  b True. This is a surgical emergency; a tracheostomy may be required before thyroidectomy.
  c True. Cosmesis is an indication for surgery.
  d True. Hyperthyroidism leads to further complications, therefore surgical intervention may be required.
  e False. The patient needs a tracheostomy rather than palliative resection.

3 a True. Cytology provides information regarding malignant and benign cells.
  b True. FNA is a safe and inexpensive procedure.
  c False. Isotope scanning detects iodine uptake in cells.
  d False. Used for diagnosis only. Treatment of thyroid lump depends on the cells found on cytology.
  e False. USS is used to assess the number of nodules in the thyroid gland.

4 a True. A dominant nodule in a multinodular goitre suggests malignancy.
  b True. This may be a symptom of medullary thyroid cancer
  c True. Rapidly growing non-tender lumps are usually associated with malignancy.
  d False. This is an obstructive sign. Other obstructive symptoms are tracheal deviation and stridor. An obstructive sign due to an enlarged thyroid gland does not suggest malignancy but further evaluation of the lump is required before surgical intervention.
  e True. Lymphadenopathy suggests malignancy. In a 60-year-old man with a neck lump and lymphadenopathy, there is a high suspicion of malignancy.
5 a False. Ultrasound will diagnose the presence of lumps including numbers and characteristics. It cannot differentiate between malignant and benign lumps.
  b False. FNA is the first-line investigation. It allows tissue to be obtained for cytology and therefore the presence of malignant and benign cells.
  c False. 15% of cold spots turn out to be malignant; therefore isotope scanning cannot confirm benign and malignant pathologies.

d True. All malignant thyroid lumps require staging CT scan to assess size and spread of disease.

e False. High TSH levels are associated with hypothyroidism, but most patients presenting with a thyroid lump are euthyroid.

6 a True. A nodule greater than 3 cm with follicular cells has a 30% chance of malignancy.

b False. Recurrent cystic nodules are more likely to be malignant and require further investigation.

c True. A 2–3 cm nodule can be observed with repeat USS and FNAC.

d False. A sudden change in size is associated with malignancy.

e True. Haematological investigations include thyroid function tests, autoantibodies, calcitonin and *RET* proto-oncogene; radiological investigations include USS, isotope scans and CT/MRI; and FNAC.

Thyroid cancers

1 a True. Any ionizing radiation.

b False. A complication of total thyroidectomy is removal of parathyroid glands and, in rare cases, hypoparathyroidism. The surgery of choice is total thyroidectomy with removal of enlarged lymph nodes, with preservation of parathyroid glands if feasible.

c True. In more than 50% cases, spread to lymph nodes is present.

d True. Patients are placed on lifelong thyroxine to suppress growth effect of TSH.

e False. It is associated with higher recurrence rates but not mortality rate.

2 a True. Makes follicular cancers distinct from other types.

b False. M/F ratio 1 : 3.

c True. A disease of 'middle' age.

d False. There is a direct relation to tumour size; tumours < 1 cm have a better prognosis.

e False Total thyroidectomy followed by radioactive iodine therapy and daily thyroxine is associated with lower recurrence rates and lower mortality in small tumours.

3 a True. There is spread to regional lymph nodes.

b False. Medullary tumour without endocrine abnormalities is the least aggressive form.

c False. Radiation exposure is a risk factor for papillary thyroid cancers.

d True. Medullary tumours originate in the parafollicular C cells which produce calcitonin. This is measured after the operation to determine if the cancer is still present or growing.

e False. Poor prognostic factors include male sex, age > 50 years, distant metastasis and association with other endocrine tumours in MEN II.

4 a True. M/F ratio 2 : 1.

b False. These tumours are rapidly growing.

c True. This is a well-recognized phenomenon.

d False. Nodal metastases are associated with a higher recurrence rate and higher mortality rate.

e True. Most cases are locally advanced at presentation and many have tracheal invasion; therefore patients need a tracheostomy to maintain their airway.

5 **a** True. Radiation is a risk factor for developing thyroid cancers.
 b True. This is one of the worrying signs.
 c True. Some thyroid cancers, e.g. medullary, rarely follicular, are familial/inherited.
 d True. Increased risk of cancer in general in the elderly, and cervical lymphadenopathy is associated with increased risk of malignancy.
 e False. This is most likely to be due to a viral infection. A sore throat and hoarseness for more than 3 weeks requires investigation.

6 **a** True. Anaplastic thyroid cancers that cannot be removed surgically are treated with external beam radiotherapy.
 b False. The side effects of radiotherapy include red sore skin, and recently operated wounds should ideally be given time to heal before exposure to radiation.
 c True. Also used to control recurrent cancer and metastatic spread to other areas of the body.
 d True.
 e True. Both papillary and follicular cancers can be treated with external radiotherapy in cases of incomplete removal with surgery. This can be used in addition to treatment with radiolabelled iodine. Radiotherapy is not routinely used for medullary thyroid cancers.

Parathyroid gland and hyperparathyroidism

1 **a** True. Hypercalcaemia causes increased acid production.
 b False. Hypercalcaemia leads to dehydration as it causes diuresis secondary to the kidneys' inability to concentrate urine.
 c False. Causes muscle weakness and loss of reflexes.
 d True. Rehydration cures this.
 e True. Long-standing hypercalcaemia is associated with calcium stones forming in the renal tract.

2 **a** True. The high PTH production from parathyroid cells is the cause of high serum calcium levels.
 b True. This is an indirect method and may be helpful if the PTH and calcium levels are only marginally raised. The calcium will be filtered out in an attempt to maintain normal calcium levels if the kidneys are functioning normally.
 c False. The various medications will not affect the parathyroid tumour; surgery is the only option in primary hyperparathyroidism.
 d False. PTH levels are normal, therefore no surgery is indicated.
 e False. This can occur in primary hyperparathyroidism. PTH levels may be only mildly elevated.

3 **a** False. The protein is only taken up by active parathyroid tumour cells; the normal parathyroid cells will be switched off when the serum calcium levels are high.

b False. This is a mild and safe radiation agent.

c True.

d True. A small radiation detecting probe is used to detect the radioactive parathyroid gland, a small incision is made over the gland, and throughout the dissection the probe is used to confirm the location of the gland. Once the gland is removed, the probe is used to confirm the right gland has been removed.

e False. It is operator dependent; many patients may have a negative scan in one hospital only to have a positive scan elsewhere.

4 a True. The parathyroids are stimulated by long-term hypocalcaemia.

b False. It is usually seen in chronic renal failure.

c True. Renal production of 1,25-dihydroxyvitamin D decreases in chronic renal failure. Vitamin D plays a role in increasing calcium absorption from the gut. When there is low level of vitamin D the absorption of calcium is decreased.

d False. Calcium levels are low to normal; therefore there are few symptoms in secondary hyperparathyroidism.

e False. The underlying condition should be treated, including medical correction of hypocalcaemia and phosphate levels. Surgery is an option if medical therapy has failed.

5 All false. Tertiary hyperparathyroidism usually occurs in chronic renal failure; the parathyroid glands become autonomous after prolonged secondary hypothyroidism. There are high calcium levels, high PTH levels and high phosphate levels, and patients complain of symptoms of hypercalcaemia. Treatment is surgical: subtotal/total parathyroidectomy.

6 a True. There may be bronchospasm due to smooth muscle contraction caused by hypocalcaemia.

b True.

c True. The peripheral nerves are affected.

d True. Hypocalcaemia causes prolonged QT interval, leading to reduced myocardial contractility. This can result in congestive heart failure, angina and hypotension.

e False. Long-term hypocalaemia leads to dry skin.

EMQS
Thyroid

1 **(i) e** Patients with medullary thyroid cancers need to have MEN II ruled out followed by total thyroidectomy with neck lymph node dissection.

(ii) d Goitre describes an enlarged thyroid gland. In pregnancy, there is hypertrophy of the thyroid gland associated with increase in total T_4 and T_3. To confirm the absence of hyperthyroidism/hypothyroidism, measure TSH and free T_4.

(iii) d Medullary thyroid cancers originate from the parafollicular C cells which produce calcitonin. After total thyroidectomy and lymph node dissection, there should be no calcitonin detected in the blood. Any rise in calcitonin indicates recurrence or incomplete excision of the thyroid gland/metastatic deposits.

(iv) a Radioactive iodine is indicated for patients with large aggressive follicular tumours. The iodine will be taken up by the remaining thyroid cells to make thyroxine. Radioactive iodine will be toxic to the cells but with minimal side effects for the patients.

(v) b Lifelong thyroxine is required to replace the hormone and suppress further growth of the gland.

(vi) c Vocal cord assessment is required before any thyroid operation as one of the complications of surgery is damage to the recurrent laryngeal nerve (1–2% risk of damage to one of the recurrent laryngeal nerves). Patients presenting with postoperative voice changes must be assessed, as complete paralysis of the vocal cords can obstruct the airway and requires tracheostomy. Damage to the superior laryngeal nerve presents with difficulty in altering the pitch of the voice; this is usually temporary.

2 (i) a De Quervain's thyroiditis affects middle-aged women. Typically presents with a painful thyroid following flu-like symptoms. There may be signs of hyperthyroidism, and blood tests reveal raised ESR and T_4, and negative autoantibodies. In the recovery phase, the patient will develop hypothyroidism that lasts a few weeks to months requiring thyroid hormone replacement.

(ii) d The symptoms of postpartum thyroiditis include fatigue, irritability, insomnia and palpitations. Hyperthyroid symptoms can be managed with medications such as beta-blockers but treatment for hyperthyroidism is not required as this condition usually resolves within a few months.

(iii) b Graves' disease is the commonest cause of hyperthyroidism, affecting more middle-aged females than males. It is an autoimmune condition with autoantibodies to thyroglobulin, TSH receptor, thyroid peroxidase and sodium-iodide symporter. There is a diffuse swelling of the thyroid gland associated with eye signs (50% of cases), and symptoms of hyperthyroidism. Treatment involves symptom relief with beta-blockers; medical treatment with antithyroid drugs (e.g. carbimazole); permanent treatment with radioactive iodine (iodine is only taken up by active thyroid cells); surgery for medical therapy. Thyroxine may be required if hypothyroidism develops after radioiodine therapy or surgery. This patient has presented late with the enlarged thyroid gland compressing the airway. She requires a tracheostomy to protect the airway, followed by further medical management of Graves' disease.

Eye signs associated with Graves' disease

Oedema, conjunctival injection, lid retraction, lid lag, exophthalmos (also known as proptosis), ophthalmoplegia (restricted ocular mobility).

(iv) g This is a medical emergency that is diagnosed clinically. It occurs in poorly controlled hyperthyroid patients after surgery, trauma or infection. Manage with aggressive resuscitation, antithyroid medication, oral iodine (Lugol's) solution, and symptom control with beta-blockers (+/− antibiotics, +/− steroids). Investigate for underlying cause: CXR, blood tests, infection screen, ECG and ABG. The mortality with treatment is 50%.

3   **(i) c** Hashimoto's thyroiditis is the commonest cause of hypothyroidism in the UK. It is an autoimmune condition with autoantibodies to thyroglobulin, thyroid peroxidase and TSH receptors. Typically affects middle-aged women with symptoms and signs of hypothyroidism: cold intolerance, hair loss, lethargy, menstrual irregularities, depression, peripheral neuropathy, bradycardia, diminished reflexes and peripheral oedema (non-pitting). USS with FNAC can be performed for histological diagnosis. Treatment is thyroxine.

  (ii) d Patients treated with radioiodine therapy should have regular thyroid function tests as many go onto develop hypothyroidism requiring lifelong throxine.

 (iii) e This patient should have thyroid function tested. Some women develop postpartum thyroiditis, which is associated with hypothyroidism after a short period of hyperthyroidism. The patient may require a short course of thyroxine for hypothyroidism.

 (iv) b This patient is in the recovery phase of De Quervain's thyroiditis. Mild cases require no treatment, but in the presence of hypothyroidism with raised TSH, a few months of thyroxine may be indicated.

4   **(i) e** This chronic renal failure patient has symptoms of hypercalcaemia. The parathyroid glands have been chronically stimulated to produce PTH, and one of the effects of increased PTH leads to increased absorption of calcium from the distal tubules and hypercalcaemia.

  (ii) d One of the complications of total thyroidectomy is removal of all parathyroid glands. This causes an immediate drop in calcium and decrease in PTH. Start IV calcium and supportive measures. Persistent hypoparathyroidism is managed with vitamin D and calcium supplements.

 (iii) b The commonest presenting symptom of hyperparathyroidism is renal colic caused by increased renal excretion of calcium.

In primary hyperparathyroidism
↑PTH → ↑calcium (bone) + ↑calcium (intestine) + ↑calcium (urine) =
hypercalcaemia

In secondary hyperparathyroidism
↑PTH and ↓/↔ serum calcium
↑ALP
↑↓Vitamin D
↑Phosphorus (in renal failure), ↓phosphorus (absorption problems)

In tertiary hyperparathyroidism
↑PTH + ↑phosphorus + ↑calcium

---

5   Thorax: answers

MCQs
Penetrating thoracic trauma
1 b

2 a True.
   b True. This is becoming the primary diagnostic tool in a lot of centres.
   c False. This plays no role in the investigation of penetrating trauma. OGD can directly visualize the oesophagus in patients with mediastinal injury.
   d True. To visualize the trachea and bronchus in patients with mediastinal injury.
   e True.

3 a True.
   b False. A high index of suspicion is required. Diagnosis is made on laparoscopy/laparotomy.
   c True. The initial injury may be missed.
   d False. Can be repaired laparoscopically.
   e True.

Blunt thoracic trauma
1 b

2 c

3 a False. Deceleration forces cause shearing within the vessel and compression of the vessel against the spinal cord.
   b True.
   c False. There are decreased peripheral pulses.
   d True.
   e True.

4 a False. It is more prevalent with penetrating trauma.
   b True. Eventually, the heart cannot contract and expand.
   c False. There is an increase in venous pressure.
   d True. There is loss of peripheral pulses during inspiration.
   e False. The mortality rate is approximately 50%.

5 a False. Massive haemothorax is the rapid accumulation of more than 1500 mL of blood in the pleural space.
   b True. Other causes include blunt trauma, rib fractures and laceration of great vessels.

   c False. There is reduced tidal volume.
   d True. The rapid blood loss results in hypovolaemia and shock.
   e True.

6 a True. Supplemental oxygen.
   b True.
   c False. Thoracostomy is indicated in haemothorax.
   d True. For very large pulmonary contusions.
   e True. To prevent further complications.

Rib fractures

1 a False. Flail chest is caused by three or more adjacent rib fractures in two or more places.
   b True. This is the definition of flail chest.
   c True.
   d False. There is poor air entry.
   e True.

2 c

3 a True. Can help to open up the airways.
   b False. Patient-controlled analgesia.
   c True. Care should be taken as intercostal nerve blocks can result in pneumothorax.
   d False. Epidural anaesthesia.
   e True. Early mobilization and chest physiotherapy help to prevent complications.

4 a True.
   b True.
   c False. Respiratory arrest is a complication.
   d True. With first rib fractures.
   e True. Fractures of the lower rib can injure the spleen, adrenals or kidneys.

Tension pneumothorax

1 a True. Air can enter but not escape.
   b False. Air continuously leaks out of the lung into the pleural space.
   c True.
   d False. The collapsed lung presses against the heart.
   e True. Death can follow rapidly.

2 b The diagnosis of tension pneumothorax is entirely clinical.

3 a False. If the opening is two-thirds the diameter of trachea, air passes through the chest defect.
   b True. This is the definition of open pneumothorax.

c True. Air replaces lung tissue.

d False. Use 100% oxygen and seal the sterile occlusive dressing.

e False. The open pneumothorax may develop tension if the chest defect is improperly sealed.

4 **e** The British Thoracic Society (BTS) advocates conservative management.

5 **a** True.

 b True.

 c False. There is hyperresonance on the affected side.

 d False. There is diminished breath sound on the affected side.

 e True.

6 **a** False. There is no non-invasive treatment for tension pneumothorax.

 b True.

 c True.

 d True. After needle decompression.

 e True. Check for lung re-expansion.

EMQS

1 **(i) i** Thoracic outlet syndrome.

 (ii) d This is a classic description of a myocardial infarction.

 (iii) j Rib fractures are common after minor trauma in elderly osteoporotic patients.

 (iv) e The classic signs of tension pneumthorax include respiratory distress, absent breath sounds on the affected side, hyperresonance on percussion of the affected side, hyperexpansion of wall on the affected side.

2 **(i) h**

 (ii) c

 (iii) a

 (iv) b

3 **(i) e**

 (ii) b

 (iii) d

 (iv) a

4 **(i) a** This sign is a hallmark of aortic injury.

 (ii) h This patient requires analgesia for his sternal fracture. Surgical intervention is rarely required.

 (iii) f Pseudoaneurysms and intimal flaps of aorta are rare injuries that can be managed conservatively.

6 Breast: answers

MCQs

1 a False. Breast lump is the commonest reason for referral to breast clinic.
  b True.
  c True.
  d False. Phyllodes tumour is a non-epithelial neoplasm.
  e True.

2 c 'Breast mice' are highly mobile.

3 e HER2-sensitive lesions are sensitive to this monoclonal antibody. It is thought to block tumour cell growth, works synergistically with chemotherapy and helps natural killer cells to detect abnormality.

4 c LCIS is not a cancer, but it increases the risk of breast cancer.

5 b In comedo intraductal carcinoma, the necrotic cells can be expressed like a blackhead on the skin when the lesion is cut. This type of DCIS is more aggressive than the non-comedo types of DCIS.

EMQs

1 **(i)** a Paget's disease of the nipple is almost always associated with underlying breast cancer.
  (ii) b The acute mastitis has developed into an abscess. Breast abscesses are common in breast-feeding females
  (iii) d Smoking is a risk factor for ductal ectasia.
  (iv) e This typically describes a fibroadenoma.

2 **(i)** a This is typical of postpartum mastitis.
  (ii) c Galactoceles are single or multiple nodules that contain milk.
  (iii) b
  (iv) f Obesity is a risk factor for developing cellulitis.

7 Acute abdomen: answers

MCQs
Necrotizing fasciitis
1 a True. Identification of necrotizing fasciitis should include the immediate resection of involved tissues and empiric administration of antibiotics.
b False. Use of hyperbaric oxygen has been controversial.
c False. Benzylpenicillin is administered in cases in which the presence of clostridial infection is possible.
d True. See (a).
e True. Gram-positive organisms are treated with vancomycin or a semi-synthetic penicillin and Gram-negative organism are treated with an aminoglycoside or a monobactam.

2 a True.
b True.
c False.
d True.
e True.
Underlying disease processes predispose patients to necrotizing fasciitis. Three common factors may include impaired immune system, compromise of fascial blood supply, and the presence of microorganisms that are able to proliferate within this environment. Infection of this type is usually polymicrobial in nature, with Gram-positive and Gram-negative enteric and Gram-negative anaerobic organisms being frequently identified.

3 a True.
b False.
c True.
d False.
e True.
Necrotizing fasciitis can be a complication of many surgical procedures.

Volvulus
1 a True.
b False. Immobile/bed-bound patients are at risk of developing sigmoid volvulus.
c False. Chronic constipation is the most important predisposing factor.
d True.
e False. Megacolon.
Other risk factors for developing sigmoid volvulus include Hirschsprung's disease and intestinal pseudo-obstructions.

2 b The management involves resuscitation and colonoscopic decompression +/− laparotomy for anaesthetically fit patients. A right hemicolectomy may be indicated in ischaemic bowel.

3 a False. Tympanic abdomen on percussion.
b True.
c True.
d True. In colonic perforation or ischaemia, features of shock may be present.
e False. Indicates ischaemia.

4 d This man has an ischaemic sigmoid volvulus. Initiate the ABCDE sequence and fully resuscitate the patient before taking him to theatre for a laparotomy.

Shock

1 a False.
b False.
c True.
d True.
e True.
SIRS is a term that was developed to describe the clinical manifestations that result from the inflammatory cascade or systemic response to infection. SIRS is diagnosed when at least two of four clinical parameters are present (for list of parameters see Chapter 7, section Septic shock).

2 b Severe sepsis is the presence of SIRS in the setting of infection. Severe sepsis is infection with evidence of end-organ dysfunction as a result of hypoperfusion. Septic shock is severe sepsis with persistent hypotension despite fluid resuscitation, resulting in tissue hypoperfusion.

3 a Shock may occur when 40% or more of the myocardium is involved.

4 a False.
b True.
c True.
d True.
e True.
Haemorrhage causes both a rapid and slower more sustained responses. The initial response to blood loss is by decreased activation of arterial baroreceptors, by a decrease in blood pressure followed by an increase in sympathetic discharge resulting in tachycardia and vasoconstriction. Release of catecholamines (adrenergic response) leads to vasoconstriction (mainly pre- and post-capillary sphincters), tachycardia and increased myocardial contractility. Transcapillary refill is a process where there is reabsorption of interstitial fluid into the vascular space following decrease in intravascular hydrostatic pressure distal to the pre-capillary sphincter. Products of anaerobic metabolism from hypoperfused cells accumulate in the extracellular compartment inducing hyperosmolarity. This extracellular hyperosmolarity drives water from the intracellular space,

increasing interstitial osmotic pressure, which in turn drives water, sodium and chloride across the capillary endothelium into the vascular space.

5 a True.
 b False.
 c False.
 d True.
 e True.

6 a False.
 b False.
 c True.
 d True.
 e False.

ATLS

1 a False.
 b False.
 c True.
 d False.
 e False.
According to ATLS principles, any trauma patient should first have their airway cleared with C-spine protection (sometimes referred to as AcBCDE). Airway remains the main priority in the primary survey, followed by ventilation and circulatory support. In this patient, the best option is endotracheal intubation with in-line cervical traction. This requires two people, one to maintain the head in a neutral position and the other to insert the tube under direct vision. Nasotracheal intubation would be a poor option due to possible facial and basal skull fracture.

2 a False. Beck's triad includes distended neck veins, hypotension and muffled heart sounds and is present in only one-third of patients with tamponade.
 b False. Accumulation of as little as 150 mL of blood will lead to significant reduction in diastolic filling to cause reduced cardiac output.
 c False. Most patients with pentrating cardiac trauma do not require cardiopulmonary bypass to repair their injuries.
 d True. 15% of needle pericardiocenteses may give a false-negative result because of a clotted haemopericardium. Therefore echocardiography prior to needle aspiration is advisable.
 e False. Penetrating trauma usually causes cardiac tamponade.

3 a False.
 b False.
 c False.
 d True.
 e False.

All listed options are possible radiological findings; however, presence of mediastinal widening is the most common (20–40% of patients). Other signs may include elevation of left main bronchus, depression of right main bronchus and shift of NGT to the left. CT aortogram remains the gold standard for imaging of the aorta.

4 a False.
   b True.
   c True.
   d True.
   Follow the ABCDE approach as part of the primary survey.

5 a True.
   b False.
   c True.
   d False.
   e True.

6 a False.
   b True.
   c False.
   d False.
   e True.

EMQS

1   (i) c Blood-stained fluid usually indicates gangrene.
  (ii) c Ongoing sepsis with rebound tenderness suggests intestinal ischaemia or perforation.
 (iii) c Correct the electrolytes and rehydrate the patient before further investigations.

2   (i) g Migratory pain towards right iliac fossa with fever and tachycardia are normally associated with acute appendicitis.
  (ii) i
 (iii) q
 (iv) a
  (v) m
 (vi) c
 (vii) p
(viii) e
 (ix) r
  (x) b
 (xi) d
 (xii) j
(xiii) d
 (xiv) k
 (xv) k

(xvi) l
(xvii) q

3   **(i) a** This boy has appendicitis until proven otherwise. Admit for blood tests, urine test and blood cultures and observe overnight.

   (ii) g This boy has inflamed mesenteric lymph nodes. It is often associated with upper respiratory tract infection, diffuse abdominal pains, fever and nausea and vomiting.

   (iii) h The history strongly suggests gallstone pancreatitis. Remember to rule out other causes of pancreatitis.

   (iv) a The appendix is inflamed on CT.

   (v) i This is typical of renal colic.

8   Foregut: answers

MCQs
Dysphagia

1 a True. This is the first phase of swallowing.
   b False. The food is actively moved from the oral cavity to the oropharynx during the oral phase of swallowing. A food bolus in the larynx would enter the airway.
   c False. Deglutition describes the act of swallowing.
   d True. This is the involuntary second phase, which requires intact cranial nerves IX (glossopharyngeal) and X (vagus).
   e True. This is the final phase of swallowing. The peristaltic movements in the oesophagus move the food bolus into the stomach.

2 a True. Patients often describe the sensation of food being stuck.
   b True. Swallowing can be associated with pain.
   c False. Dysphagia often leads to weight loss.
   d True. Sialorrhoea is excessive salivation, which is associated with problems such as microglossia, malocclusion, and disorganized tongue mobility, all of which can be the cause of dysphagia.
   e True. Patients often complain of coughing or choking on swallowing.

3 a True. In achalasia, the oesophageal muscles do not relax to allow liquids or solids to pass into the stomach.
   b True. This can lead to scarring and stricturing of the throat making swallowing difficult.
   c False. Dysphagia is not a known complication of breast radiotherapy.
   d True. Parkinson's disease is a neurological condition associated with loss of dopamine-producing nerve cells; this can affect nervous control of swallowing muscles.
   e False. In Alzheimer's disease, patients are unable to care for themselves, making them prone to health problems including malnutrition. It is not a known cause of dysphagia.

4 a True. Botulinum toxin paralyses the muscles in spasm in achalasia.
   b True. The stricture is identified on endoscopy and a balloon is carefully inflated to increase the size of the lumen.
   c False. Symptoms of Parkinson's disease can be improved with medication.
   d False. Management usually involves dietary modification, iron therapy for anaemia +/– mechanical dilation to disrupt the web.
   e False. The management of pharyngeal pouch is surgical (diverticulectomy or Dohlman's procedure).

Plummer–Vinson syndrome is also known as Paterson–Brown–Kelly syndrome in the UK. It describes a collection of symptoms and signs: post-cricoid dysphagia, upper oesophageal webs (composed of thin layer of squamous mucosa and sub-mucosa) and iron deficiency anaemia. The cause is unknown.

5 **a** True. Food, liquids and saliva may enter the airways and cause aspiration pneumonitis.
    b True.
    c True. Inability to swallow may result in malnutrition and dehydration.
    d False. This is not a complication of dysphagia, but may predispose to dysphagia.
    e False. This may predispose to dysphagia.

6 **a** True.
    b True. To exclude anaemia.
    c False. This is useful in imaging the biliary system.
    d True. Manometry assesses oesophageal dysmotility.
    e False. EUS is a useful investigation for dysphagia to exclude oesophageal cancer.

GORD

1 **a** True. Most common digestive symptom in the UK.
    b True. May be confused with ischaemic cardiac pain.
    c True. Properly termed volume reflux.
    d False. GORD does not usually present with dysphagia, but can do so rarely if it has been complicated by stricture formation.
    e False. It is not a systemic inflammatory process.

2 **a** False. GORD is ameliorated by reducing the pH of refluxate, but reflux continues.
    b True. For example weight reduction, avoidance of strong alcohol and spices, bed head raising.
    c False. *Helicobacter* infection is associated with gastric and duodenal ulcers.
    d True. When it is chronic and poorly treated.
    e True. Surgery provides long-term control but is not always 100% effective.

3 **a** True.
    b False. Oesophageal stricture.
    c False.
    d True.
    e False. This causes dysphagia in immunocompromised patients.

4 **a** False.
    b True.
    c True.

d True.

e True.

Smoking, obesity and hiatal hernia weaken the lower oesophageal sphincter. Advise lifestyle changes.

5 a True. Measure lower oesophageal pressures.

b False.

c True.

d False.

e True.

6 a True.

b False. These can cause oesophageal inflammation in those with achalasia or strictures.

c True.

d False. Prokinetic such as metoclopramide are used.

e True.

Barrett's oesophagus

1 a False. Barrett's is a metaplastic change from squamous to columnar epithelium.

b False. The overall risk is not known.

c True. The incidence of Barrett's oesophagus is rising in the Western world and this appears responsible for an increasing incidence of oesophageal cancer.

d False. 13–15% of oesophageal adenocarcinoma are associated with Barrett's oesophagus.

e False. Not all patients will progress to severe dysplasia or cancer, and the focus is on prevention or early detection.

2 a False. Male sex is a risk factor.

b True.

c True.

d False. The presence of extended segments (>8 cm) is a risk factor.

e False. A long history of reflux is a risk factor.

3 a True. There are often no symptoms as the columnar epithelium is insensitive to acid.

b True. Some may complain of indigestion.

c True. Barrett's is found in patients with GORD.

d False.

e False. This is not a known symptom of Barrett's disease.

4 b Histology is required for diagnostic accuracy.

5 a True. Symptom control followed by endoscopy with biopsy to confirm regression.

b False. This is considered for patients with high-grade dysplasia who are fit for surgery.

c False. This is suitable for those with high-grade dysplasia unfit for surgery.

d False. This is not the recommended management for Barrett's disease.

e False. Regular surveillance depends on the presence of dysplasia.

Malignant oesophageal tumours

1 a True.

   b False. Plummer–Vinson syndrome (oesophageal webs) is a risk factor squamous cell oesophageal cancer and this is associated with anaemia.

   c True.

   d True.

   e True.

2 a True.

   b True.

   c False. This is not a known presentation of oesophageal cancer.

   d False.

   e True.

3 a True. To ease symptoms of narrowed oesophagus.

   b True. To ease symptoms of narrowed oesophagus.

   c True. Used to shrink tumour before surgery.

   d True.

   e True. Palliative radiotherapy is used.

4 a True. The incidence of oesophageal cancer has been rising more rapidly over the past decades, mainly adenocarcinoma of the lower third.

   b True. Oesophageal cancer can be visualized endoscopically if the tumour is large enough, and biopsy provides a histological diagnosis. Staging and work-up requires CT and EUS, looking for signs of surgical incurability (local or distant dissemination).

   c False. Barrett's oesophagus may be complicated by adenocarcinoma.

   d False. Oesophageal cancer has a poor overall prognosis; however, resected patients do better, especially with early-stage node-negative disease, where 5-year survival approaches 50–60%.

   e False. Oesophageal cancer is more common in patients over 50 years of age.

Gastric cancer

1 a True.

   b True.

   c True.

   d True.

   e False. Male sex is a risk factor.

2 a True.

   b True.

   c False. Malaena or blood mixed with stools may be a presentation.

   d False.

   e False. Patients usually complain of lethargy.

3 a The initial diagnosis is made with endoscopy and biopsy.

4 d The rest of the tumours are rare. Fibromas are benign tumours.

5 a False. Often presents at a late stage and has a poor prognosis.
  b False. Less likely than in focal types of gastric cancer.
  c True. Mucosa may appear relatively normal but there is reduced peristalsis and air distension.
  d False. It is less common than focal gastric cancers.
  e True. These are common presenting symptoms.

6 a True.
  b True.
  c True.
  d True. Symptom control is important.
  e False.

EMQs

1 (i) a Long-standing undertreated or untreated GORD can result in benign stricture formation presenting as dysphagia. A definitive diagnosis is made at upper gastrointestinal endoscopy.
  (ii) e Oesophageal cancer is more common over the age of 50 years and dysphagia associated with weight loss in this age group is most likely to be due to oesophageal malignancy.
  (iii) b Given the young age and no other relevant history (or risk factors). globus hystericus is likely, but it is important to exclude treatable alternative pathology.
  (iv) h Cardiospasm due to achalasia or diffuse oesophageal spasm is the most likely explanation. It is often temporized with botulinum toxin (Botox) but is best treated definitively with cardiomyotomy (Heller's procedure), which is now usually performed laparoscopically.
  (v) c The history is typical of Boerhaave's syndrome, as are the clinical and radiological findings. This is often lethal due to the amount of pleural soiling at the time of presentation.

2 (i) i This story is typical of duodenal ulceration. Such patients may gain weight due to milk consumption and frequent meals.
  (ii) h Reflux oesophagitis is most likely, and this is supported by the risk factor of obesity and the exacerbating factors.
  (iii) c Viral hepatitis likely given the history of possible exposure and liver function pattern. Antibody testing will confirm.
  (iv) f The inflammatory features and persistence of pain of acute cholecystitis distinguish this from episodic biliary colic, which often precedes it as the patient describes.
  (v) d A perforated duodenal ulcer is more likely to be the cause of this patient's clinically evident peritonitis, given her consumption of

NSAIDs and steroids. (The usual differential, perforated diverticular disease, does not appear on the list of options.)

3 **(i) f** Long-term endoscopic surveillance because Barrett's oesophagus can progress to dysplasia which can only be detected by biopsy. Annual surveillance may be carried out more frequently if dysplasia worsens.

(ii) c PPIs, as H_2 receptor antagonists are usually not sufficiently effective.

(iii) g Reassurance that this is normal during pregnancy and unlikely to persist after delivery.

(iv) b A fundoplication can now be carried out safely laparoscopically, and offers a solution to the mechanical problem of gastro-oesophageal reflux.

(v) h Endoscopy to exclude serious causes for her symptoms, and is the speediest means of reaching a diagnosis and includes the ability to take biopsies.

9 Hepato-pancreato-biliary disease: answers

MCQs
Pancreatic cancer

1 a True. 95% of pancreatic tumours are malignant pancreatic adenocarcinomas.
b False. 50% of patients present to GP with painless obstructive jaundice.
c False. Its strongest association is with smoking *not* diabetes.
d False. ERCP with stenting is used to relieve biliary obstruction whereas EUS is used to stage the disease and to take diagnostic biopsy.
e False. Curative treatment is with Whipple's resection, although less than 15% of tumours are suitable for surgery.

2 a False. Tumours involving the head commonly cause biliary obstruction, therefore presenting with obstructive jaundice, steatorrhoea and dark urine.
b False. Early symptoms of patients with tumours involving the body of the pancreas include weight loss, nausea and back pain.
c True. Late symptoms of patients with tumours involving the body/tail of the pancreas include diabetes, cachexia, vomiting from duodenal obstruction and GI bleeding.
d True. See explanation in (a).
e True.

3 a True.
b False. The presence of a palpable gallbladder in the presence of obstructive jaundice is likely to be caused by a malignant pathology.
c True. The subcutaneous nodule is also known as Sister Mary Joseph nodule.
d True. This is also known as Blumer's shelf.
e True. Advanced intra-abdominal disease may also present with palpable mass, hepatomegaly from liver metastasis or splenomegaly from portal vein thrombosis.

4 a False. 85% of patients with elevated CA19-9 have pancreatic cancer.
b True.
c False. 40–45% of patients with pancreatic cancer have an elevated CEA.
d True.
e False. 85–95% of patients.

5 a True. Surgical treatment is at the forefront of pancreatic cancer treatment. However, chemotherapy plays an important role in the both the adjuvant and neoadjuvant setting in patients with unresectable disease.
b False. The combination of gemcitabine and erlotinib leads to a higher median and 1-year survival in metastatic disease *not* in adjuvant treatment.

    c False. Chemotherapy can improve the survival of pancreatic cancer.

    d True. Postprandial pain indicates an obstructed pancreatic/biliary duct so endoscopic treatment may improve the symptoms.

    e False. Only 5% of patients may develop duodenal obstruction due to pancreatic cancer.

6 **a** False. The mean survival in unresectable disease is 4–6 months, with a 5-year survival of less than 3%.

    b False. The 5-year survival in resectable disease is 15–20%.

    c False. Median survival in patients who undergo successful resection is 12–19 months.

    d True.

    e False. Successful resection occurs in only 20% of patients with pancreatic cancer.

7 **a** False. Carcinomas from the periampullary region have a much better prognosis (50% survival in 5 years), whereas generally there is a 90% mortality within 12 months.

    b True. Most commonly between 50 and 70 years of age. They are more common in men than women, with a 2 : 1 ratio and increasing incidence in the West.

    c True. Courvoisier's law states that a palpable gallbladder in the presence of jaundice is unlikely to be due to gallstones. This is usually caused by neoplastic stricture obstructing the distal CBD.

    d True. Chronic pancreatitis and smoking can predispose to this carcinoma of the pancreas.

    e False. The majority of carcinomas (90%) are ductal in origin. Only 7% are acinar.

8 **e** The strongest association with the development of pancreatic cancer has been made with cigarette smoking.

Liver abscess

1 **a** True.

    b True.

    c True. Bacterial/pyogenic abscesses are usually caused by instrumentation resulting in ascending cholangitis.

    d True.

    e False. Untreated abscesses are associated with 100% mortality.

Hepatocellular carcinoma

1 **a** False. HCC is the primary cancer of the hepatocyte.

    b True. About 80% of patients with newly diagnosed HCC have pre-existing cirrhosis.

    c False. HCC is uncommon and comprises only 2% of all malignancies.

    d True.

    e True. Tumours are normally multifocal within the liver 75% of the time.

2 a True.
  b True.
  c True.
  d False.
  e False.
  Less than 1% of cases of HCC present as a paraneoplastic syndrome, most commonly hypercalcaemia, hypoglycaemia and erythrocytosis.

3 c Associations with hormonal manipulations such as OCP and anabolic steroids have been suggested but are weak.

4 a True. 5% of patients with HCC are suitable for transplantation.
  b True.
  c True. Unfortunately HCC is a relatively chemoresistant tumour and therefore outcomes using this mode of treatment are unsatisfactory. It is also less efficacious in patients with underlying hepatic dysfunction.
  d True. Although there are no strict criteria for tumour size, many surgeons use less than 5 cm as their cut-off.
  e True. Appropriate evaluation of patients is required prior to resection since intraoperative mortality is doubled in cirrhotic versus non-cirrhotic patients.

5 a True. AFP is elevated in 75% of cases.
  b True. Also an elevation of AFP of >400 ng/mL predicts HCC with specificity greater than 95%. AFP is inadequate for screening due to the high rate of false positives in active hepatitis.
  c True. The overall sensitivity of MRI is thought to be similar to that of triphasic CT scanning, although MRI is superior in nodular cirrhotic livers.
  d False. Biopsies may be avoided in a clinical setting of an enlarging mass in a cirrhotic liver.
  e True.

6 d In the UK the most common causes are heavy alcohol drinking and infection with hepatitis C virus.

Cholangiocarcinoma

1 e Most tumours (60–80%) are found at the hepatic duct bifurcation. Other reviews state that 55% are found in the upper third of the CBD, 15% in the middle third, 20% in the lower third and 10% are diffuse.

2 e When found, most cholangiocarcinomas are incurable and only a small proportion of proximal lesions are curable. Distal lesions are more like to be resected in order to achieve cure (30% 5-year survival for periampullary tumours and 0–10% for hilar lesions). The localized nature of the disease would make one think that transplantation would be an option, although this has not been the case.

3 a False. Aggressive surgical treatment includes complete hepatic resection and transplantation, although the results have been associated with poor outcome mainly from a high rate of recurrence.

b False. Whipple is the procedure used for distal lesions.

c True. Regardless of surgical therapy, stenting of biliary anastomosis is important since postoperative strictures or recurrent tumours are common.

d True. The prognosis for patients with hilar bile duct tumours (Klatskin tumours) is poor with mortality rates of 80–90%. Hepatic lobectomy is indicated for potential cure if the bile duct lesion extends into the hepatic parenchyma.

e True. It has been shown that liver transplantation may have a survival benefit over palliative treatments especially in the early period.

4 a False. Cholangiocarcinoma is less common than gallbladder cancer.

b True.

c False. There is an association with cholangiocarcinoma and gallstones.

d True.

e True.

5 a True. 90% of patients with cholangiocarcinoma present with jaundice.

b False. Selective coeliac angiography can be helpful preoperatively to determine whether there is invasion in the major adjacent structures.

c True. PTC is preferred for proximal lesions as ERCP may fail to visualize the proximal part of the lesion.

d True. When biliary obstruction is present, further visualization is required with PTC or ERCP.

e True. Biliary catheters may help in resection and reconstruction and may allow the administration of local radiation therapy.

6 a True. 90% are adenocarcinomas and the rest are made up of squamous cell carcinoma.

b True. The annual incidence in Israel is 7.3 per 100 000 people.

c True. 90% of tumours are not resectable and so the median survival is very low.

d True.

e True.

Acute pancreatitis

1 a False. Gallstones and alcohol intake include the most common causes. Gallstone pancreatitis like gallstones is more common is women. Conversely, alcohol-induced pancreatitis is more common in men.

b False. Physical signs include dehydration, tachycardia, increased respiratory rate, mild pyrexia and epigastric tenderness. In haemorrhagic necrotizing pancreatitis both Cullen's sign (periumbilical bruising) and Grey Turner's sign (flank bruising) are classically seen.

c True. The Glasgow (Imrie) score measures eight parameters. The presence of two or more at 48 hours correctly predicts a severe attack in 85% of patients.

d True. Upper GI perforation can cause a raised amylase as well as mesenteric infarction, torsion of an intra-abdominal viscus, retroperitoneal haematoma, macroamylasaemia and renal failure.

   e False. By definition pseudocysts can only be diagnosed 6 weeks after the onset of the attack. Pseudocysts greater than 6 cm will not usually resolve spontaneously and should be treated with surgery.

2 a False.
   b False.
   c True.
   d False.
   e False.

3 d The degree of amylase rise is not a prognostic indicator in acute pancreatitis.

4 a Standard treatment for patients with acute pancreatitis includes IV fluid resuscitation, electrolyte replacement and analgesia. Prophylactic antibiotics are used in patients with evidence of pancreatic necrosis. Nasogastric decompression is reserved for patients with significant ileus who are at risk for emesis and aspiration. The use of octreotide has not been proven to benefit patients with pancreatitis.

5 e Many pharmacological agents that reduce acinar cell enzyme release have been evaluated, but show unimpressive results.

6 All true. The incidence of pancreatitis following distal gastric resection is 0.6–1.2%, and after biliary tract surgery is 0.5–3%. This occurs due to direct handling of the pancreas. About 1% may develop pancreatitis after ERCP. The risk of pancreatitis can be reduced by limiting the amount of contrast injected into the pancreatic duct. Pancreatitis after coronary artery bypass graft is thought to be due to ischaemia and hypotension.

Chronic pancreatitis

1 a False. Chronic pancreatitis is defined as persistent or recurrent abdominal pain, with endocrine or exocrine insufficiency. The common causes of chronic pancreatitis include alcohol abuse, gallstones, hyperparathyroidism, congenital abnormalities of the pancreatic duct, trauma and cystic fibrosis. While chronic pancreatitis may due to repeated insults of acute pancreatitis, not all patients with repeated attacks will develop the chronic form.
   b True. Patients with disabling symptoms who have a dilated pancreatic duct are eligible for longitudinal pancreaticojejunostomy (Peustow's procedure).
   c False.
   d False. Total pancreatectomy is avoided due to problems with brittle diabetes, weight loss and steatorrhoea.
   e False. Mesenteric angiography has no role in this case.

2 d Serum blood tests have no use in making the diagnosis. Serum amylase rises in an acute attack, whereas amylase levels may be normal or mildly elevated in chronic pancreatitis. EUS has become widely recognized as the most sensitive and reliable method for diagnosing chronic pancreatitis.

3 a, e In the UK most cases of chronic pancreatitis are as a result of alcohol abuse. Less than 5–10% of people with alcoholism develop the disease.

4 e Patients with pancreatic duct dilatation (>8 mm) may undergo decompression using longitudinal pancreaticojejunostomy. The entire pancreatic duct is opened from the pancreatic tail to 1 cm from duodenum. Following this, a side-to-side anastomosis is performed between the open pancreatic duct and a loop of jejunum; 80% have reported an improvement in symptoms.

5 d Strictures of the bile duct occur in chronic pancreatitis due to the close position of the duct with the head of the pancreas. In 66% of patients the bile duct passes through the pancreatic parenchyma. Inflammation of the pancreas can encase and compress the duct.

6 d Pain is the predominant symptom in pancreatitis. The pain is localized to the epigastrium and radiates to the lumbar vertebrae. It is aggravated by eating and relieved by abstinence and sitting forward. Steatorrhoea is observed after 90% of the pancreatic exocrine tissue has been damaged. Diabetes is present in 50–70% of patients with chronic pancreatitis.

Pancreatic pseudocyst (advanced topic)

1 d The common causes of pancreatic abscess formation are pancreatic pseudocyst and necrotizing pancreatitis. The diagnosis is suggested by persistent fever, leucocytosis and a palpable abdominal mass. Bacteraemia and sepsis are late clinical features. Percutaneous aspiration with positive cultures is a definitive preoperative test. When the abscess is diagnosed the treatment of choice is surgical debridement.

2 a A pancreatic pseudocyst can be observed for several months to allow spontaneous resolution. Simple aspiration is performed if the aspiration is sterile. If the aspiration is infected, then a large drain should be inserted or an open procedure may be required.

3 d Nealon's classification describes the relationship of the pseudocyst with the pancreatic duct.
   (i) Normal duct and no communication with pseudocyst.
   (ii) Normal duct with communication with pseudocyst.
   (iii) Normal duct with stricture and no communication with pseudocyst.
   (iv) Normal duct with stricture and communication with pseudocyst.
   (v) Normal duct with complete obstruction without communication of pseudocyst.
   (vi) Chronic pancreatitis with no communication with the pseudocyst.
   (vii) Chronic pancreatitis with communication with the pseudocyst.

4 e The most common location of pancreatic pseudocyst is the lesser sac. Although less common it is still possible that pseudocyst may develop in the greater sac, paracolic gutters, mediastinum, pelvis and scrotum.

5 a Acute infection is the most common complication of a pancreatic pseudocyst. Obstruction of the viscus is not common with pseudocysts which have been present for a long time. The presentation is less obvious and complete obstruction is not usually present. Pseudocyst may also erode into a named arterial vessel, most commonly the splenic artery. Bleeding may occur following rupture of the pseudoaneurysm.

6 d 10% of pancreatic pseudocysts become infected.

Gallstones

1 a True. *Escherichia coli* produces the enzyme β-glucoronidase, which hydrolyses soluble conjugated bilirubin to form free bilirubin, which precipitates as calcium bilirubinate (pigmented stone).

b True. Cholecystitis is inflammation of the gallbladder as a result of obstruction of the cystic duct with a stone and therefore a secondary infection. The pain is in the RUQ and may be constant and may be exacerbated by movement and breathing. When the pain radiates to the lower scapula there may be an area below the scapula which is hypersensitive; this is known as Boas' sign.

c False. The most common cause for jaundice is alcohol.

d True. Oral dissolution therapy (chenodeoxycholic acid or ursodeoxycholic acid) alone can be successful in dissolving pure cholesterol gallstones. Treatment is prolonged and requires patient compliance. Side effects include diarrhoea, which often leads to discontinuation of therapy. Recurrence of stones after cessation of treatment is also common.

e True. This is a long right subcostal (muscle-cutting) incision. The gallbladder is exposed and the cystic duct and artery dissected. The cystic duct is cannulated and a perioperative cholangiogram is performed to look for any stones in the common duct. If a filling defect is seen, the common duct can be opened and the stones extracted.

2 a False. In haemolytic jaundice the excess bilirubin production is associated with increased secretion of conjugated pigment in the bile and therefore increased production of urobilinogen by bacterial decomposition in the distal small intestine. The urine consequently contains excess amounts of urobilinogen and urobilin.

b True. Postoperative jaundice usually occurs in the first 3 weeks. The causes include the following.
- Resorption of haematomas, haemoperitoneum, haemolysis of transfused erythrocytes (especially when stored products are used), haemolysis due to glucose-6-phosphate dehydrogenase deficiency.
- Impaired hepatocellular function due to halogenated anaesthetics, sepsis, hepatic ischaemia secondary to perioperative hypotension.
- Unsuspected injury to the biliary tree.

   c True. Carotenaemia is a condition causing yellow discoloration of the skin but not the sclera or mucous membranes. There is also presence of yellow-brown pigmentation of carotenoid pigment in palms, soles and nasolabial folds. This condition is caused by excess intake of carotene-containing substances such as carrots and mangoes.

   d False. Murphy's sign is tenderness at the midpoint of the right subcoastal margin on inspiration. It is a sign of cholecystitis. Cholangitis is associated with Charcot's triad: jaundice, RUQ tenderness and fever/rigors.

   e False. Phytomenadione (vitamin K) is used preoperatively in obstructive jaundice to correct clotting abnormalities but this process takes 1–3 days. Without bile the gut cannot absorb the fat-soluble vitamins A, D, E and K. The production of four clotting factors are affected (II, VII, IX and X) resulting in an increased prothrombin time.

3 **a** False.

   b False.

   c False. Normal serum bilirubin is approximately 3–20 µmol/L. Jaundice becomes visibly apparent at levels > 35 µmol/L.

   d False. AFP levels are normally low in adult life. It can be measured in the serum and used as a tumour marker for testicular and ovarian cancer.

   e False. Amylase is not typically deranged in obstructive jaundice. Please refer to section on hyperamylasaemia.

4 **a** True. Ascending cholangitis is infection of the CBD caused by bacteria ascending from the duodenum and small bowel. It mostly occurs due to partial obstruction of the bile duct by gallstones. Other causes include benign or malignant stricturing of the CBD.

Benign and malignant causes of CBD stricture

Benign stricture
- Postoperative damage
- Anastomosis fibrosis

Malignant stricture
- Cholangiocarcinoma
- Gallbladder cancer
- Pancreatic cancer
- Ampullary cancer
- Duodenal cancer

---

   b True. Charcot's triad is a combination of three common findings in acute cholangitis, said to be reported in 15–20% of cases. These include fever, RUQ pain and jaundice. Dr Jean-Martin Charcot was a Parisian physician working at the Pitié-Salpêtrière Hospital who first described the triad in 1877.

   c False. LFTs in late stages of ascending cholangitis show an obstructive picture with raised bilirubin, ALP and GGT. Early stages may show a hepatitic picture with derangement in ALT and ASP.

   d False. Gram-negative bacilli are the most common forms of bacteria associated with cholangitis, including *E. coli* (25–50%) and *Klebsiella*

(15–20%). Patients who have had previous surgery to the CBD are more likely to be infected by anaerobes (*Bacteroides* and *Clostridium*).

e False. The most common definitive treatment for ascending cholangitis caused by gallstones is ERCP. The CBD may be cleared using many different types of instruments including a balloon or basket. Larger stones may require mechanical destruction using a lithotripter. Although becoming increasingly more common, laparoscopic surgical exploration is still rarely used, mainly because not all patients can withstand a GA and the technique itself is very specialized requiring an expert operator.

5 a Abdominal USS is the most appropriate initial investigation in the evaluation of the patient with jaundice. The presence of a dilated CBD directs the surgeon to search for a mechanical cause. Furthermore, USS is a very sensitive way of detecting gallstones.

6 a False.
  b False.
  c False.
  d True.
  e True. Cholecystectomy is indicated in patients with symptomatic gallstones disease and its complications, i.e. cholecystitis, obstructive jaundice, pancreatitis. The rate of developing symptoms in patients with asymptomatic gallstone disease is 2% per year. This rate does not exceed the possibility of morbidity and mortality from the operation and therefore an elective operation should not be offered to asymptomatic patients. An operation should not be offered until angina is well controlled as cardiac disease is the most common cause for postoperative mortality. Recent studies have confirmed that the mortality rate for patients with diabetes and those without have a similar mortality rate following acute cholecystitis and therefore these patients should not be offered an operation unless they present with symptomatic disease.

7 c Uncontrolled sepsis with multiorgan failure can be the leading events following acute cholangitis. Therefore the initial treatment should be to decompress the biliary system to avoid reflux of bacterial toxins into the venous circulation. Any cause for obstruction should be addressed following decompression of the bile duct.

EMQs

1 **(i) a** This imaging technique allows excellent visualization of liver, pancreas, spleen, lymph nodes and a lesion in the porta hepatis.
  (ii) d Visualization of the proximal or upper biliary tree for suspected intrahepatic biliary obstruction is best studied by PTC.
  (iii) d In a Tc-Iodida scan, technetium-labelled iododiethyl IDA is taken up by hepatocytes and excreted rapidly into the biliary system. Its main uses are in the diagnosis of acute cholecystitis and jaundice from biliary atresia.

(iv) b This technique outlines the biliary and pancreatic ducts. CBD stones can be removed after balloon dilatation or sphincterotomy. ERCP is preferred due to it potential therapeutic role.

2 (i) k This patient has underlying multiple myeloma as the cause for her hypercalcaemia.

(ii) b

(iii) a The most characteristic sign of pancreatic carcinoma of the head is obstructive jaundice. Patients with jaundice may have Courvoisier's sign and may have evidence of excoriations from pruritis.

(iv) c Symptoms in the history mostly consist of fever, headache, and malaise. Within 24 hours patients report ear pain aggravated by a chewing movement of the jaw. The fever usually subsides after a variable period of up to a week.

(v) d This is an autosomal recessive disease seen in white people. Cystic fibrosis is a disease of the exocrine gland involving multiple organ systems mainly resulting in recurrent chest infections, pancreatic enzyme insufficiency, and associated complications in untreated patients. End-stage lung disease is the main cause of death.

3 (i) d

(ii) f

(iii) c

(iv) b

(v) e Infectious mononucleosis caused by EBV.

4 (i) a The most characteristic sign of pancreatic cancer of the head is obstructive jaundice. Patients with jaundice may have a palpable gallbladder and have evidence of excoriations from pruritis.

(ii) f This is a chronic cholestatic disease characterized by fibrosing inflammatory destruction of both intrahepatic and extrahepatic bile ducts. In 75% of patients with PSC there is an association with IBD (commonly ulcerative colitis). Clinically these patients usually present with fluctuating pruritis, jaundice and cholangitis.

(iii) c Gilbert's syndrome.

(iv) h CBD stones.

(v) d This is a chronic progressive cholestatic disease of unknown aetiology. This pathology was described in the previous question.

5 (i) a This woman requires ERCP, attempted stone extraction and stenting to decompress the infected biliary system.

(ii) d

(iii) f The history is consistent with head of pancreas malignancy. Presence of a palpable gallbladder in the presence of jaundice is unlikely to be due to gallstones (Courvoisier's law). This patient therefore requires a pancreaticoduodenectomy, also known as Whipple's procedure.

(iv) a BSG guidelines recommend cholecystectomy in the same admission or within 2 weeks of onset of symptoms.

(v) h This elderly woman is not fit to undergo a GA for laparoscopic cholecystectomy. USS reveals a large distended gallbladder and in the presence of swinging pyrexia, which does not improve with intravenous antibiotics, this patient requires a cholecystostomy for the treatment of gallbladder empyema.

6 (i) **d** Hepatomegaly is prominent in right-sided heart failure but may occur rapidly in acute heart failure. When occurring acutely the liver is usually tender.

(ii) **b** Autoimmune hepatitis is classified as type 1 or type 2. Type 1 is the most common form in North America. It can occur at any age but most often starts in adolescence or young adulthood. About half of those with type 1 have other autoimmune disorders, such as type 1 diabetes, proliferative glomerulonephritis, thyroiditis, Graves' disease, Sjögren's syndrome and ulcerative colitis.

(iii) **i** Primary biliary cirrhosis occurs when interlobular bile ducts are damaged by chronic granulomatous inflammation. This causes progressive cholestasis, cirrhosis and portal hypertension. Often asymptomatic, diagnosis usually comes about following the discovery of a raised ALP on routine LFTs. Symptoms include lethargy and pruritis. Clinical signs include jaundice, skin pigmentation, xanthelasma, xanthomata, hepatomegaly and splenomegaly.

(iv) **a** Alcoholic liver disease can present with psoriasis.

(v) **g**

7 (i) **e** Both parotid enlargement and Dupuytren's contracture are associated with excess alcohol consumption.

(ii) **j** Clubbing and coarse crepitation at both lung bases suggest bronchiectasis. Cystic fibrosis causes liver cirrhosis and bronchiectasis.

(iii) **c** Primary biliary cirrhosis is associated with raised cholesterol and xanthelasma.

(iv) **g**

(v) **d**

8 (i) **a** This is a chronic disease of unknown cause, characterized by hepatocellular inflammation and necrosis to eventual cirrhosis.

(ii) **c** Wilson's disease is a inherited autosomal recessive disorder of copper metabolism. There is excessive deposition of copper in the liver, brain and other tissues. Most common neurological feature is asymmetric tremor, occurring in approximately half of individuals with Wilson's disease.

(iii) **b** This is a chronic progressive cholestatic disease of the liver. The aetiology is unknown, although it is presumed to be autoimmune in nature. This disease usually affects the small to medium bile ducts, which leads to progressive cholestasis and often end-stage liver failure.

(iv) **i** This syndrome is characterized by intermittent jaundice in the absence of haemolysis or underlying liver disease. Gilbert's syndrome is precipitated by dehydration, fasting, menstrual periods, or stress. These episodes resolve spontaneously, and no treatment is required.

(v) **d**

10　Spleen: answers

MCQs

1 **a** True. Only grade 1 or 2 splenic injuries can be managed conservatively.
 b True. ITP is also an indication for splenectomy but the common indications are trauma and lymphoma.
 c True.
 d True.
 e False. Not usually required unless there is iatrogenic injury intraoperatively.
 f True.

2 **a** True.
 b True.
 c True. Post-splenectomy patients are prone to developing infections, therefore vaccinations against *Haemophilus influenzae*, *Streptococcus pneumoniae* and *Neisseria meningitidis* are recommended. Long-term antibiotics are also recommended to reduce the risk of overwhelming post-splenectomy infection.
 d False.
 e False.

3 **a** True. Pathologically enlarged spleen is more likely to rupture.
 b False. 75% of ruptures occur within 2 weeks.
 c True. Ruptured spleen occasionally causes displacement of the surrounding structures resulting in a raised hemidiaphragm.
 d False. It leads to referred pain over the left shoulder in the head-down position (Kehr's sign).
 e True. Because of the anatomical location of the spleen, it is very much prone to injury following left lower rib fractures.

EMQS

1 **(i) h** This patient has sustained a splenic injury. Observe the patient: he can be transferred for a CT abdomen if haemodynamically stable.
 (ii) k A contrast CT abdomen is the investigation of choice in patients with blunt abdominal trauma.
 (iii) d This patient is very unwell with persistent vomiting. The CT confirmed a spontaneous ruptured spleen.
 (iv) g This exsanguinating patient needs to go to theatre to stop the bleeding.
 (v) d Assess the patient's ABCDE and once your assessment is complete, call your senior for advice and assistance.

2   (i) e
    (ii) b
   (iii) a
   (iv) f
    (v) c

11 Midgut: answers

MCQs
Appendicitis

1 a True. The appendix is an outpouching of the whole bowel wall which makes it a true diverticulum. False diverticulum is one which only contains part of the bowel wall.
  b False. The appendix develops as an outgrowth of the caecum.
  c False. The position of the base of the appendix remains constant; however the tip varies.
  d False. The appendix is a non-essential part of the GALT.
  e True.

2 a False. Appendicitis is the commonest surgical emergency in the UK, with 35 000 hospital admissions annually.
  b False. Dietary fibre is said to decrease transit time through the bowel and discourage faecolith formation. This reduces the risk of appendiceal lumen obstruction. It is therefore thought that dietary fibre reduces the risk of appendicitis.
  c False. Appendicitis commonly presents in the first and second decade of life; however, no age is exempt.
  d True. Perforation rates are higher among patients younger than 18 and older than 50 years. This is most likely to be due to delays in diagnosis as a result of atypical presentation.
  e False. There is a slightly higher incidence in males.

3 a True. The typical symptoms present with periumbilical/epigastric pain which radiates to the right iliac fossa.
  b False. The classical symptoms occur in 50% of patients and were first described by American physician John Benjamin Murphy (1857–1916).
  c True. 20% of appendixes may lie subcaecally and typically present with diarrhoea and urinary frequency.
  d False. Vomiting precedes pain in bowel obstruction, whereas it usually follows pain in appendicitis.
  e True. The tip of the appendix may lie near the hepatic flexure.

4 a False. In uncomplicated appendicitis the vital signs are usually unchanged.
  b False. Rovsing's sign is in fact the demonstration of pain in the right iliac fossa upon deep palpation of the left iliac fossa.
  c True. McBurney's is the most common point of maximal tenderness. It is one-third of the distance from the anterior superior iliac spine to the umbilicus.
  d True. A number of clinical and laboratory-based scoring systems have been devised to assist diagnosis.

e False. This suggests that the inflamed appendix is located along the course of the right psoas muscle.

5 a False. AXR has no role in the diagnosis of appendicitis.
  b True. Urinalysis is helpful in excluding pregnancy and urinary tract pathology (UTI or renal stones).
  c True. Inflammatory markers such as WCC and CRP are helpful in the diagnosis of appendicitis.
  d False. CT imaging is the most sensitive and specific imaging modality in the diagnosis of appendicitis.
  e True. Particularly in obese patients and those with equivocal clinical signs.

6 a False. There is no good evidence that the use of analgesia will cloud the clinical picture.
  b False. All patients should receive broad-spectrum perioperative antibiotics, as they have been shown to reduce postoperative wound infection and intra-abdominal abscess formation.
  c True. Spontaneous resolution of early appendicitis can occur, and antibiotics alone can be used to treat appendicitis if no facilities for appendicectomy are available. However, a 14–35% readmission rate was associated with antibiotic treatment, and because of the high recurrence rate and relatively low morbidity and mortality associated with appendicectomy early operative intervention remains the treatment of choice.
  d True. The longer the delay in a patient with appendicitis, the higher the risk of perforation.
  e False. The options are open or laparoscopic.

7 a True. Appendicectomy is a relatively safe procedure with a low mortality of only 0.8 per 1000 in uncomplicated appendicitis.
  b False. The rate of wound infection is dependent on intraoperative wound contamination. Rates of wound infection vary from <5% in simple appendicitis to 20% in cases with perforation and gangrene.
  c False. Abdominal ultrasound or CT scan is required to diagnose the abscess. Treatment may be radiologically assisted drain insertion or open or per rectal drainage of pelvic abscess.
  d False. The usual perforation rate on presentation is 16–30%; however it is much higher, up to 97%, in elderly and children in whom it is more difficult to diagnose.
  e False. There have been reported cases of appendicitis in the surgical stump after previous appendicectomy.

Small bowel obstruction

1 a False. Hiatal hernias are not associated with SBO.
  b True. Adhesions are the commonest cause of SBO.
  c True. A large abscess may cause extrinsic compression of the small bowel.

    d False. IBD may cause SBO.
    e True.

2 **a** True. Symptoms of gastroenteritis may be severe.
    b True. Acute and chronic pancreatitis should always be considered in patients presenting with abdominal pains.
    c True. The typical history of acute appendicitis is central abdominal pain (midgut origin) migrating to the right iliac fossa (peritonism over the region where the inflamed appendix lies).
    d True. Diabetics may present to the surgeons with an acute abdomen. Consider ketoacidosis early and rule out on preliminary blood investigations.
    e True. In all females who have not reached menopause, rule out pregnancy with urine or blood β-HCG early on in the investigations.

3 **a** False. Barium follow-through is avoided in complete SBO.
    b True.
    c False. MRI abdomen is as good as CT abdomen but not as widely available.
    d True. USS abdomen will confirm dilated loops of small bowel but has limited value in diagnosing the specific cause of SBO.
    e True. AXR is the investigation of choice and should be done first before further imaging.

4 **a** True. Ischaemia or perforation of small bowel may develop into an abscess.
    b True. SBO after abdominal surgery may result in wound dehiscence.
    c False. Patients with SBO are usually dehydrated because there is third spacing. Careful fluid management is essential to ensure adequate hydration.
    d False.
    e True. After multiple surgeries on the small bowel.

Meckel's diverticulum

1 **a** False. Meckel's diverticulum is present about 60 cm proximal to ileocaecal valve.
    b False. It is present at the antimesenteric border of the ileum.
    c True.
    d True.
    e False. It is about 5 cm in length.

2 **a** False. Not all Meckel's diverticulum are symptomatic. They become symptomatic only in the presence of complications.
    b True.
    c True. A fibrous band arising from the Meckel's diverticulum to the umbilicus may cause SBO.
    d True. Patient with intussusception will present with intermittent abdominal pain and intermittent abdominal mass.

   e True. Acute inflammation of Meckel's diverticulum may present with symptoms similar to acute appendicitis.

3 a False. Technetium-labelled scan is only helpful in the presence of bleeding from Meckel's diverticulum.
   b True.
   c True.
   d False. It should be resected if it is found to be inflamed. Some surgeons would even resect a normal Meckel's diverticulum if it has a particularly narrow neck that might later obstruct.
   e True.

4 a True.
   b False.
   c True.
   d True.
   e False.

5 a This patient had a perforated Meckel's diverticulum. Once the patient is resuscitated, plan for a laparotomy.

6 a A pregnancy test must be done before any other investigations or treatments.

EMQs

1 **(i) d** There is a pelvic abscess causing fever and bladder irritation.
   (ii) d There is a pelvic abscess causing fever and rectal irritation.
  (iii) e This patient has developed sepsis as a result of delayed presentation after a perforated appendix.
   (iv) f This patient has developed an ileus postoperatively.
   (v) b This is typical of gangrenous appendix.

2 **(i) c** This patient has postoperative ileus and hypokalaemia, which may have caused the ileus. He will need potassium supplementation and careful fluid monitoring. Start management following the ABCDE approach; insert an NGT, IV line for fluid resuscitation and catheterize to monitor UO.
   (ii) a This patient has a large paraumbilical hernia with small bowel within the hernia sac. The bowel has an increased chance of being strangulated, therefore a laparotomy is required to remove the small bowel from the hernia sac (+/– resection of small bowel) and repair the hernia.
  (iii) d This patient does not require another laparotomy. The interventional radiologist will assess the images and decide whether any collection is amenable to percutanous drainage. The collection needs to be sent for MC&S once it is drained.

12   Colorectal: answers

MCQs
Diverticular disease

1 **b** Acute management of diverticulitis includes active fluid resuscitation, analgesia and antibiotics.

2 **b** Uncomplicated diverticular disease is managed by dietary and lifestyle advice, often with addition of laxatives to keep bowels regular.

3 **c** CT abdomen is sensitive to grading extent of diverticular inflammation, to help manage the patient's condition further.

4 **b** Acute diverticular pelvic collections often need surgical intervention when the patient is not responding to conservative management. This patient needs resection of the sigmoid colon and Hartmann's procedure. Some may consider anastomosis but the general condition of the patient and blood supply to the colon in the presence of sepsis and inotropic support have to be considered when making this decision.

5 **a** True. Patients generally present with left lower quadrant pain, but some Asian patients may present with right lower quadrant pain indicating inflamed diverticula in the ascending colon.
  b False. Patients complain of nausea and vomiting-associated anorexia.
  c True. Like other inflammatory conditions, the patients may have fever and tachycardia.
  d True. There may be a large tender inflammatory mass commonly over the left iliac fossa.
  e True. Some cases are associated with rectal bleeding that is severe enough to require transfusion.

6 **a** True. Chronic inflammation can lead to fistula formation between bowel and adjacent structures, e.g. bladder, adjacent large or small bowel, and vagina.
  b True. Inflamed tissue is friable, leading to perforation.
  c True. Patients can develop a perforation, and if not contained can develop into a large pelvic abscess.
  d True. Chronic ischaemia due to recurrent diverticulitis can lead to bowel stricture.
  e True. Very tight strictures can lead to symptoms and signs of obstruction.

Colorectal cancer

1 **b** Colonoscopy helps in complete visualization of the luminal surface, and also helps in obtaining a biopsy for tissue diagnosis. Once confirmed, colorectal cancers are staged by CT scan to assess distant metastases, with MRI used to locally stage rectal cancer.

2 a Rectal cancers that are locally advanced at presentation are considered for neoadjuvant sensitizing chemotherapy and potentially curative radiotherapy prior to surgery.

3 b Presence of FAP and other hereditary colorectal cancers are part of exclusion for HNPCC. HNPCC is identified using Amsterdam II criteria.

4 c Anterior resection involves resection of the rectum and sigmoid colon. Excision of low rectal lesion with anal sphincter is termed abdominoperineal excision of rectum. Resection of ascending colon and hepatic flexure is termed right hemicolectomy; resection of splenic flexure and descending colon is left hemicolectomy. A defunctioning ileostomy is performed generally for tumours below the peritoneal reflection as leak rate increases the more distal the anastomosis in the rectum.

5 a True. Patients with regular bowel habits often complain of altered bowel habit, usually looser stools/diarrhoea. In rectal cancer, the patient often suffers tenesmus.
  b True. Particularly in rectal cancer.
  c True. More likely in advanced stages of colorectal cancer.
  d True. The tumour may be bleeding, resulting in mild microcytic anaemia.
  e False. Perianal abscess is not a known symptom of colorectal cancer; it is associated with Crohn's disease.

6 a True. Age is the biggest single risk factor for colorectal cancer. More than 80% of colorectal cancers are diagnosed in those aged above 60.
  b True. The risk of colorectal cancer is increased in those with IBD.
  c False. These are benign lesions; they may cause abdominal pain with obstruction or intussusceptions.
  d True. This rare condition is familial or sporadic and is responsible for 1% of colorectal cancers. In FAP, there are hundreds of benign polyps in the colon, and each polyp has the potential to become cancerous. Treatment for FAP is a total colectomy.
  e True. Lynch syndrome is HNPCC. The gene for HNPCC helps to repair faulty DNA. In Lynch syndrome, there is a faulty gene for HNPCC which increases the risk of several cancers.

IBD

1 c Remission of IBD is usually maintained with 5-ASA.
2 b Pancolitis and crypt abscess are hallmarks of CD.
3 a This man presents with signs of UC, which predisposes individuals to colorectal cancer.

4 d Inflammation due to UC is usually limited to mucosa and submucosa. Extension beyond these anatomical layers indicates severe disease.

5 a Typically, fistulae are treated in the following way: treat sepsis, provide good nutrition, determine the anatomy of the fistula and definitive surgical *p*rocedure (mnemonic: SNAP). Enterocutaneous fistula is an absolute indication for TPN.

6 a False. UC involves rectum and colon.
   b False. CD involves anywhere from mouth to anus.
   c True. Gross rectal bleeding is unusual in CD.
   d True. Up to one-third of CD patients have perianal lesions and fistulas/fissures.
   e True. Skip lesions are characteristic of CD.
   f False. In CD, there are crypt abscesses which progress to aphthous ulcers extending longitudinally and transversely, resulting in a characteristic cobblestone appearance of the mucosa.
   g True.
   h True.
   i False. Masses and abscesses are common in CD.
   j True. CD is often described as a transmural granulomatous disease.

7 d Panproctocolectomy is resection of the large bowel, rectum and anus. This is followed by the fashioning of an end ileostomy.

8 a False.
   b True.
   c False.
   d True.
   e True.
Panproctocolectomy can be performed in patients with HNPCC-related colon cancer.

9 a False. Ileostomies are usually formed on the right side, although they can be placed on the left side.
   b True. Ileostomy is usually formed to protect a distal anastomosis which can be reversed later.
   c False. Ileostomy has a spout to protect the skin from the liquid contents of the ileum, which contain digestive enzymes.
   d False. Stomas protect distal anastomosis.
   e False. Hartmann's procedure involves the formation of a colostomy of the proximal end of bowel.

Lower gastrointestinal bleeding

1 b Radiation proctitis presents with recurrent troublesome bleeding and telangiectasia is seen. Treatment is difficult.

2 b 'Redcurrant jelly' is the sloughed mucosa from (often) the splenic flexure. Complications are rarely seen.

3 e This is a typical presentation of acute diverticular bleeds. The patient needs admission to hospital as he requires resuscitation including blood transfusion if required. Note that bleeding is more common in diverticular disease than in diverticulitis.

4 b Anal fissures are a result of suboptimal blood supply to the mucosa of anal canal resulting in ulceration.

5 c Haemorrhoids are common.

6 b Condylomata acuminatum are the most recognizable symptom of genital HPV infection.

Haemorrhoids

1 a True. This is the definition of internal haemorrhoids.
  b False. There are three haemorrhoidal cushions.
  c True.
  d False. This is a one of the treatment options for fissures.
  e True. There is bright red blood on the toilet paper, covering the stool or in the toilet bowl.

2 a True.
  b True.
  c False. Hepatic disease is a risk factor.
  d True.
  e True. This is traditionally thought to be a risk factor for haemorrhoids.

3 a True.
  b False.
  c False. The diagnosis of haemorrhoids is made by excluding other pathologies.
  d True.
  e False. Males are equally affected.

4 c The safest option is to treat this thrombosed pile conservatively.

5 a Haemorrhoidectomy is the treatment of choice as this procedure is reserved for patients with large symptomatic grade III or IV haemorrhoids.

6 a False. Try not to strain.
  b True. Keep stools soft.
  c True. To reduce constipation.
  d False. Encourage emptying bowels when the urge occurs.
  e True.

Fissure in ano

1 a True.
  b False. Calcium channel blockers are beneficial.
  c False. Nitroglycerin ointment.
  d True.
  e False. Antibiotics are reserved for those with infected anal fistulae.

2 a True.
  b True. Constipation and faecal impaction can occur due to pain, discouraging defecation.
  c True.
  d False.
  e False.

3 c A cause of fissure in ano is thought to be sphincter spasm with accompanying ischaemia. This can prevent healing.

4 a Blind digital anal stretch is actively discouraged in modern surgical practice for the fear of occult sphincter injury resulting in incontinence.

5 b Most anal fissures are found in the posterior midline.

6 c There is a high incidence of anal fissures in Crohn's disease.

Fistula in ano

1 e Irritable bowel syndrome not associated with fistula in ano.

2 a True.
  b True.
  c True.
  d True.
  e False. This is a feeling of fullness after eating.

3 a True. A seton is a non-absorbable material placed through the fistula tract to keep the tract open. This allows continuous drainage of any infection/abscess and promotes fibrosis.
  b True.
  c False.
  d True.
  e True. Fibrin glue is only useful in the absence of infection.

4 a Drain the abscess in an emergency situation. The fistula can be dealt with once the acute episode has been treated.

5 b This patient has fistula in ano as a result of a previously incompletely drained anorectal abscess.

6 a True. The position of the trans-sphincteric fistula makes it more difficult to treat.
  b True. Incontinence is one of the complications of treatment with seton.
  c False.
  d False. Posterior fistulae are usually complex.
  e True.

13 Nutrition: answers

MCQs

1 a True. Phosphate is the most abundant intracellular anion and is important in nearly every aspect of cell function. Skeletal and smooth muscle weakness is the commonest clinical manifestation of phosphate deficiency and can range from ileus to proximal myopathy.

b True. Magnesium is important in cellular metabolism and its deficiency has been reported in up to 20% of inpatients. It is most commonly lost via the renal and GI systems, and the symptoms of hypomagnesaemia include arrhythmias, muscle cramps and fibrillation, and irritability and disorientation.

c False. Potassium is the most abundant intracellular cation and it is therefore difficult to measure the total levels. In hypokalaemia, there are muscular and cardiac symptoms (tachycardia or muscle weakness). Hyperkalaemia on the other hand is very serious as it can cause fatal cardiac arrhythmias and death.

d True. In hyponatraemia, the total body water rises, causing the cells to swell. This can in turn lead to a number of signs and symptoms: headache and confusion, muscle spasms and cramps, nausea and vomiting, seizures, fatigue, decreasing consciousness and coma.

e True. Severe hypercalcaemia causes bone pain and fractures; GI symptoms of nausea, vomiting and constipation; renal stones, polydipsia and polyuria; depression/confusion (Bones, groans, stones, psychic moans).

2 a True. Malnutrition is associated with poor wound healing and impaired immune responses, leading to more complications and delayed recovery from illness.

b True. In one study of 500 consecutive hospital admissions, malnutrition was found in 40% of patients.

c True. Eating an imbalanced diet (lack of essential nutrients) can lead to malnutrition.

d True. There are enough calories to stop hunger but there is lack of nutrients in the diet.

e True. MUST is used to identify adults (particularly elderly) who are malnourished, at risk of malnutrition and malnutrition in the obese.

3 a False. Specific indications for TPN include debilitating illnesses lasting longer than 2 weeks; loss of 10% or more of pre-illness weight; serum albumin levels <3.5 g/dL; excessive nitrogen loss from wound infection, fistula or abscess; renal or hepatic failure; non-function of the GIT lasting 5–7 days.

b True. Only patients with high caloric and nutritional needs due to illness or injury will benefit from TPN. In a patient with a healthy GIT, likely to resume normal function, the risks of TPN outweigh the potential benefits.

c False. The Liverpool care pathway is for dying patients in hospital/
community. In such cases, TPN is contraindicated as its risks outweigh its
benefits.

d True. Composition is usually tailor made to the individual's requirements
and include dextrose (15–50% solution), fat emulsions (10–20% solution),
electrolytes, vitamins and trace elements.

e True. The TPN is bypassing the GIT and therefore there is no stimulation of
the gallbladder, pancreas and small intestine.

4 a False. Once the NGT is inserted, the aspirate must be tested with litmus
paper and the stomach auscultated. If the position of the NGT is still
uncertain, a CXR must be ordered to ensure the tube is not in the right/
left main bronchus.

b True. NGTs are used to provide liquid nutrition, fluids and medications.
Nasogastric feeding can be used for 6 weeks. In stroke patients, their
impaired swallowing may resolve within this time. For those with
long-term feeding issues, a PEG is inserted.

c False. The nasogastric aspirate must be below pH 5 to confirm the fluid is
from the stomach but this does not guarantee that the NGT is in the right
place. If there is uncertainty, the location of the NGT must be checked with
a CXR.

d True. Ryles tubes are usually used for draining GI contents but can be used
for feeding. It is better to have a fine-bore NGT (less than 9Fr) as it causes
less discomfort and less risk of oesophageal erosion.

e True. In hospital, the dietician will work out how much nasogastric feed
the patient requires in 24 hours.

5 a True. TPN is administered via a central line or peripherally inserted central
catheter. There may be infection at the site of central line insertion or
bacteraemia and sepsis due to organisms in the lumen of the central line.
The line may need to be removed and the tip sent to microbiology as well
as blood cultures taken from the central line.

b True. Electrolyte management is one of the difficult aspects of TPN,
and this is why patients require daily electrolyte monitoring.

c True. These signs are due to a large blood clot forming at the tip of the
central line. The central line may need to be removed and an anticoagulant
will need to be started.

d False. Careful monitoring is required in patients receiving TPN.
Hyperglycaemia is an early complication of TPN and should be anticipated.

e False. Hiccups are spasmodic involuntary contractions of a hemidiaphragm
and are not a known complication of TPN.

6 a True. Refeeding syndrome is due to a shift from utilizing protein and fat
stores to carbohydrates, which causes a rise in insulin levels and
movement of glucose accompanied by electrolytes into the cells.

b False. Refeeding syndrome occurs in both parenteral and enteral feeding,
due to the load of carbohydrates.

c False. Potassium, magnesium and phosphate move intracellularly for
metabolism, resulting in very low concentrations in serum.

d True. There is a drop in serum electrolytes and accumulation in fluid in the extracellular space, leading to increased cardiac workload and metabolic demand. This can lead to acute cardiac failure especially in those with pre-existing cardiac disease.

e True. In a surgical patient unable to take oral nutrition due to perforated oesophagus, TPN should be started slowly after all electrolyte abnormalities have been corrected.

EMQ

1 **(i) f** This man needs nutritional support during this episode of acute pancreatitis. His duodenum is also inflamed as a consequence of his acute pancreatitis causing GOO, and therefore enteral nutrition would not be tolerated. Passing an endoscope to place a feeding tube in the duodenum/jejunum would be very difficult and placing a surgical jejunostomy is not required at this time. TPN would be most appropriate.

(ii) a Postoperative patients are encouraged to eat and drink as oral intake is more physiological, cheap and associated with fewer complications.

(iii) c The small bowel is the first part of the GIT to regain normal motility; therefore in patients with high nutritional requirements after surgery, a jejunostomy is a good route for feeding.

(iv) e This patient requires long-term support with feeding, so a PEG is most appropriate.

(v) b This patient has increased nutritional requirements not met by her oral intake and may benefit from increased nutritional support.

14   Hernias: answers

MCQs

1   **e**   Indirect inguinal hernias are the most common in both males and females; however, femoral hernias are the most common in females.

2   All true. The cremasteric fibres in the scrotum are a continuation of fibres from the internal oblique muscle. The lymphatic system to the abdominal wall includes the superficial lymphatics, which run parallel to the superficial veins, which above the umbilicus drain into the ipsilateral axillary vein and below it into the ipsilateral femoral vein. The strength of the anterior abdominal wall is maintained by transversalis fascia. Scarpa's fascia holds little strength in wound closure although contributes in accurately approximating the scar.

3   **a**   False. Femoral hernias arise below and lateral to the pubic tubercle, whereas indirect inguinal hernias arise above and medial to the pubic tubercle.
    b   True. Indirect hernias emerge lateral to the inferior epigastric vessels, whilst direct ones emerge medially.
    c   False. Hernias are defined as 'the protrusion of any organ, structure or portion thereof through its normal anatomical confines'.
    d   False. Indirect hernias are the commonest sort of hernia in both sexes and at all ages.
    e   False. The deep/internal ring is located at the midpoint of the inguinal ligament (mid way between the anterior superior iliac spine and pubic tubercle). The superficial/external ring is located above and medial to the pubic tubercle.

4   **a**   False.
    b   False.
    c   True.
    d   True.
    e   True.
    The use of a truss as an external support device to exert pressure over the defect should be avoided. They do not maintain hernias in a reduced state and have the risk of strangulating an unreduced hernia. The natural history of hernias is that the size of the defect and the sac enlarges over time and this increases the difficulty of the repair. The risk of complications from a hernia is greater the longer the exposure to a hernia and the larger the sac relative to the defect. Furthermore, there is a higher rate of morbidity and mortality associated with emergent repairs.

5   **a**   True.
    b   True.

c True.
d False.
e True.

Factors which increase the likelihood of recurrence include closure under tension, failure to identify an adequately strong musculo-aponeurotic tissue and wound infection. Recurrence of hernia should be infrequent and varies from 1 to 9%. Sensory nerve injury may lead to disabling symptoms from neuromas or nerve entrapment. Although vascular injuries are uncommon, injury of the femoral vein is the most common.

6 a True.
  b True.
  c False.
  d False.
  e True.

Incarceration is common in large hernias with a small neck. Most adult henias are acquired and are called paraumbilical hernias. Patients with increased intra-abdominal pressure with concomitant chronic abdominal distension (i.e. from ascites) are also at increased risk of developing paraumbilical hernias as are multiparous women. The repair is advocated in patients with ascites to avoid serious complications.

15   Gynaecology: answers

MCQs
Ectopic pregnancy
1 a True.
   b False.
   c False.
   d True.
   e True.

2 a True.
   b True.
   c False.
   d True.
   e False. Can be abdominal or cervical.

3 a True.
   b False.
   c True.
   d True.
   e True.

4 a False.
   b True.
   c False.
   d True.
   e True.

5 a True.
   b True.
   c False.
   d False.
   e True.

6 a False.
   b True.
   c False.
   d False.
   e True.

PID
1 a True.
   b False.
   c False.

   d True.
   e True.

2 **a** True.
   b False.
   c True.
   d True.
   e True.

3 **a** True.
   b True.
   c False.
   d True.
   e True. Oral antibiotics can be just as effective.

4 **a** True.
   b True.
   c False.
   d False.
   e True.

5 **a** False.
   b True.
   c True.
   d True.
   e True.

6 **a** True.
   b False.
   c True.
   d True.
   e False.

Ovarian cyst

1 **a** True.
   b True.
   c False.
   d True.
   e True. These are formed as part of the normal menstrual cycle.

2 **a** True.
   b True.
   c True.
   d True.
   e True. Large cysts can cause abdominal bloating.

3 **a** False.
   b True.
   c True.
   d True.

e False. This tumour marker is measured in females with suspected ovarian cancer.

Brief summary of ovarian cancer

- Most are epithelial cancers
- Known as the 'silent killer' due to the lack of symptoms
- Affects women after the menopause
- Risk factors include hormone-replacement therapy, endometriosis, family history and smoking, *BRCA1* and *BRCA2* genes
- Treatment is surgical +/– chemotherapy

---

4 a False.
 b True.
 c True.
 d True. Malignant ovarian cysts need to be removed by laparotomy.
 e False. These need surgery.

5 a False.
 b False.
 c False.
 d True.
 e False.

6 a True. Usually unexplained weight gain.
 b True. There can be pain during sexual intercourse.
 c True. This is a rare presentation.
 d True.
 e False. There is loss of appetite.

EMQs

1 **(i) f** This is a condition associated with polycystic ovarian syndrome after treatment with ovulation-inducing drugs like clomifene citrate. There is maturation of multiple follicles at the same time producing multiple ovarian cysts. The result is enlarged ovaries with abdominal pain and ascites.

 (ii) b Dermoids are benign cysts that are very mobile due to their long pedicles. Typically, sudden movement causes the cysts to twist around its pedicle. This causes occlusion of venous flow in the presence of continuous arterial flow, which results in congestion and stretching of the capsule. The patient experiences sudden abdominal pain and often requires surgery.

 (iii) c This is a sexually transmitted disease due to *Chlamydia*, *N. gonorrhoeae* and *Trichomonas*. This condition is typically seen in females with multiple sexual partners. Symptoms include lower abdominal pain associated with foul-smelling discharge and cervical excitation on vaginal examination. Many young females with PID are asymptomatic.

2   (i) d This is associated with infection within 2 weeks of insertion of IUCD. The infection ascends from cervix to fallopian tubes and peritoneal cavity. Severe infection leads to the collection of pus in the pouch of Douglas giving rise to swinging pyrexia and boggy mass in posterior fornix. Treatment is IV antibiotics and drainage of the abscess, which can be done transvaginally under ultrasound guidance.

    (ii) a This condition is associated with implantation of the fertilized ovum in the fallopian tube. The zygote grows, ruptures through the tube and causes intra-abdominal bleeding. There is referred pain to the shoulder caused by blood irritating the diaphragm. The treatment is resuscitation with fluids and removal of the tube containing the pregnancy.

   (iii) g This is associated with sudden onset of abdominal pain caused by bleeding in the cyst which leads to distension and stretching of the cyst capsule. The management is essentially conservative as most of the haemorrhagic cysts resolve spontaneously.

   (iv) e This condition is due to spontaneous bleeding into the fibroid and is commonly seen with pregnancy due to increased vascularity of the fibroid. The treatment is essentially conservative with analgesia.

3   (i) c
     (ii) d
Obstetric emergencies may present as surgical emergencies.

16 Urology: answers

MCQs
UTI
1 f *Escherichia coli* causes 80% of all UTIs. *Enterobacter* and *Klebsiella* are common causes of hospital-acquired UTI. *Pseudomonas* and *Candida* found in immunosuppressed patients or after treatment with antibiotics. *Proteus* spp. associated with urinary stones. *Staphylococcus saprophyticus* is responsible for 10% of symptomatic lower UTIs in sexually active young females.

2 a Initial bacterial resistance is the commonest cause of unresolved bacteriuria.

3 a True. Creation of false passages is common in large-prostate males where excessive force, repeated catheterization or inexperienced use of an introducer is used. If a patient cannot be catheterized by a junior doctor, seek senior help.
  b True. Infection from non-sterile technique can lead to urethritis, cystitis, pyelonephritis and transient bacteraemia.
  c True. Trauma from inflation of the balloon in the urethra or prostate. Can lead to urethral perforation.
  d True. Paraphimosis is commonly caused by failure to reduce the foreskin after catheterization.
  e True. Urethral strictures can result from improper catheterization and recurrent infections of the urethra.
  f True. Any urethral instrumentation will lead to a raised PSA.
  g True. Bleeding can commonly occur in large prostates and in decompression haematuria following rapid large bladder volume drainage.
  h True. Large bladder drainage can result in diuresis post drainage especially volumes greater than 1–2 L.
  i False. Rectal perforation is a risk of suprapubic catheterization not urethral catheterization.

Renal colic
1 a True. Often intercurrent UTI.
  b True. Sympathetic response.
  c True. Irritation of trigone of bladder and of ureters.
  d True. In an obstructed system this feature may indicate a pyonephrosis and requires urgent action to drain an obstructed kidney.
  e False. This is a common sign in peritonitis. Patients with renal colic often cannot keep still.
  f True. Rarer cause but can occur in patients with comorbidities such as diabetes. Staghorn calculi or calculus in a single functioning kidney.

Impaired renal function may also represent dehydration secondary to vomiting and reduced fluid intake.

2 a False. Calcium oxalate stones make up most renal calculi, and due to calcium content show up on X-ray if larger than 3–4 mm.
   b False. Struvite stones form from chronic UTI; uric acid results from breakdown of protein.
   c False. Rarely.
   d False. Both protect against stone formation and so a deficit will cause stones to form.
   e False. The bleeding needs to occur within the kidney or ureter for obstruction to cause renal colic. Clots in the bladder can cause retention of urine.
   f False. Assess the patient clinically and if dry start IV fluids. Otherwise, IV fluids may increase distension of the renal capsule and ureter proximal to an obstructed system and exacerbate the pain.
   g False. The majority of patients present with the classical colic pain radiating from loin to groin/genitals and analgesia should be given early.
   h False. NSAIDs are contraindicated in renal impairment; if unsure/elderly patient await U&E results. NSAIDs are a useful analgesic.
   i False. Calcium oxalate stones make up the majority of renal calculi and show up well on KUB X-ray if larger than 3–4 mm and not lying over a bony prominence, giving an 80% sensitivity.

3 a–c All are causes of RUQ pain so should be thought of for right loin to groin pain.
   d, e Can also cause RUQ pain but more likely to be epigastric.

4 a True.
   b True.
   c True.
   d False. Acute diverticulitis is usually left lower quadrant pain.
   e True.

5 a True.
   b False.
   c True.
   d False.
   e True.

The stone can obstruct anywhere but at these three points there is a decrease in the luminal diameter from distal to proximal.

Prostate cancer

1 a False.
   b False. The incidence is rare in the under forties and increases with age, so that in the ninth decade there is an 85% incidence.

c True. The Afro-Caribbean has the highest risk with often a more aggressive disease. Although Asians and Orientals often have a lower risk in their countries of origin, these risks increase as they migrate to Western countries. This indicates not only genetic but environmental causes.

d True. Often microscopic or macroscopic haematuria is present. This may be confused as BPH. There is often an intercurrent UTI.

e False. Prostate cancer spreads most commonly to bone, lymph nodes, liver, brain and skin; 30–40% of patients often present with metastatic disease such as bone pain, pathological fractures and abnormal liver function.

2 a False. TNM classification in used but Gleason score is used for histology. The Gleason grade is given to the microscopic appearances of cancer: A, most common pattern (scored from 1 to 5); B, second most common pattern (scored from 1 to 5). Gleason score is sum of A and B. Increasing score indicates increasing severity of disease and worse prognosis.

b True. Results are awaited from the ProtecT (Prostate Testing for Cancer and Treatment) study comparing surgery, radiotherapy and active surveillance with regard to the best treatment for localized prostate cancer.

c True. Active surveillance can be offered for low-grade localized disease where the risk of clinically significant prostate cancer is low. It can also be used in asymptomatic metastatic disease where the PSA is still relatively low.

d False. Both surgery and radiotherapy have excellent curative rates in confined disease; however both have risks, including incontinence, erectile dysfunction and impotence (less in nerve-sparing surgery). Risks from radiotherapy include cystitis, proctitis and haematuria; risks from brachytherapy (implanted radioactive seeds), cryotherapy (implanted ice) and high-intensity focused ultrasound (HIFU) include fistula formation. For prostate-confined disease in a patient with life expectancy greater than 10 years, treatment is aimed at curative intent. In a surgically fit patient this is radical prostatectomy (open, laparascopic or robotic). In a less fit patient, radical radiotherapy is treatment of choice. Other options include brachytherapy, cryotherapy or HIFU or active surveillance.

BPH

1 a True.

b True.

c False. PSA is specific for prostate cells but not the pathology behind the enlargement.

d False. The prostate continues to enlarge with age in a hormonally dependent manner.

e False. The initial outflow obstruction leads to a thickening of the bladder wall.

f False. Only the superficial posterior surface (posteromedial part of lateral lobes which correlates to peripheral zone) can be felt.

Initially conservative measures such as reducing bladder irritants (tea/coffee) and lifestyle changes (reduction in fluids late at night) can help. If this is ineffective, then medical management can help.

2 **f** Bleeding is common, but significant bleeding can require termination of the procedure, blood transfusion, or a prolonged hospital stay. Irrigating fluid may also be absorbed by cut veins in large amounts leading to transurethral resection (TUR) syndrome, which is a hyponatraemic, hypochloraemic metabolic acidosis. This is a potentially fatal complication and requires immediate resuscitative measures and the involvement of both surgeons and anaesthetists. The large working sheath combined with the use of electrical energy may also result in stricturing of the urethra. The cutting of the prostate also results in a partial resection of the urinary sphincteric mechanism, causing the muscle along the bladder outlet to become weak or incompetent. As a result, when the individual ejaculates, this sphincteric mechanism cannot keep the bladder adequately closed. Consequently, the ejaculate is forced backwards into the bladder (i.e. retrograde ejaculation) rather than from the end of the penis. The nerves associated with erection run along the outer rim of the prostate, and the high-energy current and/or heat generated by such may damage these nerves, resulting in erectile dysfunction.

RCC

1 **a** False. Less than 10% present with this triad.
  b False. Night sweats, fever, fatigue and pyrexia are present in one-quarter of patients at diagnosis and are signs of metastatic spread.
  c False. The right testicular vein drains into the IVC directly and is less likely to be blocked by RCC extension then extension of RCC into the left renal vein which is joined by the left testicular vein. Unilateral left varicocele needs renal USS to ensure no left RCC is present.
  d False. Paraneoplastic syndromes can occur at any stage and are present in up to 40% of patients with RCC at presentation. These may manifest as anaemia, polycythaemia, hypertension, hypoglycaemia, Cushing's disease and hypercalcaemia.

Bladder cancer

1 **a** False. Microscopic haematuria is not often due to bladder cancer in the under fifties but in the over fifties it can represent bladder cancer in up to 14% of patients.
  b False. Although macroscopic haematuria in the over fifties can be caused by bladder cancer in up to 50% of patients, abdominal pain as a result of bladder cancer is not that common as the obstructive pathology develops gradually.
  c False. Although colovesical fistula symptoms include haematuria, pneumaturia and recurrent UTIs, they are more commonly the result of diverticulitis and Crohn's disease.
  d True. Suprapubic mass is palpable or found on DRE (above the prostate). Signs of pallor and fatigue can result from anaemia secondary to blood loss or renal failure. Anuria results from bilateral ureteric obstruction and lower limb oedema from lymphatic/venous obstruction.

Miscellaneous

1 a True. Use ice packs until detumescence acheived.

b False.

c True. Sympathomimetics vasocontrict and reduce blood flow into the corpora. Caution in high-flow priaprism as this can lead to hypertension. High-flow priaprism will show up on blood gas analysis with well-oxygenated corporal blood. If this fails, senior help is required to aspirate the corpora with butterfly needle and syringe. Failing this, a surgical diversion procedure involves shunting blood from the corpora to the glans penis (Winter's procedure).

d False. Sildenafil is a phosphodiesterase inhibitor which increases cavernosal blood flow and would exacerbate the situation.

Paraphimosis results when the foreskin becomes trapped behind the corona of the glans penis. The glans therefore swells, with the foreskin forming a constrictive band. This is common after catheterization. Treatment is lidocaine (LA penile block), compression of the glans and pulling back foreskin. If recurrent, circumcision is recommended once swelling subsides.

2 a False. This is really a lump extending from the inguinal region into the scrotum. It can be painful. Always check that you can get above a scrotal lump as a large indirect inguinal hernia can be difficult to differentiate from scrotal originating pathology.

b True. A hydrocele is a collection of peritoneal fluid within the parietal and visceral layers of the tunica vaginalis. This can encompass the testicle making it difficult to palpate – imagine feeling for a squash ball in a tense balloon. They are tense lumps that are fluctuant and transilluminate. They can be treated with aspiration and sclerosis or surgical removal of the layers.

c True.

d True. Feels similar to epididymal cyst.

e True. Feels like a 'bag of worms'. Often gives greater symptoms towards the end of the day, with an ache or dragging sensation.

f False. Tumours can develop quickly and unilaterally. They are hard and irregular painless lumps in the scrotum, often making the testes difficult to recognize. Urgent ultrasound is required to positively identify a suspicious testis. Tumour markers include β-HCG, AFP and lactate dehydrogenase. Surgery is always indicated to remove the testicle to gain a pathological diagnosis. With teratoma and seminoma, the commonest tissue types, imaging to the pelvis also helps stage the tumour and plan if further adjuvant treatment (chemotherapy or radiotherapy) is required.

g True. This can also be painful. There is often related trauma or recent surgery especially inguinal.

EMQs
UTI

1 **(i) a** Females are 20 times more likely to have UTI due to a shorter urethra and closer proximity of urethra to anus.

(ii) c

(iii) b Or secondary to wet nappies, should be investigated to prevent long-term damage.

(iv) d

2 (i) d Infection is with IV antibiotics due to the risk of sepsis.

(ii) b Treatment with IV antibiotics, then a prolonged course of oral antibiotics to prevent abscess formation.

(iii) c Long-term oral antibiotics.

(iv) a Treatment is with oral antibiotics

3 (i) a This common and often painful condition requires immediate catheter insertion.

(ii) a These patients often have painless and large bladder residuals often greater than 1 L. They should be catheterized especially in the presence of hydronephrosis. They need close monitoring of UO for diuresis and decompression haematuria. They may actually go home with intermittent self-catheterization if they are not eligible or suitable for surgery for the obstructive pathology.

(iii) e UTIs are not an indication for catheterization and it can be painful to do so. Only catheterize if the patient has gone into retention as a result.

(iv) a Patients who present unwell or become unwell during the course of their hospital stay require catheterization so that their UO can be closely monitored (hourly) as a measure of renal perfusion/function.

(v) e Males do not need to be catheterized to get an uncontaminated urine specimen. This can be done with intermittent self-catheterization in females to avoid contamination by skin flora.

(vi) a Intravesical chemotherapy is a treatment that requires urethral catheterization for its insertion and drainage.

(vii) b A neurogenic bladder is often chronic as a result of diseases like diabetes and multiple sclerosis. In these cases patients can learn to self-catheterize (with training and only if dexterous enough) and so avoid the problems of long-term catheterization.

(viii) e Patients undergoing an LA or day-case GA procedure often do not require catheterization. Those undergoing major surgery will require catheter insertion prior to the procedure to monitor UO during the procedure and for monitoring postoperatively until the patient is ambulatory.

(ix) d After radical prostatectomy, catheter insertion should not be attempted at all by non-urological staff as there is a risk of avulsing the vesicourethral anastomosis. Call the urology registrar or consultant immediately.

Prostate cancer

1 (i) b

(ii) b

(iii) a

(iv) e Largely replaced by gonadotrophin-releasing hormone analogues.

(v) c Shown in clincal trials to have survival benefit in hormone-responsive prostate cancer.

(vi) d

BPH

1 **(i) a** They block α_{1a}-adrenergic receptors in the prostate stroma, urethra and bladder neck.

(ii) c

(iii) b

(iv) d

Note that 5α-reductase inhibitors can reduce PSA by up to 50%. This has implications for monitoring of PSA in patients. An increase in PSA while taking 5α-reductase inhibitors often implies pathology other than BPH.

RCC

1 **(i) b** Oncocytomas are radiologically difficult to distinguish from RCC. Hence treatment is radical or partial nephrectomy. Biopsy is not useful as it can often still leave doubt about the diagnosis.

(ii) a,c,e RCC is also known as Grawitz tumour, hypernephroma or clear cell carcinoma. Hypernephroma was originally believed to originate from the adrenal gland.

(iii) d,f Angiomyolipomas, also known as renal hamartomas, are benign tumours that can occur anywhere in the body. There is an association with the autosomal dominant condition tuberous sclerosis. Due to the fat content they appear bright on USS (reflective property of fat) and low density on CT. Unfortunately they can be symptomatic, giving rise to flank pain +/– haematuria. Rarely, the life-threatening condition of Wunderlich's syndrome (massive retroperitoneal bleeding) requires emergency embolization or nephrectomy. Generally, angiomyolipomas can be monitored with imaging and if asymptomatic left alone.

Miscellaneous

1 **(i) a** Tender swollen testicle and epididymis associated with infective signs clinically +/– biochemically. Treatment is with antibiotics. In patients under the age of 40, think STI; for the over forties, think bladder outflow obstruction and UTI.

(ii) c Often discovered over weeks and months. It is usually irregular and firm. There may be weight loss and loss of appetite. Appearances on USS are often indicative of tumour. Treatment is orchidectomy via a groin approach (to clamp the cord structures and prevent tumour seeding).

(iii) d Sudden twisting of the testicle results in ischaemic pain to the affected side. There is severe pain with exquisitely tender testicle. Sympathetic system activation gives symptoms of nausea, vomiting, sweating, and tachycardia and palpitations. Other differential is renal colic. USS is not indicated as this can delay treatment. Testicular ischaemia for more than 6 hours will lead to necrosis and death of that testicle.

(iv) b Often patient has pre-existing groin or scrotal lump.

17 Vascular: answers

MCQs
AAA

1 **a** False. The definition of AAA is a diameter of greater than 3 cm.
  b False. It is commoner in males over the age of 65.
  c True. Approximately 90% of AAA are located below the renal arteries.
  d True. Marfan's syndrome is the most common genetic disorder of connective tissue caused by a variety of missense mutations in the gene encoding fibrillin 1 on the long arm of chromosome 15. These individulas have an increased risk of cardiovascular complications including AAA.
  e True. Atherosclerosis causes 80% of AAA. Plaque deposition narrows and hardens the vessel wall which eventually becomes weak and expands from the high intraluminal pressure.

2 **a–d** True. There is an increased risk of AAA in male siblings of known patients.
  e False. Respiratory disease is associated with increased RAAA.

3 **a** True. Retroperitoneal RAAA develop a self-contained haematoma which tamponades the leak, preventing rapid exsanguination. Intra-abdominal leaks have a worse prognosis.
  b True. Half the patients with AAA will also have PAA.
  c False. RAAA will present with haemodynamic instability and shock. Leaking AAA is more likely to present with abdominal pain radiating to the back.
  d False. EVAR can be used in patients with suitable aneurysm morphology and involves transfemoral or transiliac placement of prosthetic graft. It is associated with reduced morbidity as it does not involve cross-clamping the aorta or GA.
  e True. An open AAA repair involves cross-clamping the aorta and distal vessels. Clots can form within the prosthetic graft/clamped vessels and may go on to occlude distal vessels, becoming apparent only hours after the operation. Embolectomy may be required.

4 **a** True. Approximately 15% of AAA will rupture.
  b False. Half of patients reach hospital and the overall mortality associated with RAAA is up to 95%.
  c False. RAAA must be excluded first. The patient will exsanguinate, rapidly deteriorate and die.
  d False. Hardman index used to calculate prognosis after emergency open surgery for RAAA. The presence of three or more variables is uniformly fatal.

Hardman index

Score 1 point for each criterion present.
- Age > 76 years
- Serum creatinine > 190 μmol/L
- Hb < 9 g/dL
- Ischaemia on ECG/significant cardiorespiratory disease
- History of loss of consciousness

---

   e False. The CXR can be done after the patient has been stabilized. The ABC approach is needed in all emergency situations. Call your seniors immediately. In a conscious patient who has a clear airway, place 15 L/min oxygen via a non-rebreathing mask, insert two large-bore cannulas in the antecubital fossa to obtain blood (FBC, U&E, lactate, G&S) and infuse adequate intravenous fluid and catheterize to monitor end-organ function. Make sure that you warn blood bank (you may need O-negative blood) and theatres (may need to transfer the haemodynamically unstable patient straight here).

5 a True. Aorto-intestinal fistula may have formed and resulted in massive lower GI bleeding.
   b True. Loss of consciousness due to hypovolaemic shock.
   c True. Bilateral lower limb ischaemia may result from a large embolus in the abdominal aorta lodging at the bifurcation and hence occluding the flow of blood into the lower limbs.
   d False. This is associated with aortic dissection.
   e True. Grey Turner's sign is bruising in the flanks and is a sign of retroperitoneal haemorrhage as a consequence of RAAA. If the blood leaks into the abdominal cavity and travels with gravity, the patient may complain of groin pain, scrotal bruising and penile pain. These symptoms can easily be mistaken for renal colic, and therefore any elderly males with 'renal colic' and relevant risk factors for AAA should have RAAA excluded first.

6 a False. Approximately 60% of AAA are suitable for EVAR.
   b False. There is reduced physiological stress in EVAR as there is no need for GA or cross-clamping of aorta. The specific complications for EVAR are graft migration, graft kinking, endovascular leak and graft occlusion.
   c True. There is still a 1% risk of AAA rupture after EVAR.
   d True. Graft occlusion is one of the complications.
   e False. There are three main types of graft: aorto-aorto, bifurcated aorto-iliac, aorto-uni-iliac.

PAA

1 a True.
   b True. PAAs account for up to 80% of peripheral aneurysms.
   c False. Approximately 50% of patients with PAAs have associated AAA but only 2% of patients with AAA have associated PAA.

d False. Approximately 5% rupture, and the risk of mortality post rupture is low.

e True. Around 50% of patients with PAA present with thrombosis, with up to 25% of patients presenting with associated distant embolic episode. Bypass surgery is indicated for all symptomatic PAA due to the high risk and morbidity related with thromboembolism.

2 a True. PAA is usually bilateral in half the cases.
b True. Foot drop is one of the presentations of PAA.
c True. A venous graft is preferred when performing a PAA bypass procedure.
d False. There is a 1% risk of amputation due to PAA thrombosis.
e True. Rest pain suggests progressive thrombosis of PAA.

3 a False. PTFE grafts are used when vein grafts have failed.
b False. Lower and higher limb veins may be used as grafts.
c False. PTFE grafts have a higher risk of failure than vein grafts.
d True. Prophylactic antibiotics are given to prevent infection.
e False. Fine vicryl sutures are used to anastomose the graft.

Carotid artery stenosis

1 a False. Obesity and lack of sedentary lifestyle is associated with carotid artery disease.
b True.
c False. The risk is associated with hypertension.
d True.
e False. Dysrhythmias are associated with increased risk of CVAs.

2 All true: a–d are symptoms of TIAs.
3 a False.
b True.
c True.
d True.
e False.

4 a Doppler ultrasound will measure the thickness of the carotid arteries and blood flow using sound waves. A tilt table test is used to diagnose neurally mediated syncope in patients who suffer repeated fainting episodes.

5 b It is very important to modify the lifestyle and start medical management for comorbidities but in symptomatic cases of severe carotid artery stenosis, carotid endarterectomy is recommended. Surgery is not recommended for those with less than 70% stenosis or complete carotid artery blockage.

6 e In a post-operation scenario, always think of complications related to surgery. The possible complications of surgery include haematoma, infection, cranial nerve damage, stroke, death and restenosis. The common symptoms of temporary nerve damage include hoarse voice (vagus or recurrent/superior laryngeal nerve damage), difficulty swallowing (vagus), numbness in skin of neck and earlobe (greater auricular nerve damage), and tongue weakness/paralysis (hypoglossal nerve). These symptoms usually clear up in a few months.

Amputations

1 a False. It is an irreversible procedure.
   b False. There are many types of amputations in the lower limb.
   c False. Try conservative measures first.
   d True. Trauma is the commonest reason for an amputation in the UK.
   e False. Complications associated with amputations include infection, DVT and pulmonary embolism, contractures and pressure ulcers.

2 a False. The mortality associated with AKA is higher than that with BKA.
   b True.
   c True. Flexion contracture is one of the complications associated with BKA.
   d True.
   e True.

3 a False. BKA is the procedure of choice for EPVD but this depends on the vascular collateral supply to the lower limb.
   b False. The 5-year survival is worse than those with Dukes B colon cancer.
   c True. The majority of patients will become wheelchair bound.
   d True. 'Phantom limb' is one of the complications associated with AKA.
   e False. Involves greater metabolic stress and is therefore better than BKA.

Varicose veins

1 a False. Patients usually complain of a burning or throbbing sensation.
   b False. The affected leg(s) ache.
   c False.
   d True.
   e True.

2 a True. There are many small communicating veins emptying into the larger veins. Therefore, if these veins are not identified and tied off, they provide a route to the superficial veins and there is rapid recurrence of varicose veins. In some cases, there is vein regrowth (neovascularization).
   b True. The surgery for saphenofemoral junction incompetence involves making two incisions, one near the saphenofemoral junction (SFJ), in the groin, and one further down the vein, near the knee. All the veins draining into the SFJ are identified and tied off before disconnecting the saphenous vein from the femoral vein. A wire is introduced through the top of the saphenous vein and carefully pulled out the incision made near the knee. The whole vein is then stripped from the thigh.
   c False. Varicose vein surgery usually involves GA.
   d True. The patient can usually go home the same day.

3 a False.
  b False.
  c True.
  d True.
  e False.

4 a True.
  b True. A chemical is injected into the medium-sized varicose veins under LA.
  c False.
  d False.
  e True.

5 a True.
  b True.
  c False. Varicose veins can cause phlebitis.
  d True.
  e True. Minor trauma can cause bleeding.

6 All true. The operation is on the veins, so bleeding can occur and some cases require re-exploration to stop the bleeding. Some patients (diabetics) are at increased risk of wound infections, and if there is a small collection of blood (haematoma) this is a nidus for infections. A proportion of patients are left with an area of numbness near the scars due to damage to a small cutaneous sensory nerve. There are rare cases of DVT and pulmonary embolism, and this risk is increased in patients on the OCP. All patients who have GA are at potential risk of cardiorespiratory complications, because most GA agents cause vasodilatation and severe hypotension can cause cardiac strain.

Diabetic foot

1 a True. Any trauma resulting in abrasions or bruising can result in infection.
  b True. Callus, clawed toes and hallux rigidus are just some of the foot deformities that can cause trauma and infection.
  c True. May be ill-fitting, causing trauma.
  d True.
  e False. Regular examinations will alert the patient to any suspicious areas. The primary reasons for developing diabetic foot ulcers and infection are the development of peripheral neuropathy, peripheral vascular disease and abnormal WBC function.

2 a True.
  b True. Charcot's foot can occur in both types of diabetes.
  c False. Charcot's foot results when diabetic neuropathy goes unnoticed.
  d True. Pressure/trauma within the foot goes unnoticed in those with peripheral neuropathy and results in internal fractures that fail to heal properly.
  e False. It is often difficult to diagnose until advanced disease develops.

Charcot's foot is seen in diabetics with abnormal neurovascular supply to the foot. Stress fractures and foot trauma combined with weak bones results in the hypertrophic osteoarthropathy seen in Charcot's foot.

3 e This elderly man with known PVD has chronic foot ulcers that may require surgical débridement and antibiotics, but pain indicates ischaemia and therefore a procedure will be required to aid ulcer healing. An angiogram with angioplasty will be a better option than bypass surgery under GA for this ischaemic ulcer.

4 a A duplex scan to assess the distal circulation and locate the lesion.

5 e There will be healthy granulation tissue under the necrotic tissue in neuropathic ulcers.

6 c This patient will only get better once the abscess has been drained by the surgical team.

Peripheral vascular disease

1 a False. Non-invasive investigations should be employed first. DSA is the gold standard investigation because it provides a complete map of the lower limb circulation that is easy to interpret and is easier for intervention, but duplex USS or MRA should be used to identify the problem first.

b True. The stenosis or blockage is identified using non-invasive investigations before DSA and angioplasty is performed.

c False. DSA involves puncturing a large artery, which can develop a pseudoaneurysm and bleeding post procedure. It is therefore important to apply adequate pressure dressing over the puncture site to prevent these complications.

d False. Duplex USS combines B-mode ultrasound (conventional imaging) and colour Doppler ultrasound to show how blood is flowing through the vessels and measures the velocity of the flow of blood. It is used to estimate the diameter of a blood vessel as well as the amount of obstruction in the blood vessel.

e True. An MRI machine comprises a large magnet which would attract metallic implants in patients. The strong magnetic field causes the protons of hydrogen atoms to align in a particular direction, and these are then exposed to a beam of radio waves. This spins the various protons of the body, and they produce a faint signal that is detected by the receiver portion of the MRI scanner. The receiver information is processed by a computer and an image is produced. The advantages of MRA are that it is non-invasive, faster and easier than DSA.

2 a True. The ischaemic limb has a reduced perfusion pressure and therefore the blood pressure at the ankle will be less than that measured from the brachial artery.

b False. Rest pain, indicative of critical ischaemia, is worst at night in bed when there is a loss of hydrostatic pressure. As a result the patient seeks to relieve this by hanging the leg over the side of the bed.

c False. Ischaemic ulcers are found over pressure areas such as the heels, heads of first and fifth metatarsals, and the toes.

d True. This is useful in diabetic patients with high ABPIs. There is less calcification in toe arteries, and toe–brachial index can be measured.

e False. There are several drugs licensed for symptomatic relief of intermittent claudication but only cilostazol and naftidrofuryl have been shown to have any benefits.

3 a True. A large atrial thrombus can be a source of emboli that can partially or completely block the blood vessel at any point in the circulation.

b True. An example of autoimmune vasculitis is Buerger's disease that affects male smokers.

c True. Syphilis is caused by *Treponema pallidum*, and this infects and damages large arteries.

d True. An example of acquired PVD is Takayasu's disease. This is a chronic inflammatory condition of unknown cause, seen in Asian females. There is destruction of the artery wall of the large arteries in the body, aorta and its branches.

e True. Trauma from a road traffic collision or fall can cause a number of injuries.

4 All true. This young man has a classic history of Buerger's disease, a condition in young Asian/white males aged 20–40 who are heavy smokers. They usually have a history of claudication indicating arterial disease, before rest pain. Some present with gangrene in fingers and toes, and redness and swelling in the extremities, and infection should be excluded. There is a very strong association with smoking, and it is thought that tobacco triggers an autoimmune response. Imaging will reveal a 'corkscrew' appearance of the affected arteries near the hands and feet, and multiple areas of stenosis and blockages. Stopping smoking is the only effective treatment in Buerger's disease; those who continue to smoke go on to require amputations.

5 a True. Smoking is the most important risk factor in this patient.

b False. Abdominal USS will not assess the blood flow or blood vessel anatomy. A duplex scan would be better.

c True. This eman has Leriche's syndrome (aorto-iliac disease) caused by atheromatous occlusion of the aorta at the bifurcation into the iliac arteries. MRA or CTA is the investigation of choice.

d False. Atheromatous aorto-iliac disease is a slowly progressing disease, and there is usually development of collaterals, so there is no need for immediate surgical intervention. Elective surgery will involve bypassing the aorto-iliac disease.

e True. Change in diet and exercise should be advised and risk factors should be minimized to improve the patient's symptoms.

6 a True. Antiplatelet therapy is recommended for all patients with symptomatic PVD.

b True. There is strong evidence for treating hypertension in patients with PVD.

c False. Folic acid and vitamin B_6 are cofactors of homocysteine, a factor associated with increased atherosclerotic risk, but there is not enough evidence for routine treatment of hyperhomocysteinaemia.

d False. Insulin is only indicated for optimal glycaemic control in diabetic patients with PVD.

e True. Lipid-lowering medications, statins, are recommended for patients with PVD.

7 a Chronic lower limb ischaemia can often be wrongly diagnosed in patients with nerve root compression. Without a thorough history and examination, you cannot ask for the appropriate investigations. The finding of a pulsatile abdominal mass is an indication for abdominal USS; on eliciting a straight leg test of only 15°, think about sending the patient for an MRI to rule out sciatica.

Ischaemic limb

1 a Sudden limb pain that is present during rest is associated with ischaemia; if it has been present less than 2 weeks, it is classified as acute ischaemia. This patient has shortness of breath due to a large left ventricular infarct and an embolus from his inactive left ventricle has lodged in his leg, resulting in acute leg ischaemia.

2 a True. This is part of the 6 Ps.

b True.

c False. Persistent hypotension is not a sign of acute limb ischaemia.

d True. This is a very late stage of acute limb ischaemia that indicates the need for emergency intervention.

e False. The ischaemic limb may be mottled +/− bluish discoloration due to venous congestion but acutely ischaemic limbs are generally pale/marble white.

3 a False. Hypotension predisposes to acute thrombosis.

b False. Thrombophilia patients have an increased tendency to blood clotting. Tests are available to diagnose thrombophilia.

Some examples of thrombophilia tests

- Protein C deficiency: protein C is part of the anticoagulant regulatory system. Activated protein C (APC) inactivates activated factor V and factor VIII.
- Free protein S deficiency: free protein S is a vitamin K-dependent cofactor for anticoagulant activity of APC.
- Antithrombin (AT) deficiency: AT is a very important inhibitor of coagulation; it inhibits coagulation proteases.

c True. There is increased hypercoagulability in malignancy.

d True. Polycythaemic blood has increased viscosity and increased tendency to thrombosis.

e False. Cardiovascular causes of thrombosis include AF, MI, heart failure, metallic heart valves.

4 a False. Obese patients are at increased risk of thrombosis but obesity itself is not a cause of acute limb ischaemia.

b True. Shaft of femur fracture may damage the superficial femoral artery and its branches.

c True. A common presenting symptom of popliteal aneurysm is acute ischaemia due to embolic/thrombotic episode.

d True. Any major vessel may become damaged during surgery.

e True. Embolus and thrombotic occlusions are the commonest causes of acute limb ischaemia.

5 a This patient has critical ischaemia, therefore admit for analgesia and plan for an amputation. There is no advantage in trying to revascularize the left ischaemic limb as the patient has contractures and is immobile.

6 a This man has acute exacerbation of chronic leg ischaemia. He requires admission for duplex scanning to diagnose location of lesion +/- angioplasty (if amenable to angioplasty).

EMQs

1 **(i) a** This man is a smoker and has a tender pulsatile mass in the epigastric region; therefore, until proven otherwise, he needs to be treated as a possible leaking AAA. Only then, can renal colic be excluded, as patients with leaking AAA can also have coexisting haematuria secondary to developing coagulopathies.

(ii) c Abdominal USS is a non-invasive method for assessing the AP diameter of the AAA and is therefore a useful tool for monitoring the size of the aorta.

(iii) b PAA tend to thrombose and this explains his symptoms and signs. A patient with factor IX deficiency (Christmas disease) will require factor IX when he has a bypass operation to improve his distal circulation. Liaise closely with the haematologists.

(iv) d There is high suspicion of a rapidly expanding abdominal aorta, which may be slowly leaking; therefore make sure the patient is haemodynamically stable. Stable patients with a suspected leak can have CT scans for diagnosis. However, if the patient becomes haemodynamically unstable, he must be taken to theatre immediately for repair.

(v) e This patient requires a bypass operation to heal his foot ulcer and relieve his symptoms. MRA will reconstruct the vascular system to assess the quality of the proximal and distal blood supply, so that the right operation is planned.

2 **(i)** **b** One of the complications of a total knee replacement is damage to the popliteal artery. In this case, the artery has been cut and a contained haematoma has formed, which continues to communicate with the popliteal artery, forming a pseudoaneurysm (a false aneurysm, not surrounded by the vessel wall). On examination, there will be features of compartment syndrome (pressure in the compartment exceeds the blood pressure within the veins and capillaries causing their collapse). This disrupts the supply of oxygen and nutrients to nerve and muscle cells, leading to damage and death. This patient will need a bypass operation as soon as possible.

(ii) **f** Cancer patients have an increased risk of DVT due to increased hypercoagulability. This is a specific paraneoplastic phenomenon, as a result of factors excreted by cancer cells or factors produced by the body against the cancer cells. The patient has an extensive acute DVT involving the iliac and femoral veins, which has caused his symptoms and signs, and is an indication of recurrence and/or spread of cancer.

(iii) **f** This patient has presented late with extensive acute DVT. The symptoms and signs are of venous gangrene, and this requires an amputation. The patient should be started on anticoagulation in order to decrease the chance of developing pulmonary embolism, and an extensive investigation should be carried out to exclude the diagnosis of cancer.

(iv) **a** This patient has critical ischaemia, and an ABPI of less than 0.6 will support the diagnosis. Mr T. has Buerger's disease (thromboangiitis obliterans), which usually affects young male smokers. Buerger's disease is probably an autoimmune disease, causing inflammation and thrombosis of arteries and veins.

(v) **d** This is wet gangrene (infected dead tissue) with ascending cellulitis due to occlusion of the blood supply. If left alone, the patient may develop septicaemia.

3 **(i)** **b** Angioplasty +/– stenting is the management option for short segments of femoral artery stenosis.

(ii) **c** For those with an occlusion of a stented femoral artery, a femoral endarterectomy is the next option.

(iii) **a** To re-establish circulation to the right leg, this patient needs a graft (vein or synthetic) from the left femoral artery to right femoral artery.

(iv) **e** This patient requires an operation to help her ulcers to heal. The axillary artery is used to supply blood to the femoral arteries and bypass the diseased segments.

(v) **d** This man needs a bypass from the proximal femoral artery to below the popliteal artery aneurysm.

All these patients require contrast arteriography, CTA or MRA to assess their vasculature and to plan the operation.

4 **(i)** **a** Perthes' test (tourniquet around the mid-thigh) examines the deep venous system by occluding the superficial system (SFJ). Pain and engorgement of the legs after light exercise indicates that the deep venous system is diseased as the increased arterial blood flow required during exercise cannot be carried back through the femoral vein.

(ii) c This patient has saphenofemoral incompetence as demonstrated by the tourniquet test. If there is deep venous disease, the patient will not benefit from the operation as the only source of venous drainage back to the main circulation will have been removed. Therefore, a duplex scan should be performed in all patients being considered for the operation outlined.

(iii) e This lady has damaged the valves in the femoral vein because of a previous DVT. This valvular incompetence leads to venous insufficiency resulting in early filling of the venous pool after muscle contraction (pumps venous blood back to the main circulation). Venous hypertension eventually develops with capillary dilatation and plasma protein leakage. Elastic compression stockings provide graduated compression and produce alteration of microvascular haemodynamics, thus protecting the skin from the effects of venous hypertension. Severe arterial disease should be excluded before using compression bandaging, as 1 in 10 leg ulcers are due to mixed arteriovenous disease.

(iv) d Sclerotherapy involves injecting sclerosants into the empty vein and then applying pressure to the area for 4–6 weeks. The vein will scar and disappear. It is in increasing use, and is suitable for recurrent or persistent varicose veins below the knees.

(v) c Superficial thrombophlebitis occurs in varicose veins and usually settles in 2–6 weeks but may develop complications such as infection. Recurrent superficial thrombophlebitis is an indication for surgery.

18 Orthopaedics: answers

MCQs
Brachial plexus injuries
1 a True. Can be caused by penetrating injuries to the neck.
  b False. It is usually caused by high-energy trauma, commonly high-speed motor vehicle accident.
  c True. Can be caused by blunt injuries.
  d True. Due to stretching during delivery.
  e True. Low- and high-velocity gunshot wounds can result in brachial plexus injuries.

2 a False. Not relevant here, and uncommon in elderly.
  b False. Cell bodies are avulsed from the cord.
  c True. Cell bodies still in continuity with axons, so chance of recovery or successful surgical reconstruction better.
  d False. Not relevant.
  e False. Not relevant, although fewer females are injured.

3 e Pain syndromes (burning/shooting/crushing pain) are commonly reported in patients with preganglionic brachial plexus injury. In reality, all the options are possible causes in this scenario, but a brachial plexus injury must be excluded. An MRi scan is required to examine his brachial plexus.

Radial nerve injury or entrapment
1 a False. There is typically wrist drop.
  b False. The triceps is spared.
  c False. This is lost.
  d True. Not at this level of injury.
  e True. The radial nerve is responsible for extending fingers, wrists and elbow and sensation to the hand.

2 a True.
  b True.
  c True.
  d True.
  e True. There may be non-union of the humerus due to infection.
  As with all types of surgery, infection, iatrogenic injury, incomplete recovery and wound dehiscence are complications.

3 a This patient describes 'Saturday night' palsy but this must first be confirmed by examination, looking for other possible causes.

Ulnar nerve palsy

1 a True.
  b False. Compression can occur while administering or during GA but anaesthetic drugs are not causative.
  c True.
  d True. There is a high rate of post-surgical ulnar nerve palsies.
  e True.

2 a True.
  b True. This allows real-time evaluation of the nerve.
  c True.
  d True. This is a helpful adjunct to USS and nerve conduction studies.
  e True. Characteristic features are seen in nerve compression.

3 a False. Deformity of the hand.
  b True.
  c False. There is difficulty moving the digits only.
  d True.
  e True.

4 a False. Older age is associated with poor prognosis.
  b False.
  c False. The presence of ulnar nerve responses is associated with better surgical prognosis.
  d True.
  e True. If a neuropathy is responsible.

Carpal tunnel syndrome

1 a True. The carpal tunnel can be involved by fracture-related oedema and haematoma.
  b True. Usually disappear after birth.
  c True. Repetitive work, mechanics and assembly-line workers are at increased risk.
  d False. Females are more likely to develop carpal tunnel syndrome than males.
  e False. More likely to associated with obesity.

2 a True.
  b True.
  c True.
  d True. These are common symptoms of carpal tunnel syndrome.
  e False. Sometimes the hand can change colour but there is no ischaemia.

3 a True. But condition may still exist if negative.
  b False. But may be needed to exclude radiological features, e.g. rheumatoid arthritis.
  c True. Ideally confirms diagnosis before surgery is performed.
  d False. No relevant scan exists.
  e True. Can detect impaired movement of the median nerve.

4 a True. To reduce pain and inflammation within the carpal tunnel.
b True. Reduces swelling from inflammation.
c False. Will not help as elbow movements do not contribute.
d False. Wrist physiotherapy, mainly stretching exercises, may help.
e True. Used to reduce the compression by preventing prolonged wrist flexion.

5 a True. This could well be carpal tunnel syndrome but requires confirmation.
b False. The question stated it was already well controlled.
c False. The diagnosis should first be confirmed.
d False. She has clumsiness, i.e. functional impairment, and surgical decompression will be required if carpal tunnel syndrome is proven.
e False. As for (d). A diagnosis is first required.

6 c Try conservative measures first. The symptoms may improve after delivery. If the symptoms are constant and severe after delivery, referral to a specialist hand surgeon is warranted.

Shoulder dislocation

1 All true. Greater than 95% of shoulder dislocations are caused by trauma but in rare cases harmless movements can result in dislocations. This may be due to an inherited disorder of soft tissues such as Marfan's syndrome and Stickler's syndrome, an autosomal dominant genetic disorder affecting connective tissues. Epileptic fits can result in anterior or posterior dislocations.

2 d Consider acromioclavicular subluxation as this also causes shoulder pain. There is widening of the acromioclavicular space on AP view.

3 a True. This is typical in anterior dislocation.
b False.
c True. This is typical in posterior shoulder dislocations.
d False.
e False.

4 a True. Rotator cuff muscles surround the shoulder joint adding stability.
b True.
c True. You can also damage the axillary artery; look for axillary haematoma.
d False. Most sternal fractures occur in older patients after blunt anterior chest trauma (e.g. hitting the steering wheel during a road traffic accident). Care must be taken to rule out associated injuries such as cardiac contusion, aortic disruption and lung contusion.
e False. This typically happens in male athletes with worn biceps tendon. With strong action of the biceps muscle (e.g. heavy lifting), they feel a pop in the elbow associated with pain. There may be bruising at the elbow and the biceps muscle may retract up, resulting in a prominent bump in the upper arm ('Popeye' sign).

5 e The patient will need to be initially assessed using the ABCDE approach, but it is important to ensure she is comfortable before examining/radiologically assessing the right limb. In this case, the patient had a fracture in the upper third of her humerus associated with an anterior dislocation.

6 a More than 90% of shoulder dislocations in patients under the age of 20 years will recur.

Colles' fracture

1 a True. As for all fractures.
  b True Although most Colles' are sustained in a fall.
  c False. Not a known risk factor.
  d False. Not a known risk factor.
  e True. A known risk factor common to all fractures.

2 a True. A reaction to inflammation.
  b True. 'Dinner fork'.
  c True. Often reported by the patient.
  d False. Usually exquisitely tender.
  e False. The initial discoloration is ecchymosis (bruising).

3 a True.
  b True.
  c True.
  d False.
  e True.

4 a True. Caused by ischaemia of the forearm muscles.
  b True. Carpal tunnel syndrome can occur.
  c False. Not at correct anatomical level.
  d True. As for (b).
  e False. Post-traumatic (secondary) osteoarthritis.

5 c Splinting the wrist will provide the best form of analgesia. Record observations and neurovascular status before calling the orthopaedic registrar and booking theatres.

6 c This is a Barton's fracture (fracture dislocation of radiocarpal joint). It will need fixation with K-wires before applying a plaster cast.

7 d Using plates and screws to fix such fractures in position can be technically challenging.

Fractured neck of femur

1 a True. Especially in postmenopausal women.
  b False. Sedentary inactive lifestyle is a risk factor.

    c True. As a result of osteoporosis.

    d False. Low body weight is a risk factor.

    e True. Risk of falls and increased chance of developing osteoporosis.

2 **a** False. Not universally available.

    b True. If high suspicion of hip fracture not seen using other investigations, MRI may help.

    c True. Ideally, both AP and lateral X-ray views are obtained to assess the hip fracture.

    d True. If high suspicion and not seen on other techniques, increased tracer uptake at fracture site.

    e False. PET has an important role in detecting primary and secondary malignancies.

3 **a** False. Usually carried out for displaced fractures.

    b False. May be an option for undisplaced fractures.

    c False. Not usually required for minimal displacement.

    d True. The native hip joint should be maintained in young patients. In this case, an urgent (<6 hours) left DHS is the operation of choice. The side to be operated on must be clearly marked, the anaesthetist contacted and informed consent obtained before theatre.

    e False.

4 **a** The operation that will restore former function is a right hemiarthroplasty.

5 **a** False. Garden I and II fractures would be treated with a DHS.

    b True. Hemiarthroplasty or total arthroplasty will avoid the late complications of non-union and AVN.

    c False. Indicated in patients with restricted mobility.

    d False. Medically unfit patients have a higher risk of AVN.

    e True. Total hip replacement may also be an option.

6 **a** True. Replacement will require revision within 15–20 years, therefore salvage of the patient's own joint is better.

    b True. As the risk is not justified.

    c False. This would only be carried out if the joint has a low risk of AVN.

    d False. Internal fixation is not generally performed for subcapital fractures. Sometimes internal fixation can be performed for undisplaced basicervical fractures.

    e True. Heals well with a low risk of AVN.

7 **a** False. Gait disturbance rather than central distrubance.

    b False. However the sciatic nerve may be bruised or damaged.

    c True. A general complication of trauma and/or surgery.

    d True. DVT is a risk.

    e True. Especially as a foreign body is inserted.

> **Surgical sieve for students**
>
> VITAMIN C: Vascular, Iatrogenic, Trauma, Anatomical/Autoimmune, Metabolic, Inflammatory, Neoplastic, Congenital

8 d Many elderly patients have comorbidities. All other causes of the patient's fall should be excluded such as pneumonia, UTI and so on. In reality, history-taking, examination, resuscitation and investigation will be carried out simultaneously by a team.

OA of knee

1 a True.
   b True. Increased loading of joints (hip, knees, ankles).
   c False. This is not a known risk factor for OA.
   d False.
   e True. OA often 'runs' in families.

2 a True. A painless soft lump that can develop behind the knee joint.
   b False. One-third of patients improve; rapid deterioration in 1 in 20 people.
   c True. Light exercise is advised to avoid this problem.
   d True.
   e False. This is not a complication.

3 c Send the fluid for microscopy, Gram staining and culture. Take the patient to theatre if the effusion is positive for microorganisms or there is high clinical suspicion of septic arthritis.

> **Septic arthritis**
>
> • Patient is unwell with rigors and fevers; joint painful, inflamed and swollen; all movements restricted.
> • X-ray is usually normal, USS may show joint effusion. Diagnosis: aspirate affected joint under aseptic conditions, send aspirate to microbiology for Gram staining, microscopy and culture. Send blood for inflammatory markers.
> • Differential diagnosis includes acute inflammatory monoarthritis.
> • Treatment: surgical washout for confirmed sepsis. If microbiology normal: splint, rest and NSAIDs.

4 b This patient has a haemarthrosis. Check the INR before attempting to aspirate the joint as the blood will reaccumulate if it is high.
5 a This patient has an acute meniscal injury causing locked knee. With analgesia and rest the locked knee will unlock. Follow up with an orthopaedic referral as necessary.
6 e This is symptomatic Baker's cyst. Once the Baker's cyst is confirmed on USS, aspirate the fluid and administer intra-articular corticosteroid injection.

EMQs

1 **(i) d** This is a typical injury after hitting a hard surface with a clenched fist.
   (ii) f The crescent-moon shape of the lunate bone becomes obvious on X-ray.
   (iii) h
   (iv) b
   (v) c This is the commonest fracture in osteoporotic females.

2 **(i) g**
   (ii) e
   (iii) f
   (iv) d

3 **(i) b,c,f** The blood will track down from the proximal humeral fracture site.
   (ii) d Middle third humeral shaft fractures are associated with radial nerve damage.
   (iii) d Middle third humeral shaft fracture can be treated with U-slabs, hanging cast or internal fixation.
   (iv) d Non-union is most frequently seen in middle third fractures.

4 **(i) a**
   (ii) b
   (iii) e
   (iv) d or b Epileptic patients may sustain anterior or posterior shoulder dislocations.

19 Burns and plastics: answers

MCQs

1 a True. The most appropriate donor sites include the anterior, lateral or medial part of the thigh; the buttock; or the medial aspect of the arm.

b True. Partial-thickness wounds will heal by granulation and epithelialization will take 7–21 days. Therefore split-thickness skin grafts are not placed on tendon, bone or cartilage.

c True. The graft is trimmed to fit the donor site and secured using staples or interrupted sutures.

d False. Presence of microorganisms is a contraindication to graft application. Group A β- haemolytic *Streptococcus* can destroy the whole graft.

e False. Split-thickness skin grafts obtain nutrition by imbibition of plasma from the wound bed; after 48 hours fine anastomotic connections develop.

2 a True. When considering full-thickness graft donor sites, skin similar to the area surrounding the wound/defect should be sought. The colour, texture and sebaceous qualities are some of the features considered.

b False. Dark necrotic/black patches indicate partial or complete rejection.

c True. Elliptical incisions are easier to close.

d True. Donor site can usually be approximated by primary closure. However, if the defect is large this may need a split-thickness graft.

e True.

f False. It is best to remove any underlying fat so as to avoid graft rejection

3 a True. In an emergency, the patient must be assessed following the ATLS guidelines, which always starts with A for airways. The airways together with C-spine should be cleared before moving on to breathing (gas exchange) and circulation.

b False. Haemoglobin should be checked before transfusing blood. Intravenous fluid resuscitation with crystalloids is urgently required as fluid loss is likely to be great.

c False. The Parkland formula (warm isotonic fluids 2–4 mL/kg per %BSA for second- and third-degree burns) will guide intravenous fluid resuscitation required in the 24-hour period. The first half of the calculated 24-hour fluid volume is given in the first 8 hours since the burn.

d False. Blood pressure is often difficult to obtain due to the burns. A urinary catheter is inserted to guide fluid balance.

e True. All electrolytes should be kept within physiological range to prevent complications associated with abnormal electrolytes.

4 a True. Burn wound cellulitis is typically caused by *Streptococcus pyogenes*; treatment involves excising the burnt tissue and IV antibiotics.
  b True. A sweet smell from the burnt tissue indicates a *Pseudomonas aeruginosa* infection.
  c True. A blue/green discharge from the wound associated with increasing pain indicates infection of the wound and the surrounding soft tissue. The common cause of infection is *Pseudomonas aeruginosa* and other Gram-negative species.
  d True. Full-thickness grafts have more tissue, therefore require better conditions for survival and more time to heal. The necrotic patches indicate partial or complete loss of the graft. This is most likely to be caused by infection.
  e False. This describes a full-thickness burn.

5 All true. The commonest cause of graft failure is haematoma and seroma (both prevent graft adherence to underlying structures), trauma (disrupt attachments) and bacterial infection (toxic substances produced).

6 a False. Burns patients have great fluid requirements from the time of thermal injury because of the increased capillary permeability resulting in fluid loss, hypovolaemia, shock and acute renal failure.
  b True. This is caused by SIRS in burns.
  c True. Circumferential burns have a high risk of developing compartment syndrome, which leads to myoglobin-related renal failure. Treat with escharotomy or fasciotomy.
  d True. Fourth-degree burns include full-thickness skin, subcutaneous fat, fascia and muscle. Common causes are electrical, contact burns, and immersion burn in an unconscious patient.
  e False. The burns patient is in a state of hypermetabolism with negative nitrogen balance, therefore early enteral feeding is recommended.

EMQs

1 **(i) d** This is a clean wound. The results need to be cosmetically acceptable, therefore subcuticular skins stitches will be appropriate after cleaning the wound and inspection for foreign body.
  (ii) h Thiersch graft from right thigh, split-thickness skin graft with splintage, and postoperative physiotherapy would be appropriate. The donor site of thigh is preferable to arms for cosmetic reasons.
  (iii) a Composite skin graft with fat will enable appropriate cover of the exposed phalanx.
  (iv) j Transpositional flap from the forehead would adequately cover a large defect at the inner canthus. Wolfe graft is suitable for smaller lesions.
  (v) f Trapezius myocutaneous graft would be the most appropriate flap to cover the extensive area after wide local excision for recurrence.

2 **(i) e** 5.6 L are required in the first 24 hours.

   (ii) a The fluid required in the first 8 hours is half the total fluid requirement in 24 hours.

  (iii) b The fluid required in the next 16 hours is half the total fluid requirement in 24 hours.

  (iv) d In children, each leg represents 14% BSA, therefore 14% × 20 kg × 4 mL.

   (v) f The anaesthetist must be contacted; unconscious patients need to have their airways protected.

20 Useful procedures: answers

MCQs

1 **a** False. Abscesses are caused by bacterial infection.
   b False. They can develop in the body.
   c True.
   d False. Abscesses are typically tender.
   e True.

2 **a** True.
   b False. Abscesses feel warm to hot.
   c True. As the abscess progresses, it starts to point.
   d True. Small cutaneous abscesses and large intra-abdominal abscesses can cause fever and rigors.
   e True.

3 **a** True.
   b True.
   c True.
   d False. Commoner in sedentary occupations.
   e False. Incision and drainage is the treatment of choice.

21 Clinical scenarios: answers

1a b The history and examination is highly suggestive of neck of femur fracture.

1b e The AP and lateral view of the left hip is required to assess the fracture.

1c b It is important to keep the patient comfortable.

2a a Blisters and erythema suggests first-degree burn.

2b a The patient's palm area is roughly 1% of their total BSA.

3a b The right actions to take include administration of high-flow (15 L/min) oxygen and bronchodilators, obtain ABG including carbon monoxide, and contact anaesthetists for early airway intervention. *Cautions*: do not give oral fluids, minimal intravenous access, avoid pulse oximetry and keep patient cool.

3b d Patients with facial burns develop oedema and their airways can obstruct. Do not wait, call the anaesthetist to assess the airway and intubate the patient.

4a b Cholangiocarcinoma typically presents with painless jaundice and palpable distended gallbladder, and a very high CA19-9 strongly suggests cancer.

4b b ERCP allows stenting of the bile duct and histological diagnosis.

4c c An INR is essential before an invasive procedure in patients with liver dysfunction.

4d a CT abdomen and chest is part of cancer staging.

5a b, d, e and f Leaking AAA, peptic perforation and acute pancreatitis require prompt diagnosis and emergency surgical management. MI is a medical emergency that may present to surgeons.

5b a, c, f, g and h In an emergency, one needs to exclude all serious life-threatening problems. An erect CXR may show a pneumoperitoneum or calcified enlarged aorta; arterial gases can indicate the metabolic status of the patient (acid–base); glucose is required to exclude DKA, a medical emergency that can be incorrectly referred to the surgical team; ECG to exclude ST elevation MI; blood test to investigate inflammatory responses. In surgical specialties, one should G&S in emergency situations, in case cross-matching of blood is required.

5c e Deranged liver function tests, raised inflammatory markers and hyperamylasaemia suggest acute pancreatitis. There are other causes of raised serum amylase levels: salivary amylase, ectopic pregnancy, perforated viscus, ischaemic bowel and renal failure

5d a, c, e and g.

5e a USS abdomen is the best investigation for gallstones.

6a b, c, d and f These differential diagnoses should be considered in a patient with an acute abdomen with pyrexia and tachycardia. Biliary colic, gastritis and mucocele are not usually associated with sepsis.

6b d Laparoscopic cholecystectomy and CBD exploration would remove the gallbladder and remove any gallstones in the CBD. ERCP is the best option for removing the obstruction and decompressing the biliary system but there is a theoretical risk of cholangiocarcinoma later on in life. There are also other risk factors associated with ERCP: acute pancreatitis, bleeding from the sphincterotomy site (may be life-threatening) and aspiration.

6c b In the UK, gallstones are twice as common as alcohol-induced pancreatitis

7a g All the above questions are important for establishing a differential diagnosis. Remember the mnemonic SOCRATES for assessing pain: Site, Onset, Character, Radiation, Alleviating factors, Timing, Exacerbating factors, Severity. Other factors that may help include the following.

- Bowel habit may help one to decide if there is an acute change. If this is associated with weight loss, there will be a high suspicion of malignancy.
- The absence of bowel action and flatus indicates complete bowel obstruction.
- The presence of blood in the vomitus or stools hints to gastrointestinal bleeding.
- History of foreign travel can point towards infectious causes.

7b a This is typical of SBO. Gastroenteritis can be associated with colicky abdominal pains and vomiting but is not usually associated with absence of flatus. The examination did not reveal any specific areas of peritonism, therefore it is unlikely to be appendicitis or inflamed Meckel's diverticulum; there was minimal abdominal distension, therefore it is unlikely to be a volvulus. The waves of pain indicate a colicky type of pain from the bowel and relief on vomiting suggests bowel obstruction.

7c g None of the above. A plain AXR may be sufficient to establish a diagnosis of obstruction but cannot definitively exclude any of the above diagnoses.

7d a, c, d, e and f It is important to keep the patient comfortable, resuscitate the patient and measure the input and output. There is no need for transfusion.

7e c Repeating the AXR may help but the following should be taken into consideration: approximately 20% of AXR are non-specific, 30% suggestive of SBO and only 50% of SBO can be seen. Abdominal USS will only confirm dilated loops of bowel. A CT scan is greater than 90% sensitive for SBO. The advantage of CT is that the cause of the obstruction can often be seen and this will help the surgeon to plan the operation.

7f c Adhesions are the commonest cause of SBO followed by hernias and then tumours.

8a h There are lots of differential diagnoses for RUQ pain.

8b b Mesenteric angiography may diagnose this condition.

8c c Mesenteric ischaemia is caused by SMA or SMV occlusion. It usually affects the bowel from the second part of the duodenum to the transverse colon.

9a d The most relevant examination in this scenario would be to feel the peripheral pulses in both lower limbs followed by Doppler examination.

9b a This patient has no history of trauma and is complaining of acute right leg pain with associated cold foot. The first and most important differential diagnosis is acute right leg ischaemia as delay in diagnosis can result in loss of the limb.

9c a The clotting profile is useful before starting heparin infusion.

9d a This patient is likely to have an embolism from the left atrium.

Appendix 1 Commonly used surgical equipment

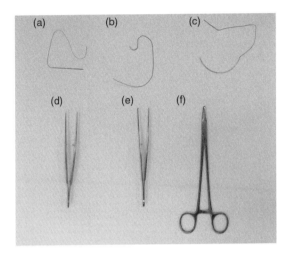

(a) Straight needle commonly used for subcuticular skin closure. (b) J needle for deep closure (deep bite of tissue), e.g. laparoscopic port incision closure or hernia repair. (c) Large curved needle, e.g. for closure of burst abdomen or for securing a drain. (d) Atraumatic non-toothed forceps for delicate tissue handling.
(e) Toothed forceps generally used for holding skin or muscle. (f) Needle holder.

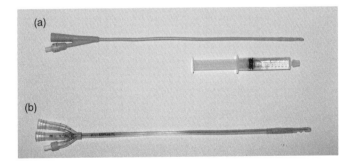

(a) Foley two-way urethral catheter for males. (b) Foley three-way urethral catheter for irrigation, e.g. haematuria.

EMQs and MCQs for Surgical Finals, 1st edition. © Hye-Chung Kwak, Imran Bhatti, Jaskarn Rai, Farhan Rashid, Bachittar Singh Jassar, Murthy Nyasavajjala, Viren Asher, Jon Lund and Mike Larvin. Published 2011 by Blackwell Publishing Ltd.

Appendix 2   Normal ranges for blood tests

AFP	$<10\,\mu g/L$
Albumin	34–38 g/L
ALP	40–129 U/L
ALT	0–40 U/L
Amylase	28–100 U/L
APTT	25–37 s
Bilirubin	0–21 μmol/L
CA125	<30 U/L
CA19-9	40 U/mL
CEA	<2.5 ng/mL
Creatinine	70–120 μmol/L
CRP	0–5 mg/L
Fasting glucose	3.5–6 mmol/L
GGT	11–51 IU/L
Hb	13.5–18 g/dL (slightly lower ranges for females)
HbA_{1c}	4.5–9%
INR	0.8–1.2
K	3.5–5.3 mmol/L
Na	133–145 mmol/L
Platelets	$150–450 \times 10^9/L$
Protein	59–82 g/L
Prothrombin time	9–13 s
PSA	0–4 ng/mL
Troponin	<0.4 ng/mL
Urea	2.5–6.6 mmol/L
WBC	$4.5–11 \times 10^9/L$

EMQs and MCQs for Surgical Finals, 1st edition.   © Hye-Chung Kwak, Imran Bhatti,
Jaskarn Rai, Farhan Rashid, Bachittar Singh Jassar, Murthy Nyasavajjala, Viren Asher,
Jon Lund and Mike Larvin. Published 2011 by Blackwell Publishing Ltd.

Appendix 3   Orthopaedic examination

LOOK, FEEL, MOVE and X-RAY

Typical muscles tested

Elbow flexion (C5, C6)
Elbow extension (C7, C8)
Wrist extension (C7, C8)
Finger flexion (distal phalanx of middle finger) (C8/T1)
Finger abduction, little finger (T1)
Hip flexion (L1, L2)
Knee flexion (L5, S1)
Knee extension (L3, L4)
Ankle dorsiflexion (L4, L5)
Ankle plantar flexion (S1, S2)
Long toe extension (S1)

Assess power using MRC classification

Total paralysis	0
Visible contraction (flicker or contraction)	1
Movement with gravity eliminated	2
Movement against gravity	3
Movement against gravity and resistance	4
Normal power	5

Nerve injuries

Important dermatomes

C5	Clavicle
C6, C7, C8	Hand (thumb, middle finger, little finger)
C6	Thumb
C7	Tip of middle finger
C8	Little finger
T4	Nipples
T10	Umbilicus

EMQs and MCQs for Surgical Finals, 1st edition.   © Hye-Chung Kwak, Imran Bhatti, Jaskarn Rai, Farhan Rashid, Bachittar Singh Jassar, Murthy Nyasavajjala, Viren Asher, Jon Lund and Mike Larvin. Published 2011 by Blackwell Publishing Ltd.

T12	Groin
S2, S3	Genitalia
S2, S3, S4	Perineum
S5	Anus

Root lesions

C4–C5	Absent pectoral jerk
C6	Absent biceps jerk
C7	Wasting small muscles of hand
	Absent triceps jerk
C8	Wasting hypothenar muscles
	Wasting small muscles of hand
L4	Wasting quadriceps
	Absent knee jerk
L5	Hypoaesthesia lateral side of great toe
	Weak extensor hallucis longus and tibialis anterior
S1	Hypoaesthesia lateral side of foot
	Absent ankle jerk
	Wasting calf muscles

Further reading and useful websites

3 ENT
UK Sjögren's association. Available at www.bssa.uk.net

6 Breast
Sainsbury, J.R., Anderson, T.J. & Morgan, D.A. (2000) ABC of breast diseases: breast cancer. *BMJ* **321**, 745–50.

Tan, P.H., Lai, L.M., Carrington, E.V. *et al.* (2006) Fat necrosis of the breast: a review. *Breast* **15**, 313–18.

7 Acute abdomen
Goldberg, R.J., Gore, J.M., Alpert, J.S. *et al.* (1991) Cardiogenic shock after acute myocardial infarction. Incidence and mortality from a community-wide perspective, 1975 to 1988. *N Engl J Med* **325**, 1117–22.

Guly, H.R., Bouamra, O. & Lecky, F.E. (2008) The incidence of neurogenic shock in patients with isolated spinal cord injury in the emergency department. *Resuscitation* **76**, 57–62.

Hasham, S., Matteucci, P., Stanley, P.R. & Hart, N.B. (2005) Necrotising fasciitis. *BMJ* **330**, 830–3.

Lieberman, P., Camargo, C.A. Jr, Bohlke, K. *et al.* (2006) Epidemiology of anaphylaxis: findings of the American College of Allergy, Asthma and Immunology Epidemiology of Anaphylaxis Working Group. *Ann Allergy Asthma Immunol* **97**, 596–602.

Martin, G.S., Mannino, D.M., Eaton, S. & Moss, M. (2003) The epidemiology of sepsis in the United States from 1979 through 2000. *N Engl J Med* **348**, 1546–54.

Nguyen, H.B., Rivers, E.P., Abrahamian, F.M. *et al.* (2006) Severe sepsis and septic shock: review of the literature and emergency department management guidelines. *Ann Emerg Med* **48**, 28–54.

9 Hepato-pancreato-biliary disease
British Society of Gastroenterology. Guidelines for the management of patients with pancreatic cancer. Available at www.bsg.org.uk/clinical-guidelines/pancreatic/index.html

12 Colorectal
British Society of Gastroenterology. Guidelines for the management of IBD in adults. Available at www.bsg.org.uk

EMQs and MCQs for Surgical Finals, 1st edition. © Hye-Chung Kwak, Imran Bhatti, Jaskarn Rai, Farhan Rashid, Bachittar Singh Jassar, Murthy Nyasavajjala, Viren Asher, Jon Lund and Mike Larvin. Published 2011 by Blackwell Publishing Ltd.

NHS Bowel Cancer Screening Programme. Further information available at www.cancerscreening.nhs.uk/bowel/

13 Nutrition in surgical patients

British Nutrition Foundation. Available at www.nutrition.org.uk

16 Urology

Fisher, R.I., Rosenberg, S.A. & Fyfe, G. (2000) Long-term survival update for high-dose recombinant interleukin-2 in patients with renal cell carcinoma. *Cancer J Sci Am* **6** (Suppl. 1), S55–S57.

Lara, P.N. Jr & Meyers, F.J. (1999) Treatment options in androgen-independent prostate cancer. *Cancer Invest* **17**, 137–44.

Reynard, J., Brewster, S. & Biers, S. (2009) *Oxford Handbook of Urology*, 2nd edn. (Oxford Handbooks Series). Oxford: Oxford University Press.

Tannock, I.F., de Wit, R., Berry, W.R. *et al.* (2004) Docetaxel plus prednisone or mitoxantrone plus prednisone for advanced prostate cancer. *N Engl J Med* **351**, 1502–12.

Wein, A.J, Kavoussi, L.R., Novick, A.C., Partin, A.W. & Peters, C.A. (eds) (2006) *Campbell-Walsh Urology*, 9th edn. Saunders.

For further information on urological cancer, see www.cancerresearchuk.org

17 Vascular

Lederle, F.A., Johnson, G.R., Wilson, S.E. *et al.* (2000) The aneurysm detection and management study screening program: validation cohort and final results. Aneurysm Detection and Management Veterans Affairs Cooperative Study Investigators. *Arch Intern Med* **160**, 1425–30.

Powell, J.T., Brown, L.C., Forbes, J.F. *et al.* (2007) Final 12-year follow-up of surgery versus surveillance in the UK Small Aneurysm Trial. *Br J Surg* **94**, 702–8.

Rutherford, R.B., Baker, J.D., Ernst, C. *et al.* (1997) Recommended standards for reports dealing with lower extremity ischemia: revised version. *J Vasc Surg* **26**, 517–38.

Further information on AAA screening.

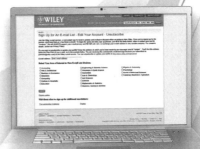
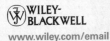

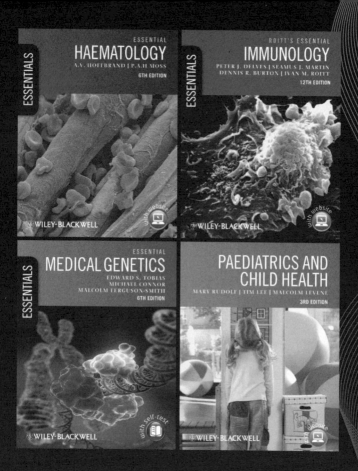
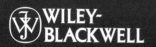